ITLS

SIXTH EDITION

Edited by John Emory Campbell, MD, FACEP

Alabama Chapter
American College of Emergency Physicians

PEARSON

Prentice
Hall

Upper Saddle River, New Jersey 07458

Library of Congress Cataloging-in-Publication Data

ITLS: international trauma life support for prehospital care providers / edited by John Emory Campbell; Alabama Chapter, American College of Emergency Physicians. —6th ed.
    p.; cm.
    Rev. ed. of BTLS. 5th ed. c2004.
    Includes bibliographical references and index.
    ISBN 978-0-13-237982-3 (pbk. : alk. paper) 1. Traumatology. 2. Medical emergencies. 3. Emergency medical technicians. I. Campbell, John E., (1943–). II. American College of Emergency Physicians. Alabama Chapter. III. International Trauma Life Support. IV. BTLS. V. Title: International trauma life support for prehospital care providers.
    [DNLM: 1. Emergency Medical Services—methods. 2. Life Support Care—methods. 3. Wounds and Injuries—therapy. WX 215 189 2008]
    RC86.7.B3775 2008
    617.1'026—dc22

                           2007014973

Publisher: Julie Levin Alexander
Publisher's Assistant: Regina Bruno
Executive Editor: Marlene McHugh Pratt
Senior Acquisitions Editor: Stephen Smith
Senior Managing Editor for Development: Lois Berlowitz
Development Editor: Jo Cepeda
Associate Editor: Monica Moosang
Editorial Assistant: Patricia Linard
Executive Marketing Manager: Katrin Beacom
Marketing Coordinator: Michael Sirinides
Marketing Assistant: Wayne Celia, Jr.
Managing Production Editor: Patrick Walsh
Production Liaison: Julie Li
Production Editor: Amy Gehl
Media Product Manager: John Jordan
New Media Project Manager: Tina Rudowski
Manufacturing Manager: Ilene Sanford
Manufacturing Buyer: Pat Brown
Senior Design Coordinator: Christopher Weigand
Interior Designer: Lee Goldstein
Cover Designer: Rob Aleman
Cover Photo: Mark Ide
Composition: S4Carlisle Publishing Services
Printing and Binding: Courier Kendallville
Cover Printer: Phoenix Color

Notice on Care Procedures

It is the intent of the authors and publisher that this textbook be used as part of an education program taught by qualified instructors and supervised by a licensed physician. The procedures described in this textbook are based upon consultation with paramedics, nurses, and physicians. The authors and publisher have taken care to make certain that these procedures reflect currently accepted clinical practice; however, they cannot be considered absolute recommendations.

The material in this textbook contains the most current information available at the time of publication. However, federal, state, and local guidelines concerning clinical practices, including, without limitation, those governing infection control and universal precautions, change rapidly. The reader should note, therefore, that new regulations may require changes in some procedures.

It is the responsibility of the reader to familiarize himself or herself with the policies and procedures set by federal, state, and local agencies as well as the institution or agency where the reader is employed. The authors and the publisher of this textbook and the supplements written to accompany it disclaim any liability, loss, or risk resulting directly or indirectly from the suggested procedures and theory, from any undetected errors, or from the reader's misunderstanding of the text. It is the reader's responsibility to stay informed of any new changes or recommendations made by any federal, state, and local agency as well as by his or her employing institution or agency.

Notice on Gender Usage

The English language has historically given preference to the male gender. Among many words, the pronouns, *he* and *his* are commonly used to describe both genders. Society evolves faster than language, and the male pronouns still predominate our speech. The authors have made great effort to treat the two genders equally, recognizing that a significant percentage of EMS providers are female. However, in some instances, male pronouns may be used to describe both males and females solely for the purpose of brevity. This is not intended to offend any readers of the female gender.

Pearson Education LTD.
Pearson Education Singapore, Pte. Ltd
Pearson Education, Canada, Ltd
Pearson Education–Japan
Pearson Education Australia PTY, Limited

Pearson Education North Asia Ltd
Pearson Educaçion de Mexico, S.A. de C.V.
Pearson Education Malaysia, Pte. Ltd
Pearson Education, Upper Saddle River, New Jersey

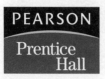

10 9 8 7
ISBN-13: 978-0-13-237982-3
ISBN-10:   0-13-237982-1

The Sixth Edition of ITLS
is dedicated to
EMS educators over the world.

It has been written that, "Those who can, do. Those who can't, teach."
This should read, "Educators are those who by doing have mastered their craft
and now pass their knowledge on so that others can do."
Because of your dedication and your influence on
those who practice and teach our craft,
you will still be saving lives
long after yours is spent.

Contents

JOHN E. CAMPBELL, MD, FACEP

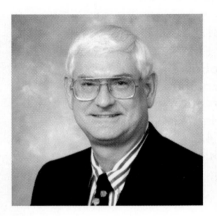

Dr. Campbell received his B.S. degree in pharmacy from Auburn University in 1966 and his medical degree from the University of Alabama at Birmingham in 1970. He has been in the practice of Emergency Medicine for 36 years, practicing in Alabama, Georgia, New Mexico, and Texas. He became interested in prehospital care in 1972 when he was asked to teach a basic EMT course to members of the Clay County Rescue Squad. He is still an honorary member of that outstanding group. Since then he has served as medical director of many EMT and paramedic training programs. He now serves as the Medical Director for EMS and Trauma for the State of Alabama.

From the original basic trauma life support course developed an international organization of teachers of trauma care called "International Trauma Life Support, Inc.," or ITLS. Dr. Campbell has served as its president since the inception of the organization.

Dr. Campbell is the author of the first edition of the *Basic Trauma Life Support* textbook and has continued to be the editor through to this new edition, now entitled *International Trauma Life Support for Prehospital Care Providers.* He also is the co-author of *Homeland Security and Emergency Medical Response.*

He was a member of the first faculty of Emergency Medicine at the School of Medicine, University of Alabama at Birmingham. In 1991 he was the first recipient of the American College of Emergency Medicine's EMS Award for outstanding achievement of national significance in the area of EMS. In 2001 he received the Ronald D. Stewart Lifetime Achievement Award from the National Association of EMS Physicians. He and his wife, Jackie, and their four dogs currently reside on their farm in Camp Hill, Alabama.

ITLS FOR PREHOSPITAL CARE PROVIDERS

Roy L. Alson, PhD, MD, FACEP, FAAEM
Associate Professor of Emergency Medicine, Wake Forest University School of Medicine, Winston-Salem, North Carolina
Medical Director, Forsyth County EMS
Associate Medical Director, NC Baptist AirCare

Jim Augustine, MD, FACEP
Clinical Faculty, Department of Emergency Medicine, Emory University, Atlanta, Georgia
Medical Director, Atlanta Fire Department
Editorial Boards, *JEMS* and *EMS*
Executive Editor, *ED Management Journal*

Jere F. Baldwin, MD, FACEP, FAAFP
Chief, Department of Emergency Medicine and Ambulatory Services, Mercy Hospital, Port Huron, Michigan

Russell Bieniek, MD, FACEP
Medical Director of Emergency Services, Saint Vincent Health System, Erie, Pennsylvania

William Bozeman, MD, FACEP, FAAEM
Associate Professor, Department of Emergency Medicine, and Associate Research Director, Wake Forest University School of Medicine, Winston-Salem, North Carolina

Walter J. Bradley, MD, MBA, FACEP
Director, Trauma and Emergency Services, Trinity Medical Center, Rock Island, Illinois

John E. Campbell, MD, FACEP
Medical Director, EMS and Trauma, State of Alabama

Leon Charpentier, EMT-P
Fire Chief, Harker Heights Texas (Retired)
Editorial Board, International Trauma Life Support

James H. Creel Jr., MD, FACEP
Chief of Emergency and Disaster Medicine, Erlanger Health System, Chattanooga, Tennessee
Assistant Clinical Professor of Surgery—UTCOM

Ann M. Dietrich, MD, FAAP, FACEP
Professor of Pediatrics, Ohio State University
Director of Risk Management, Section of Emergency Medicine, Columbus Children's Hospital, Columbus, Ohio
Pediatric Medical Advisor, Medflight of Ohio

Raymond L. Fowler, MD, FACEP
Associate Professor of Emergency Medicine, Surgery, and Allied Health and Co-Chief in the Section on EMS, Disaster Medicine, and Homeland Security, The University of Texas Southwestern, Dallas, Texas
Chief of Operations for the Dallas Area BioTel EMS System

Pam Gersch, RN, CLNC
Program Director, AirMedTeam, Rocky Mountain Helicopters, Redding, California

Martin Greenberg, MD, FAAOS, FACS
Chief of Hand Surgery, Advocate Illinois Masonic Medical Center
Chief of Orthopedic Surgery, Our Lady of the Resurrection Medical Center, Chicago
Reserve Police Officer, Village of Tinley Park
Tactical Physician, South Surburban Emergency Response Team
ITOA Co-Chair, TEMS Committee

Jonathan I. Groner, MD, FACS, FAAP
Trauma Medical Director, Children's Hospital, Columbus, Ohio

Donna Hastings, EMT-P
Vice President, Health and Research, Heart and Stroke Foundation of Alberta, NWT & Nunavut, Calgary, Alberta, Canada

Leah J. Heimbach, JD, RN, EMT-P
General Counsel, WVU Hospitals, Inc., Morgantown, West Virginia

Davis E. Hill, EMT-P
Program Director, Managing Agricultural Emergencies

David V. Maatman, NREMT-P/IC
Educator, American Medical Response—West Michigan, Grand Rapids, Michigan

Kirk Magee, MD, MSc, FRCPC
Royal College Program Director and Associate
  Professor, Dalhousie Department of Emergency
  Medicine, Halifax, Nova Scotia, Canada

Richard N. Nelson, MD, FACEP
Professor and Vice Chair, Department of Emergency
  Medicine, The Ohio State University College of
  Medicine

**Jonathan G. Newman, MD, MMM, EMT-P,
FACEP**
Assistant Medical Director, Department of Emergency
  Medicine, United Hospital Center, Inc., Clarksburg,
  West Virginia
Assistant Professor, Department of Emergency
  Medicine, West Virginia University, Morgantown,
  West Virginia

Bob Page, AAS, NREMT-P, CCEMT-P, I/C
Director of Emergency Care Education, St. John's EMS
  Education Programs, Springfield, Missouri
President, Edutainment!

Paul M. Paris, MD, FACEP, LLD (Hon)
Professor and Chairman, Department of Emergency
  Medicine, University of Pittsburgh School of
  Medicine

Andrew B. Peitzman, MD, FACS
Professor of Surgery, Vice-Chairman, Department of
  Surgery, and Chief of General Surgery, University of
  Pittsburgh Medical Center

Paul E. Pepe, MD, MPH, FCCM, FACEP
Professor of Surgery, Medicine, Public Health and Riggs
  Family Chair in Emergency Medicine, University of
  Texas Southwestern Medical Center and the Parkland
  Health and Hospital System, Dallas, Texas
Director, City of Dallas Medical Emergency Services for
  Public Safety, Public Health and Homeland Security

William Pfeifer, MD, FACS
Col. MC USAR (Trauma Surgery)

Jonathan M. Rubin, MD, FAAEM
Associate Professor of Emergency Medicine, Medical
  College of Wisconsin

S. Robert Seitz, MEd, RN, NREMT-P
Assistant Professor, School of Health and Rehabilitation
  Sciences, Emergency Medicine Program, University
  of Pittsburgh
Assistant Program Director, Office of Education and
  International Emergency Medicine, University of
  Pittsburgh Center for Emergency Medicine

Continuing Education Editor, *Journal of Emergency
  Medical Services*
Board of Directors, International Trauma Life Support

Corey M. Slovis, MD, FACP, FACEP
Professor of Emergency Medicine and Medicine, and
  Chairman, Department of Emergency Medicine,
  Vanderbilt University Medical Center, Nashville,
  Tennessee
Medical Director, Nashville Fire Department and
  International Airport

John T. Stevens, NREMT-P
Firefighter/Paramedic, Douglas County Fire/EMS
EMT/Paramedic Instructor, Westcentral Technical
  College, Douglasville, Georgia

**Ronald D. Stewart, OC, MD, FRCPC, FACEP,
DSC (Hon)**
Professor of Emergency Medicine and Professor of
  Community Medicine and Epidemiology, Dalhousie
  University, Halifax, Nova Scotia, Canada

Arlo Weltge, MD, MPH, FACEP
Clinical Associate Professor EM, University of Texas,
  Houston Medical School
Medical Director, Program in EMS, Houston
  Community College

Howard A. Werman, MD, FACEP
Professor of Clinical Emergency Medicine, The Ohio
  State University
Medical Director, MedFlight of Ohio

Katherine H. West, BSN, MS Ed, CIS
Infection Control Consultant, Manassas, Virginia

Melissa White, MD, MPH
Associate Professor, Emory University, Section of
  Prehospital and Disaster Medicine, Atlanta, Georgia

Janet M. Williams, MD
Professor of Emergency Medicine, University of
  Rochester (New York) Medical Center

John Wipfler III, MD, FACEP
Associate Clinical Professor, University of Illinois
  College of Medicine, Department of Emergency
  Medicine, OSF Saint Francis Medical Center

Arthur H. Yancey II, MD, MPH, FACEP
Deputy Director of Health for EMS, Fulton County
  Department of Health and Wellness, Atlanta, Georgia
Associate Professor, Department of Emergency
  Medicine, Emory University School of Medicine,
  Atlanta, Georgia

What's New in This Edition

The sixth edition of the ITLS textbook, *International Trauma Life Support for Prehospital Care Providers,* has been updated and refined to reflect the latest and most effective approaches to the care of the trauma patient. The text also has been made to conform to the newest AHA guidelines for artificial ventilation and CPR. Other general changes include the repositioning of the "Pearls" feature so that it consistently appears in the margins beside relevant text and many of the illustrations have been redrawn for a more up-to-date look. Important chapter-by-chapter changes are listed below.

■ In Chapter 1, the term *standard precautions* is used for the first time instead of body substance isolation (BSI). This change is reflected throughout the text. A new photo of a tactical flashlight has been added as well.

■ In Chapter 2, the description of the ITLS patient assessment plan has been revised so that it now consistently addresses it as a three-step plan composed of the ITLS Primary Survey, the ITLS Secondary Survey, and the ITLS Ongoing Exam. The patient assessment algorithm has been updated to reflect that change and new Primary and Secondary Survey flowsheets have been added. Up-to-date scoop stretchers are now shown. Hemostatic agents and tourniquets have been added to the equipment that may be needed by EMS personnel.

■ Chapter 3 reflects the new description of the ITLS patient assessment plan. A table identifying "Critical Trauma Situations" has been added.

■ In Chapter 4, the KING LT-D airway is included as another example of a blind insertion airway device. A table on "Estimating Difficulty of Intubation," which describes the Mallampati Score, has been added. A new illustration that describes the response to difficult bag-mask ventilation is also included.

■ In Chapter 5, the use of capnography to confirm placement of the endotracheal tube has been added.

■ In Chapter 6, flowsheets for the signs of tension pneumothorax, open pneumothorax, flail chest, and cardiac tamponade are included.

● In Chapter 8, the use of hemostatic agents for uncontrolled extremity hemorrhage has been added, as has the topic of capnography. Also included are new flowsheets on absolute hypovolemia, relative hypovolemia, and mechanical shock.

■ Chapter 10 has been updated to reflect the new second edition Brain Trauma Foundation guidelines.

■ In Chapter 11, new photos of removing a helmet's face guard from a possible spine-injured patient have been added, and so has a discussion of the practical tools needed to do so.

■ In Chapter 12, an airway management kit has been added to the essential components of a full spinal motion restriction system.

■ In Chapter 14, there are new photos showing an example of a hemostatic agent and a rigid scoop stretcher.

- In Chapter 15, photos on the stabilization of pelvic fractures have been added.
- In Chapter 16, the topic of radiation burns is included.
- In Chapter 17, the topic of capnography and x-rays of broken bones have been added.
- In Chapter 18, the topic of capnography has been included.
- In Chapter 21, guidelines for the unsalvageable patient have been added.
- New appendices are Appendix J, Agricultural Rescue Course Overview; Appendix K, ITLS Access Overview; and Appendix L, Tactical EMS.
- In Appendix A, the KING LT-D airway and rapid sequence intubation have been added as optional skills with illustrations. The topic of capnography is included. And the topics of the antishock garment and esophageal gastric tube airway as optional skills have been deleted.
- In Appendix I, illustrations for the on-scene incident command structure, medical incident command, and the ITLS triage decision tree have been added.

Acknowledgments

Special thanks to these friends of ITLS who provided invaluable assistance with ideas, reviews, and corrections of the text. This was such a big job, and there were so many people who contributed, that I am sure I have left someone out. My apologies in advance.

Roy Alson, MD, FACEP
Jere Baldwin, MD, FACEP
J. David Barrick, BS, NREMT-P
David Burkland, MD, FACEP
Jackie Campbell, RN
Leon Charpentier, EMT-P
David Effron, MD, FACEP
Kyee H. Han, MD, FRCS, FFAEM
Donna Hastings, EMT-P
Leah Heimbach, JD, RN, NREMT-P

Eduardo Romero Hicks, MD
David Maatman, NREMT-P/IC
Jonathan Newman, MD, FACEP
Randy Orsborn, EMT-P
William Pfeifer, MD, FACS
Mary M. Radanovich RN, BSN, EMT-P
John T. Stevens, EMT-P
Ron Stewart, MD, FACEP
Arlo Weltge, MD, FACEP
Brian J. Wilson, NREMT-P

We wish to thank the EMS professionals who reviewed material especially for this 6th Edition of International Trauma Life Support for Prehospital Care Providers. *Their assistance is appreciated.*

Chris Cousar, BS, NREMT-P, EMS Educator, University of New Mexico EMS Academy
Steve Creech, EMT-P, Training Officer, Washington County EMS, Plymouth, North Carolina
John S. Molnar, NREMT-P, Manager, CPR/CTC; Instructor, Cleveland Clinic Health System; Adjunct IPRN, BTLS affiliate faculty at School of EMS, Euclid, Ohio

Tim Swaim, Paramedic Instructor, Rockingham Community College, Wentworth, North Carolina
Jason P. Zielewicz, MS, NREMT-P, EMS Supervisor and Instructor, Office of EMS, The Pennsylvania State University

Another special thanks goes to the following photographers who donated their work to help illustrate the text.

Roy Alson, MD, FACEP
Brant Burden, EMT-P
Anthony Cellitti, NREMT-P
Leon Charpentier, EMT-P
Buddy Denson, EMT-P
Pamela Drexel, Brain Trauma Foundation
David Effron, MD, FACEP
Ferno Washington, Inc.
KING Airway Systems
Kyee H. Han, MD, FRCS, FFAEM

Eduardo Romero Hicks, MD
Jeff Hinshaw, MS, PA-C, NREMT-P
Bonnie Meneely, EMT-P
Nonin Medical, Inc.
Bob Page, NREMT-P
William Pfeifer, MD, FACS
Don Resch
Sam Splints
Surefire Tactical Lights
Z-Medica Corporation

Thanks to Southern Union State Community College EMS Department, Opelika, Alabama, and to the Opelika Fire Department for their help in photographing spinal immobilization scenes.

F. F. Kenny Allen
A. O. Keith Burnett, EMT-P
Lt. Lynn Callahan Jr.
Herbie Clark, EMT-P

Buddy Denson, EMT-P
F. F. Steve Miller
Capt. James C. Morgan Jr., EMT-P
Josh Stevens, EMT-P

International Trauma Life Support is a global not-for-profit organization dedicated to preventing death and disability from trauma through education and emergency trauma care. Founded in 1985 as Basic Trauma Life Support, ITLS adopted its new name in 2005 to better reflect its global role and impact.

The ITLS framework is a global standard that enables providers to master the latest techniques in rapid assessment, appropriate intervention, and identification of immediate life-threatening injuries. ITLS is accepted internationally as the standard training course for prehospital trauma care. It is used as a state-of-the-art continuing education course and as an essential curriculum in many paramedic, EMT, and First Responder training programs.

Today, ITLS has more than 70 chapters and training centers worldwide. Through ITLS, hundreds of thousands of trauma care professionals have learned proven techniques endorsed by the American College of Emergency Physicians and the National Association of EMS Physicians.

ITLS LEADERSHIP

Board of Directors

John E. Campbell, MD, FACEP
President
Camp Hill, Alabama

Walter Bradley, MD, MBA, FACEP
Chair
Moline, Illinois

Peter Gianas, MD
Vice Chair
Starke, Florida

Sabina Braithwaite, MD, FACEP
Secretary Treasurer
Charlottesville, Virginia

Neil Christen, MD, FACEP
Member-at-Large
Anniston, Alabama

Russell Bieniek, MD, FACEP
Erie, Pennsylvania

Amy Boise, NREMT-P
Phoenix, Arizona

Anthony Connelly, BhSc, PGCE Ed
Edmonton, Canada

Martin Friedberg, MD, CCFP(EM)
Toronto, Ontario, Canada

Anthony Cellitti, NREMT-P
Rockford, Illinois

William Pfeifer III, MD, FACS
Littleton, Colorado

S. Robert Seitz, MEd, RN, NREMT-P
Pittsburgh, Pennsylvania

ITLS LEADERSHIP
Editorial Board

Donna Hastings, EMT-P
Chair
Calgary, Alberta, Canada

John E. Campbell, MD, FACEP
Chair Emeritus
Camp Hill, Alabama

Roy L. Alson, PhD, MD, FACEP
Winston-Salem, North Carolina

Kyee H. Han, MBBS, FRCS, FFAEM
Middlesbrough, England

Eduardo Romero Hicks, MD
Guanajuato, Mexico

William Pfeifer, MD, FACS
Littleton, Colorado

Arthur Proust, MD, FACEP
St. Charles, Illinois

S. Robert Seitz, MEd, RN, NREMT-P
Pittsburgh, Pennsylvania

J. T. Stevens, NREMT-P
Douglasville, Georgia

Executive Director

Virginia Kennedy Palys, JD
Oakbrook Terrace, Illinois

WHAT MAKES ITLS BETTER?

Since its beginnings more than 25 years ago as Basic Trauma Life Support, ITLS has become a global force for excellence in trauma education and response, with more than 75 chapters and training centers worldwide. What makes ITLS a better choice for trauma training? Here are just a few of the reasons.

- *Evidence-based.* ITLS is based on current science and research.
- *Practical.* ITLS training is a realistic, hands-on approach proven to work in the field "from scene to surgery."
- *Dynamic.* ITLS content is current, relevant, and responsive to the latest thinking in trauma management.
- *Flexible.* ITLS courses are taught through a strong network of chapters and training centers that customize content to reflect local needs and priorities.
- *Recognized.* ITLS is an internationally recognized certification that is the standard for prehospital trauma education.
- *Team centered.* ITLS emphasizes a cohesive team approach that works in the real world and recognizes the importance of the emergency care provider's role.
- *Grounded in emergency medicine.* Practicing emergency physicians—medicine's front-line responders—lead ITLS's efforts to deliver stimulating content that has its base in solid emergency medicine.
- *Challenging.* ITLS course content raises the bar on performance in the field by integrating classroom knowledge with practical application of skills through interactive stations.
- *Confidence building.* The unique ITLS course format builds confidence in new providers and knowledge in experienced providers.

FOCUSED CONTENT THAT DELIVERS

ITLS is accepted internationally as the standard training course for prehospital trauma care. It is taught not only as a continuing education course, but also used as essential curricula in many paramedic, EMT, and First Responder training programs.

ITLS courses combine classroom learning and hands-on skill stations. They also challenge the student with scenario assessment stations where learning is put to work in simulated trauma situations. ITLS courses are designed, managed, and delivered by course directors, coordinators, and instructors experienced in EMS, prehospital care, and the ITLS approach.

ITLS is synonymous with training EMS personnel in providing optimal care for the injured in the prehospital setting. The program provides a variety of training options to suit the requirements of all levels and backgrounds of prehospital emergency personnel around the world.

ITLS BASIC AND ADVANCED

These comprehensive courses are designed for trauma care providers who are first to assess and initiate treatment for the trauma patient. The courses provide complete training in the skills needed for rapid assessment, resuscitation, stabilization, and transportation of trauma patients. The ITLS Basic course provides the core of knowledge and skills appropriate for all levels of EMS personnel, including EMT-Bs, First Responders, and other technicians. The ITLS Advanced course builds on that knowledge, emphasizing assessment steps and sequencing as well as treatment interventions and packaging patients for transport. ITLS Advanced is appropriate for advanced EMTs, paramedics, trauma nurses, physicians, and other advanced EMS personnel. Frequently, the Basic and Advanced courses are combined, with students participating in the skill stations appropriate for their level of training.

Hands-on skill stations include:

- Patient assessment and management
- Basic and advanced airway management
- Needle chest decompression and fluid resuscitation
- Spinal motion restriction, including rapid extrication, short backboard, helmet management, log-roll, and long backboard/scoop stretcher utilization
- Extremity immobilization and traction splint application

ITLS INSTRUCTOR COURSES

Instructor courses prepare EMS professionals to teach ITLS courses. To participate, potential instructors must successfully complete the provider course they want to teach, demonstrate instructor potential, and meet local ITLS requirements.

ITLS REFRESHER COURSES

ITLS offers refresher courses for experienced ITLS providers and instructors to keep them up to date with the ITLS curriculum and skills.

ITLS PEDIATRIC

Pediatric ITLS continues the training of the Basic and Advanced courses with an emphasis on understanding and responding to trauma in children. The eight-hour course teaches the proper assessment, stabilization, and packaging of pediatric trauma patients. It also highlights techniques for communicating with young patients and their parents. Hands-on stations include:

- Patient assessment and management
- Airway management and chest decompression
- Fluid resuscitation
- Spine motion restriction, including pediatric immobilization devices

ITLS ACCESS

ITLS Access gives EMS crews and First Responders the training they need to reach, stabilize, and extricate patients trapped in motor-vehicle collisions. The updated course includes techniques for hybrid vehicles, trucks, buses, and small aircraft in addition to its primary focus on traditional vehicles. The eight-hour course is built around the concept of using hand tools commonly carried on an ambulance or first responder unit.

ITLS MILITARY

ITLS offers a custom edition of a stand-alone military edition text, edited by a military surgeon. The scenarios are military based and cater to military personnel.

ENROLLING IN AN ITLS COURSE

ITLS provides its courses through its chapters and training centers. Each chapter is based on a geographic region, with the exception of the U.S. military. Training centers are established for proprietary training organizations to educate their own personnel in ITLS.

For information about your local chapter, contact International Trauma Life Support at 888-495-ITLS (or 630-495-6442 for international callers). ITLS staff will put you in touch with a chapter—or help you start a chapter in your area. You can also find a listing of all ITLS chapters and contact information online at http://www.itrauma.org

International Trauma Life Support

1 South 280 Summit Avenue, Court B-2

Oakbrook Terrace, IL 60181 USA

Phone: 888-495-ITLS (U.S. and Canada)

630-495-6442 (International)

Fax: 630-495-6404

Web: http://www.itrauma.org

E-mail: info@itrauma.org

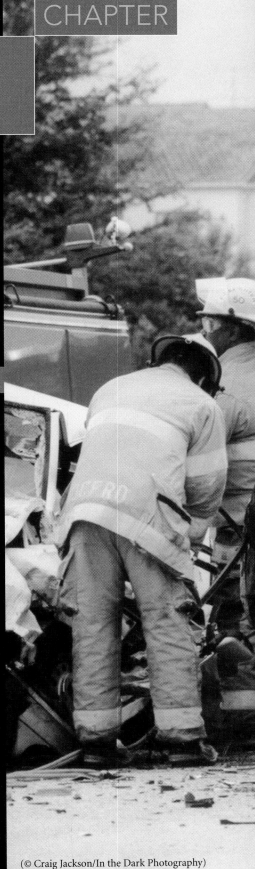

Scene Size-up

James H. Creel, Jr., MD, FACEP

OBJECTIVES

Upon completion of this chapter, you should be able to:

1. Explain the relationship of time to patient survival and explain how this affects your actions at the scene.

2. Discuss the steps of the Scene Size-up.

3. List the two basic mechanisms of motion injury.

4. Discuss mechanisms and settings for blunt versus penetrating trauma.

5. Identify the three collisions associated with a motor-vehicle crash (MVC) and relate potential patient injuries to deformity of the vehicle, interior structures, and body structures.

6. Name the five common forms of MVCs.

7. Describe potential injuries associated with proper and improper use of seat restraints, headrests, and air bags in a head-on collision.

8. Differentiate lateral-impact collision from head-on collision based on the three collisions associated with a MVC.

9. Describe potential injuries from rear-end collisions.

10. Explain why the mortality rate is higher for victims ejected from vehicles in MVCs.

11. Describe the three assessment criteria for falls and relate them to anticipated injuries.

12. Identify the two most common forms of penetration injuries and discuss associated mechanisms and extent of injury.

13. Relate three factors involved in blast injuries to patient assessment.

(© Craig Jackson/In the Dark Photography)

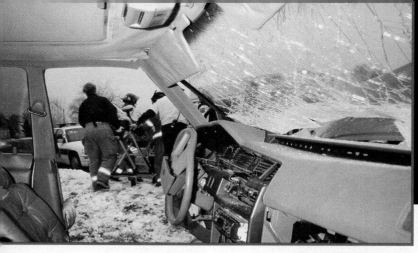

(Photo © Jeff Forster)

Dan, Joyce, and Buddy of the Emergency Transport Service (ETS) have been dispatched to a two-car collision in which one auto ran into the side of the other. They are informed that a rescue truck is on-scene and attempting to extricate one of the drivers. *How do they go about sizing up the scene when they arrive? What should they do before they approach the patients? What equipment should they carry with them as they approach the patient(s)? What injuries should they expect in a collision of this type?* Keep these questions in mind as you read the chapter. Then, at the end of the chapter, find out how the rescuers completed this call.

INTRODUCTION

Trauma, the medical term for *injury*, continues to be the most expensive health problem in the United States and most other countries. In the United States, trauma is the fourth leading cause of death for all ages and the leading cause of death for children and adults under the age of 45 years. For every fatality, there are 10 more patients admitted to hospitals and hundreds more treated in emergency departments. The cost of injury in the United States is estimated to be over $210 billion annually. This represents a cost twice that of cardiovascular disease and cancer combined. The price of trauma, in both physical and fiscal resources, mandates that all emergency medical personnel learn more about this disease to treat its effects and decrease its incidence. (See Appendix H, "Injury Prevention and the Role of the EMS Provider.")

PHILOSOPHY OF ASSESSMENT
AND MANAGEMENT OF THE TRAUMA PATIENT

For the severely injured patient, survival is time-dependent. The direct relationship between the timing of definitive (surgical) treatment and the survival of trauma patients was first described by Dr. R. Adams Cowley of the famous Shock-Trauma Center in Baltimore, Maryland. He discovered that when seriously injured patients were able to gain access to the operating room within an hour of the time of injury, the highest survival rate was achieved (approximately 85 percent). He referred to this as the "Golden Hour."

The Golden Hour begins at the moment the patient is injured, not at the time you arrive at the scene. Rarely is there much of the hour left when you begin your assessment, so you must be well organized in what you do. In the prehospital setting you do not have a Golden Hour, rather a "platinum 10 minutes" in which to identify live patients, make treatment decisions, and begin to move patients to the appropriate medical facility. This means that every action must have a lifesaving purpose. Any action that increases scene time but is not potentially life saving must be omitted. Not only must you reduce evaluation and resuscitation to the most efficient and critical steps, you must also develop the habit of assessing and treating every trauma patient in a planned logical and sequential manner so you do not forget critical actions.

When performing patient assessment, it is best to proceed in a "head-to-toe" manner so that nothing is missed. If you jump around during your assessment, you will inevitably forget to evaluate something crucial. Working as a team with your partner is also important, because many actions must be done at the same time.

It has been said that medicine is a profession that was created for obsessive-compulsive people. Nowhere is this more true than in the care of the trauma patient. Often the patient's life depends on how well you manage the details; and, remember, not all of the details are at the scene of the injury.

You or a member of your team must:

- Know how to maintain your ambulance or rescue vehicle so that it is serviced and ready to respond when needed.
- Know the quickest way to the scene of an injury.
- Know how to size up a scene in order to recognize dangers and identify mechanisms of injury.
- Know which scenes are safe and, if not safe, what to do about them.
- Know when you can handle a situation and when to call for help.
- Know when to approach the patient and when to leave with the patient.
- Know your equipment and maintain it in working order.
- Know the most appropriate hospital and the fastest way to get there. (Organized trauma systems and transfer/bypass guidelines can shorten the time it takes to get a trauma patient to definitive care.)

As if all that were not enough, you also have to:

- Know where to put your hands, which questions to ask, what interventions to perform, when to perform them, and how to perform critical procedures quickly and correctly.

If you think the details are not important, then leave the profession now. Our job is saving lives, a most honorable profession. If we have a bad day, someone will pay for our mistakes with suffering or even death. Since the early beginnings of Emergency Medical Services (EMS), patients and even rescuers have lost their lives because attention was not paid to the details listed above. Many of us can recall patients that we might have saved if we had been a little smarter, a little faster, or a little better organized. Make no mistake, there is no "high" like saving a life, but you will carry the scars of your failures all of your life.

Your mindset and attitude are very important. You must be concerned but not emotional, alert but not excited, quick but not hasty. Above all, you must continuously strive for what is best for your patient. When your training has not prepared you for a situation, always fall back on the question: *What is best for my patient?* When you no longer care, burnout has set in and your effectiveness is severely limited. When this happens, seek help (yes, all of us need help when the stress overcomes us) or seek an alternative profession.

Since 1982, the International Trauma Life Support (ITLS, formerly BTLS) organization has been identifying the best methods to get the most out of those few minutes that prehospital EMS providers have to save the patient's life. Not all patients can be saved, but our goal is never to lose a life that could have been saved. The knowledge in this book can help you make a difference. Learn it well.

SCENE SIZE-UP

Scene Size-up is the first step in the ITLS Primary Survey (Table 1-1). It is a critical part of trauma assessment and begins before you approach the patient. If you fail to perform the preliminary steps of Scene Size-up, you may jeopardize your life and the life of your patient. Scene Size-up includes taking standard precautions to prevent exposure to blood and other potentially infective material, evaluating the scene for dangers, determining the total number of patients, determining essential equipment needed for this particular scene, and identifying the mechanisms of injuries (Table 1-2).

Scene Size-up actually begins at dispatch, when you anticipate what you will find at the scene. At that time, you should think about what equipment you will need and whether other resources (more units, special extrication equipment, multicasualty incident [MCI] protocols) may be needed. Although information from dispatch is useful to begin to think about a plan, do not overrely on this information. Such information given to the dispatcher is often exaggerated or even completely wrong. Be prepared to change your plan depending on your own survey of the scene.

Standard Precautions

Trauma scenes are among the most likely to subject the rescuer to contamination by blood or *other potentially infectious material (OPIM)*. This subject will be covered in more detail in Chapter 22. Not only are trauma patients often bloody; they frequently require airway management under adverse conditions. Personal protective equipment (PPE) is always needed at trauma scenes. Protective gloves are always needed, and many situations will require eye protection. It is wise for the rescuer in charge of airway management to have a face shield or eye protection and mask. In highly contaminated situations, impervious gowns with mask or face shield may also be needed. Remember to protect your patient from body fluids by changing gloves between patients.

Scene Safety

Begin sizing up the scene for hazards as you approach. Your first decision is to determine the nearest safe place to park the ambulance or rescue vehicle. You would like the vehicle

TABLE 1-1 *ITLS Patient Assessment*	
ITLS Primary Survey	Perform a Scene Size-up.
	Perform Initial Assessment.
	Perform a Rapid Trauma Survey or Focused Exam.
	Make Critical Interventions and Transport Decision.
	Contact medical direction.
ITLS Secondary Survey	Repeat Initial Assessment.
	Repeat vital signs and consider monitors.
	Perform a neurological exam.
	Perform a Detailed (head-to-toe) Exam.
ITLS Ongoing Exam	Repeat Initial Assessment.
	Repeat vital signs and check monitors.
	Reassess the abdomen.
	Check injuries and interventions.

TABLE 1-2 *Steps of the Scene Size-up*

1. Standard precautions (personal protective equipment)
2. Scene safety
3. Initial triage (total number of patients)
4. Need for more help or equipment
5. Mechanism of injury

as close as possible, and yet it must be far enough away from the scene for you to be safe while you are performing the scene size-up. Try to park facing away from the scene, so if dangers arise you can load the patient and leave quickly. Next, determine if it is safe to approach the patient(s). Perform a "windshield survey" before leaving your response vehicle. Consider the following:

■ *Crash/rescue scenes.* Is there danger from fire or toxic substances? Is there danger of electrocution? Are unstable surfaces or structures present such as ice, water, slope, or buildings in danger of collapse? Areas with potential for low oxygen levels or toxic chemical levels (sewers, ship holds, silos, and so on) should never be entered until you have the proper protective equipment and breathing apparatus. You should never enter a dangerous area without a partner and a safety line attached.

■ *Crime scenes.* Danger may exist even after a crime has been committed. Be alert for persons fleeing the scene, for persons attempting to conceal themselves, and for persons who are armed or who are making threatening statements or gestures. Do not approach a known crime scene if law enforcement personnel are not present. Wait for law enforcement, not only for the safety of you and the victims, but also to help preserve evidence. Do not approach the scene if you see that law enforcement personnel are in defensive positions or have their weapons drawn.

■ *Bystanders.* You and the victim(s) may be in danger from bystanders. Are bystanders talking in loud, angry voices? Are people fighting? Are weapons present? Is there evidence of the use of alcohol or illegal drugs? Is this a domestic-violence scene? You may not be recognized as a rescuer, but as a symbol of authority and thus attacked. Are dangerous animals present? Request law enforcement personnel at any sign of danger from violence.

Consider whether the scene poses a continued threat to the patient. If there is danger of fire, water, structure collapse, toxic exposure, and so on, the patient may have to be moved immediately. This does not mean that you should expose yourself or your partners to unnecessary danger. You may need to call for special equipment and proper backup from the police, fire services, or the power company. If the scene is unsafe, you should make it safe or try to remove the patients from the scene without putting yourself in danger. Sometimes there is no clearly good way to do this. Use good judgment. You are there to save lives, not give up your own.

Total Number of Patients

Determine the total number of patients now. If there are more patients than your team can effectively handle, call for backup. Remember that you usually need one ambulance for each seriously injured patient. If there are many patients, establish medical command and initiate multicasualty incident (MCI) protocols. Are all patients accounted for? If the patient(s) is unconscious, and there are no witnesses to the incident, look for clues (schoolbooks or diaper bag, passenger list in a commercial vehicle) that other patients

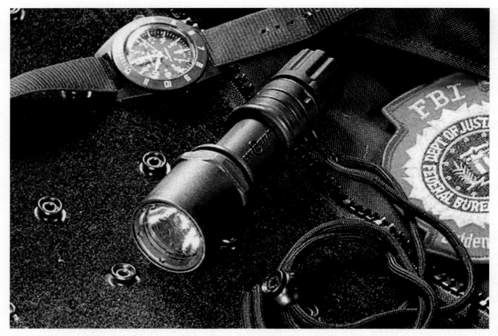

FIGURE 1-1 **Example of a small but powerful tactical flashlight.** *(Photo courtesy of SureFire™ Tactical Lights)*

might be present. Carefully evaluate the scene for other patients. This is especially important at night or if there is poor visibility. It is wise to invest in a high-intensity tactical light (Figure 1-1). They are small enough to carry in your shirt pocket but are many times brighter than regular flashlights.

Essential Equipment and Additional Resources

If possible, carry all essential medical equipment to the scene. This prevents loss of time returning to the vehicle. Remember to change gloves between patients. The following equipment is always needed for trauma patients.

- Personal protection equipment (See previous discussion.)
- Long backboard with effective strapping and head motion-restriction device
- Appropriately sized rigid cervical extrication collar
- Oxygen and airway equipment (Suction equipment and a bag-valve mask [BVM] should be included.)
- Trauma box (bandage material, blood pressure cuff, stethoscope)

If special extrication equipment, more ambulances, or additional personnel are needed, call now! You are less likely to call for help when involved in patient care. Be sure to tell additional responders exactly where to respond.

Mechanism of Injury

Once you determine that it is safe to approach the patient, begin to assess for the *mechanism of injury*. This may be apparent from the scene itself but it may require questioning the patient or bystanders. Energy transmission follows the laws of physics; therefore, injuries present in predictable patterns (Table 1-3). Knowledge and appreciation of the mechanism of injury is very helpful in your evaluation of the patient. Missed or overlooked injuries may be catastrophic, especially when they become known only after the compensatory mechanisms are exhausted.

TABLE 1-3 *Mechanisms of Injury and Potential Injury Patterns*	
Mechanisms of Injury	**Potential Injury Patterns**

Frontal impact
  Deformed steering wheel
  Dashboard knee imprints
  Spider deformity of windscreen
	• Cervical-spine fracture
	• Flail chest
	• Myocardial contusion
	• Pneumothorax
	• Aortic disruption
	• Spleen or liver laceration
	• Posterior hip dislocation
	• Knee dislocation

T-bone	• Contralateral neck sprain • Cervical-spine fracture • Lateral flail chest • Pneumothorax • Aortic disruption • Diaphragmatic rupture • Laceration of spleen, liver, kidney • Pelvic fracture
Rear impact	• Cervical-spine injury
Ejection	• Exposure to all mechanisms and mortality increased
Pedestrian vs. car	• Head injury • Aortic disruption • Abdominal visceral injuries • Fracture lower extremities and pelvis

Remember that patients who are involved in a high-energy event are at risk for severe injury. Despite normal vital signs and no apparent anatomic injury on the initial assessment, 5 to 15 percent of these patients will later exhibit severe injuries that are discovered on repeat examinations. Therefore, a high-energy event signifies a large release of uncontrolled energy, and you should consider the patient injured until you have proven otherwise.

It is important to be aware of whether the mechanism is *generalized* (MVC, fall from a height, and so on) or *focused* (stab wound of abdomen, hit in head by hammer). Generalized mechanisms require a rapid trauma survey, whereas focused mechanisms may only require a more limited exam of the affected areas or systems. Factors to be considered are direction and speed of impact, patient kinetics and physical size, and the signs of energy release (e.g., major vehicle damage). A strong correlation exists between injury severity and automobile velocity changes, as measured by the amount of vehicle damage. It is important that you consider these two questions: *What happened? How was the patient injured?*

Mechanism of injury is also an important triage tool and is information that you should report to the emergency physician or trauma surgeon. Severity of vehicle damage has also been suggested as a nonphysiologic triage tool.

Motion (mechanical) injuries are by and large responsible for the majority of the mortality from trauma in the United States. This chapter reviews the most common

TABLE 1-4 *Basic Mechanisms of Motion Injury*	
Blunt Injuries	**Penetrating Injuries**
• Rapid forward deceleration (collisions) • Rapid vertical deceleration (falls) • Energy transfer from blunt instruments (baseball bat, blackjack)	• Projectiles • Knives • Falls upon fixed objects

mechanisms of motion injuries and stresses the injuries that may be associated with these mechanisms. It is essential to develop an awareness of mechanisms of injury and thus have a high index of suspicion for occult injuries. Always consider the potential injury to be present until it is ruled out in a hospital setting.

There are two basic mechanisms of motion injury, *blunt* and *penetrating* (Table 1-4). Patients may have injuries from both at the same time.

MOTOR-VEHICLE COLLISIONS

Various injury patterns will be discussed in the following examples, which include automobiles, motorcycles, all-terrain vehicles (ATVs), personal watercraft, and tractors. The important concept to appreciate is that the kinetic energy of motion must be absorbed, and this absorption of energy is the basic component in producing injury. Motion injury may be blunt or penetrating. Generally, blunt trauma is more common in the rural setting, and penetrating trauma is more common in the urban setting. Rapid forward deceleration is usually blunt but may be penetrating. The most common example of rapid forward deceleration is the motor-vehicle collision (MVC). You should consider all MVCs to occur as three separate events (Figure 1-2).

- Machine collision
- Body collision
- Organ collision

Consider approaching an MVC in which an automobile has hit a tree head-on at 40 miles per hour. The tree brings the auto to an immediate stop by transferring the energy into damage to the tree and the automobile. The person inside the auto is still traveling at 40 miles per hour until he strikes something that stops him (such as steering wheel, windshield, dashboard). At that point, energy transfers into damage to the person and to the surface struck. The organs inside the person are also traveling at 40 miles per hour until they are stopped by striking a stationary object (such as inside of skull, sternum, steering wheel, dashboard) or by their ligamentous attachments (aorta by ligamentum arteriosum, and so on). In this auto-versus-tree example, appreciation of the rapid forward decelerating mechanism (high-energy event) coupled with a high index of suspicion should make you concerned that the victim may have possible head injury, cervical-spine injury, myocardial contusion, any of the "deadly dozen" chest injuries, intra-abdominal injuries, and musculoskeletal injuries (especially fracture or dislocation of the hip).

To explain the forces involved, consider Sir Isaac Newton's first law of motion: "A body in motion remains in motion in a straight line unless acted upon by an outside force." Motion is created by force (energy exchange), and therefore force will stop motion. If this energy exchange occurs within the body, damage of the tissues is produced. This law is well exemplified in the automobile crash. The kinetic energy of the vehicle's forward motion is absorbed as each part of the vehicle is brought to a sudden halt by the impact. Remember that the body

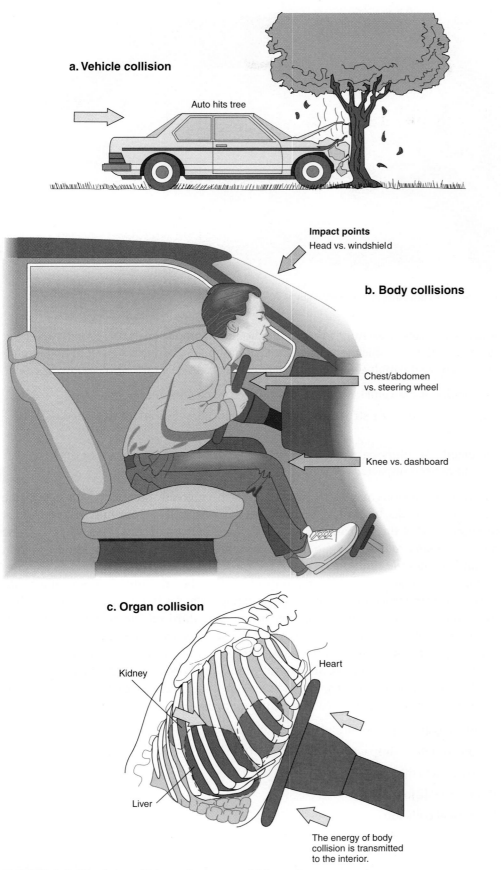

a. Vehicle collision

Auto hits tree

Impact points
Head vs. windshield

b. Body collisions

Chest/abdomen
vs. steering wheel

Knee vs. dashboard

c. Organ collision

Kidney

Heart

Liver

The energy of body
collision is transmitted
to the interior.

FIGURE 1-2 The three collisions of a motor-vehicle crash.

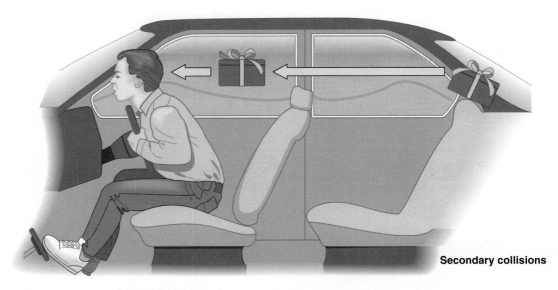

Secondary collisions

FIGURE 1-3 Secondary collisions in a deceleration MVC.

of the occupant is also traveling at 40 miles per hour until impacted by some structure within the car such as the windshield, steering wheel, or dashboard. With awareness of this mechanism, one can see the multitude of injuries that may occur. Be aware of the following clues.

- Deformity of the vehicle (indication of forces involved—energy exchange)
- Deformity of interior structures (indication of where the patient impacted—energy exchange)
- Deformity or injury patterns of the patient (indication of what parts of the body may have been impacted)

Additional collisions may occur other than the three already mentioned. Objects inside the automobile (books, bags, luggage, and other persons) will become missiles traveling at the original speed of the auto and may strike persons in front of them (Figure 1-3). These are called *secondary collisions*. A good example of this is when a parent is holding a child in her lap and crushes the child between her and the dashboard in a deceleration collision.

In many auto collisions, additional impacts occur when the auto strikes another auto and is then in turn struck by an auto following. Also, vehicles frequently deflect from hitting one object and then collide with a second or even third vehicle or stationary object. These are much like a rollover collision in that the persons inside the vehicle are subjected to energy transfer from multiple directions. It is often more difficult to predict injuries in these cases and you must quickly but carefully look for clues inside the vehicle.

MVCs occur in several forms, and each form is associated with certain patterns of injury. The five common forms of MVCs are the following:

- Head-on collision (frontal)
- T-bone or lateral-impact collision (lateral)
- Rear-impact collision (rear)
- Rollover collision
- Rotational collision

Head-on Collision

In a MVC involving a head-on collision, an unrestrained body is brought to a sudden halt, and the energy transfer is capable of producing multiple injuries.

Windshield injuries occur in the rapid forward-decelerating type of event, in which the unrestrained occupant impacts forcefully with the windshield (Figure 1-4). The possibility for injuries is great under these conditions. Of utmost concern is the potential for serious airway and cervical-spine injury.

Remembering the three separate collision events, note the following:

> *Machine collision*—deformed front end
>
> *Body collision*—spiderweb pattern of windshield
>
> *Organ collision*—coup/contracoup brain, soft-tissue injury (scalp, face, neck), hyperextension/flexion of cervical spine

From the spiderweb appearance of the windshield and an appreciation of the mechanism of injury, you should maintain a high index of suspicion for possible occult injuries of the cervical spine. The head usually strikes the windshield, resulting in direct trauma to the face and head. External signs of trauma include cuts, abrasions, and contusions. These may be quite dramatic in appearance; however, the key concern is airway maintenance with motion restriction of the cervical spine and evaluation of level of consciousness.

Steering wheel injuries most often occur to an unrestrained driver of a vehicle in a head-on collision. The driver may subsequently also impact with the windshield. The steering wheel is the vehicle's most lethal weapon for the unrestrained driver, and any degree of steering wheel deformity (check under collapsed airbags) must be treated with a high index of suspicion for face, neck, thoracic, or abdominal injury. The two components of this weapon are the ring and column (Figure 1-5). The ring is a semi-rigid, plastic-covered metal ring attached to a fixed inflexible post—a battering ram.

Utilizing the three-collision concept, check for the presence of the following:

> *Machine collision*—front-end deformity
>
> *Body collision*—ring fracture/deformity, column normal/displaced
>
> *Organ collision*—traumatic tattooing of skin

The head-on collision is entirely dependent upon the area of the body that impacts with the steering wheel. Signs may be readily visible, with direct trauma such as lacerations of mouth and chin, contusion/bruises of the anterior neck, traumatic tattoos of the chest wall, and bruising of the abdomen. These external signs may be subtle or dramatic in appearance, but more important, they may represent the tip of the iceberg. Deeper structures and organs may harbor occult injuries due to *shearing forces*, *compression forces*, and *displacement of kinetic energy*. Organs that are susceptible to shearing injuries due to their ligamentous attachments are the aortic arch, liver, spleen, kidneys,

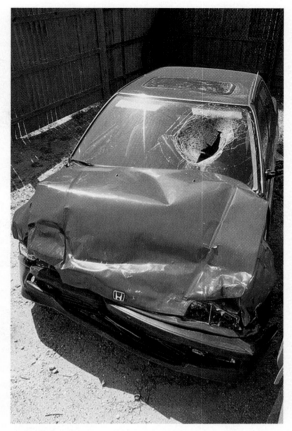

FIGURE 1-4 In a head-on collision, most injuries are inflicted by the windshield, steering wheel, and dashboard.

Steering Wheel Injuries

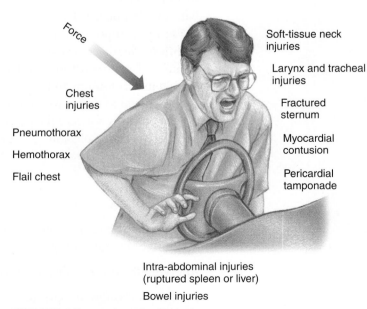

Force

Chest injuries

Pneumothorax

Hemothorax

Flail chest

Soft-tissue neck injuries

Larynx and tracheal injuries

Fractured sternum

Myocardial contusion

Pericardial tamponade

Intra-abdominal injuries (ruptured spleen or liver)

Bowel injuries

FIGURE 1-5 Steering wheel injuries.

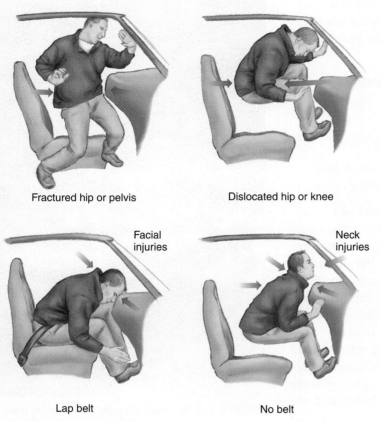

Fractured hip or pelvis

Dislocated hip or knee

Facial injuries

Neck injuries

Lap belt

No belt

FIGURE 1-6 Dashboard injuries.

and bowel. With the exception of small-bowel tears, these injuries are sources for occult bleeds and hemorrhagic shock. Compression injuries are common with the lung, heart, diaphragm, and urinary bladder. An important sign is respiratory distress, which may be due to pulmonary contusions, pneumothorax, diaphragmatic hernia (bowel sounds in chest), or flail chest. Consider a bruised chest wall as a myocardial contusion that requires monitoring of cardiac rhythm and, if available, a 12-lead EKG.

In short, the steering wheel is a lethal weapon capable of producing devastating injuries, many of which are occult. Steering wheel deformity is a cause for alarm and must heighten your index of suspicion. You must also relay this information to the receiving physician.

Dashboard injuries occur most often to an unrestrained passenger. The dashboard has the capability of producing a variety of injuries, depending upon the area of the body that strikes the dashboard. Most frequently, injuries involve the face and knees; however, many types of injuries have been described (Figure 1-6).

Applying the three-event concept of collision, you will note:

Machine collision—deformity of the car

Body collision—fracture/deformity of the dash

Organ collision—facial trauma, coup/contracoup brain, hyperextension/flexion of the cervical spine, pelvis, hip, and knee trauma

Facial, brain, and cervical-spine injuries have already been discussed. Like chest contusion, knee trauma may represent only the tip of the iceberg. Knees commonly impact with the dashboard. This may range from the simple contusion noted about the patella to the severe compound fracture of the patella. Frank dislocation of the knees can occur. In addition, kinetic energy may be transmitted proximally and may result in fracture of the femur or fractured/dislocated hip. On occasion, the pelvis can impact with the dash, resulting in acetabulum and pelvic fractures. These injuries are associated with hemorrhage that may lead to shock. Maintain a high index of suspicion and always palpate the femurs as well as gently squeeze the pelvis and palpate the symphysis pubis.

Deceleration collisions are the most common to have secondary collisions from people or objects in the back of the vehicle. These secondary missiles can cause deadly injuries.

T-Bone or Lateral-Impact Collision

The mechanism of the T-bone collision is similar to that of the head-on collision, with the addition of lateral energy displacement (Figure 1-7).

Applying the three-collision concept, look for the presence of the following:

Machine collision—primary deformity of the car—check the impact side (driver/passenger)

Body collision—degree of door deformity (e.g., armrest bent, outward or inward bowing of door)

Organ collision—cannot be predicted by external exam alone; consider organs underneath areas of external injury

Look for the following common injuries.

■ *Head.* Coup/contracoup is due to lateral displacement.

■ *Neck.* Lateral displacement injuries range from cervical-muscle strain to fracture or subluxation with neurological deficit.

■ *Upper arm and shoulder.* Injuries appear on the side of the impact.

■ *Thorax/abdomen.* Injury is due to direct force either from inward bowing of door on the side of the impact or from unrestrained passenger being propelled across seat.

■ *Pelvis/legs.* Occupants on the side of the impact are likely to have pelvic, hip, or femur fractures.

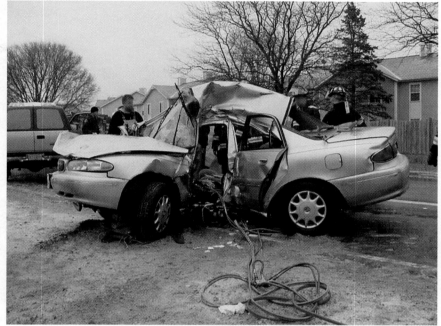
a.

Injuries of the thorax vary from soft-tissue injuries to flail chest, lung contusion, pneumothorax, or hemothorax. Abdominal injuries include those of solid or hollow organs. Pelvic injuries may include fracture/dislocation, bladder rupture, and urethral injuries. Shoulder girdle or lower extremity injuries are common, depending on the level of the impacting force.

Rear-Impact Collision

In the most common form of rear-impact collision, a stationary car is struck from the rear by a moving vehicle (Figure 1-8). Or a slower moving car may be impacted from the rear by a faster moving car. The sudden increase in acceleration produces posterior displacement of the occupants and possible hyperextension of the cervical spine if the headrest is not properly adjusted. If the seat back breaks and falls backward into the rear seat, there is greater chance of lumbar-spine injury.

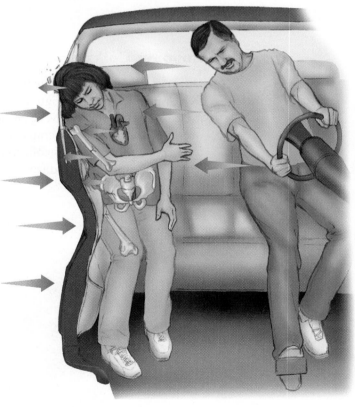
b.

FIGURE 1-7 In a lateral-impact collision, most injuries are inflicted by intrusion of the door, arm rest, side window, or door post. *(Photo courtesy of Anthony Cellitti, NREMT-P)*

Rapid forward deceleration may also occur if the car suddenly strikes something in the front or if the driver applies the brakes suddenly. Note deformity of the auto anterior and posterior as well as interior deformity and headrest position. The potential for cervical-spine injuries is great (Figure 1-9). Be alert for associated deceleration injuries as well.

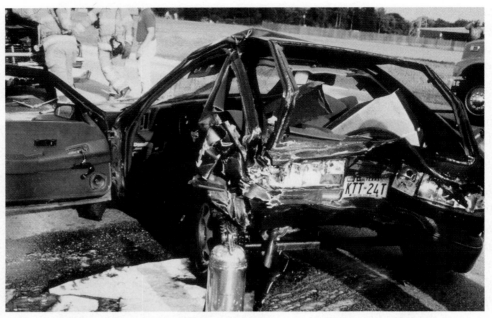

FIGURE 1-8 In a rear-impact collision, the potential exists for neck and back injury. *(Photo courtesy of Bonnie Meneely, EMT-P)*

Rollover Collision

During a vehicle rollover, the body may be impacted from any direction; thus, the potential for injuries is great (Figure 1-10). The chance for axial-loading injuries of the spine is increased in this form of MVC. Rescuers must be alert for clues that suggest the car turned over (such as roof dents, scratches, debris, and deformity of roof posts). Lethal injuries often occur in this form of collision because of the greater likelihood of occupants being ejected. Occupants ejected from the car are 25 times as likely to be killed.

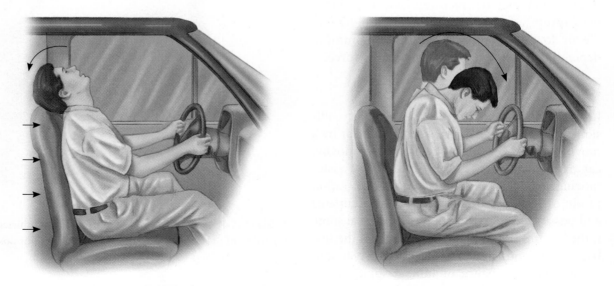

a. Victim moves ahead while head remains stationary. Head rotates backward. Neck extends.

b. Head snaps forward. Head rotates forward. Neck flexes.

FIGURE 1-9 Mechanism of cervical-spine injury in a rear-impact collision.

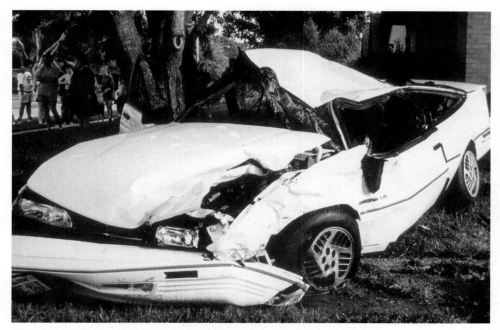

FIGURE 1-10 A rollover collision has a high potential for injury. Many mechanisms are involved, and unrestrained victims are frequently ejected. *(Photo courtesy of Bonnie Meneely, EMT-P)*

Rotational Collision

A rotational mechanism is best described as what occurs when one part of the vehicle stops and the rest of the vehicle remains in motion. A rotational collision usually occurs when a vehicle is struck in the front or rear lateral area. This converts forward motion to a spinning motion. The results are a combination of the frontal-impact and the lateral-impact mechanisms with the same possibilities of injuries of both mechanisms.

Occupant Restraint Systems

Restrained occupants are more likely to survive a collision, because they are protected from much of the impact inside the auto and are unlikely to be ejected from the auto. These occupants are, however, still susceptible to certain injuries.

A lap belt is intended to go across the pelvis (iliac crests), not the abdomen. If the belt is in place and the victim is subjected to a frontal deceleration crash, his body tends to fold together like a clasp knife (Figure 1-11). The head may be thrown forward into the steering wheel or dashboard. Facial, head, or neck injuries are common. Abdominal injuries also occur if the lap belt is positioned improperly. The compression forces that are produced when a body is suddenly folded at the waist may injure the abdomen or the lumbar spine.

The three-point restraint or cross-chest lap belt (Figure 1-12) secures the body much better than a lap belt alone. The chest and pelvis are restrained, so life-threatening injuries are much less common. The head is not restrained, and therefore the neck is still subjected to stresses that may cause fractures, dislocations, or spinal cord injuries. Clavicular fractures (at the point where the chest strap crosses) are common. Internal organ damage may still occur due to organ movement inside the body.

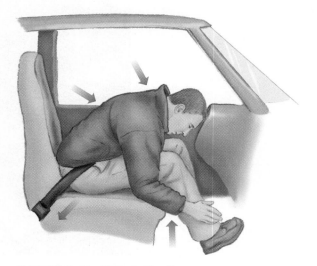

FIGURE 1-11 Clasp-knife effect.

Like belt restraints, air bags (passive restraints) will reduce injuries in victims of MVCs in most but not all situations. Air bags are designed to inflate from the center of the steering wheel and the dashboard to protect the front-seat occupants in case of a frontal deceleration crash. If functioning properly, they cushion the head and chest at the instant of impact, thus effectively decreasing injury to the face, neck, and chest. Be sure to stabilize the neck, however, until it has been adequately examined. Air bags deflate immediately, so they protect against only one impact. The driver whose car hits more than one object is unprotected after the initial collision. Air bags also do not prevent "down and under" movement, so drivers who are extended (tall drivers and drivers of small, low-slung autos) may still impact with their legs and suffer leg, pelvis, or abdominal injuries.

It is important for occupants to wear chest and lap belts even when the car is equipped with air bags. Researchers have recently shown that some drivers who appear uninjured after deceleration crashes have been found to have serious internal injuries. A clue to which driver may have internal injuries is the condition of the steering wheel. A deformed steering wheel is just as important a clue in an auto equipped with an air bag as in those that are not. This clue may be missed, because the deflated air bag covers the steering wheel. Thus, a quick "lift and look" under the air bag should be part of the routine examination of the steering wheel (Figure 1-13).

Many autos are now equipped with side air bags in the doors. Some have air bags that come down from the roof to protect the head and at least one make of auto has air bags under the dash to protect the legs. These obviously give much needed extra protection.

Certain dangers are associated with air bags. Small drivers who bring the seat up close to the steering wheel may sustain serious injuries as the bag inflates. Infants in car seats placed in the front seat may be seriously injured by the air bag.

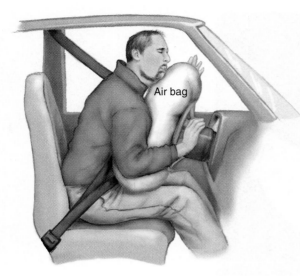

Air bag and three-point restraint prevents collisions 2 and 3.

FIGURE 1-12 Air bag and three-point restraint.

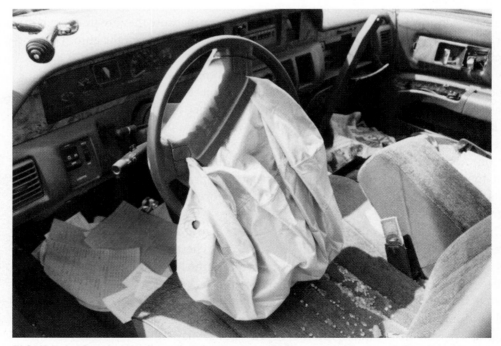

FIGURE 1-13 Lift the collapsed air bag to note whether or not there is a deformity of the steering wheel. (*Photo courtesy of Robert S. Porter*)

In summary, when at the scene of a MVC, note the type of collision and the clues (such as deformities of the vehicle) that imply high kinetic energy has been spent. Maintain a high index of suspicion for occult injuries and thus keep scene time to a minimum. These observations and clues are essential to quality patient care and must be relayed to medical direction and the receiving physician.

Tractor Accidents

Another large motorized vehicle with which you must be familiar is the tractor. The U.S. National Safety Council reports that one-third of all farm accident fatalities involve tractors. The two basic types of tractors are the two-wheel drive and the four-wheel drive. In both, the center of gravity is high, and thus the tractors are easily turned over (Figure 1-14). The majority of fatal accidents are due to the tractor turning over and crushing the driver. Most overturns (85 percent) are to the side; these are less likely to pin the driver because he has a chance to jump or be thrown clear. Rear overturns, although less frequent, are more likely to entrap and crush the driver because there is almost no opportunity to jump free. The primary mechanism is the crush injury, and the severity depends on the part of the anatomy involved. Additional mechanisms are chemical burns from gasoline, diesel fuel, hydraulic fluid, or even battery acid. Thermal burns from hot engine parts or ignited fuel are also common.

Management consists of scene stabilization followed quickly by the primary survey and resuscitation. The following questions are used as a checklist in scene stabilization.

- Is the engine off?
- Are the rear wheels locked?
- Have the fuel situation and fire hazard been addressed?

While you are assessing the patient, other rescuers must stabilize the tractor. The center of gravity must be identified before any attempt is made to lift the tractor. The center of gravity of the two-wheel-drive tractor is located approximately 10 inches above and 24 inches in front of the rear axle. The center of gravity of a four-wheel-drive tractor is

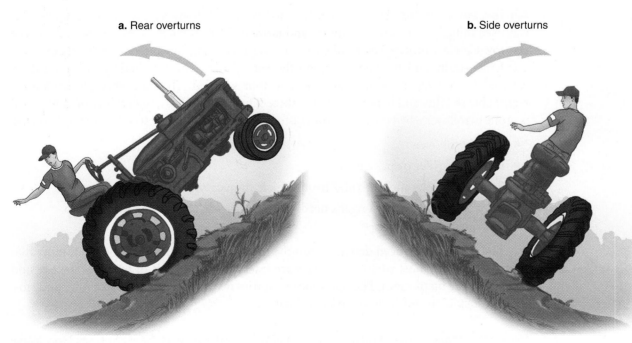

a. Rear overturns **b.** Side overturns

FIGURE 1-14 Tractor accidents.

closer to the midline of the machine. Because tractors usually overturn on soft ground and their centers of gravity are tricky to determine, great care must be taken during lifting to avoid a second crush injury. Because of the tractor weight and length of time (usually prolonged) the driver is pinned, anticipate serious injuries. Often, the patient will go into profound shock as the compressing weight of the tractor is removed—similar to what happens when antishock trousers are suddenly deflated.

Rapid, safe management of tractor accidents requires special exercises in lifting heavy machinery as well as good trauma management. To obtain additional information and training opportunities related to tractor incidents and other agricultural emergencies, please refer to Appendix J in the back of this book.

Small-Vehicle Crashes

Other small vehicles that fall into the motion injury category include the motorcycle, ATV, personal watercraft (PWC), and snowmobile. The operators of these machines are not encased within them, and, of course, wear no restraining devices. When the operator is subjected to the classic head-on, lateral-impact, rear-end, or rollover collision, the only forms of protection are the following:

- Evasive maneuvering
- Helmet usage
- Protective clothing (such as leather clothes, helmet, boots)
- Use of the vehicle to absorb kinetic energy (such as bike slide)

Motorcycles: It is extremely important for motorcycle riders to wear helmets. Helmets help prevent head injury (which causes 75 percent of motorcycle deaths). Regardless, helmets give no protection to the spine. The operator of a motorcycle involved in a crash is much like an ejected automobile occupant and severe injuries are common. Injuries depend on the part of the anatomy subjected to kinetic energy. The lack of protective encasement leads to a higher frequency of head, neck, and extremity injuries. Important clues include deformity of the motorcycle, distance of skid, and deformity of stationary objects or cars.

All-Terrain Vehicles: The ATV was designed as a vehicle to traverse rough terrain. The ATV was used initially by ranchers, hunters, and farmers. Unfortunately, some people view it as a fast toy. Careless misuse has resulted in an ever-increasing morbidity and mortality from accidents—sadly and frequently among the very young. The two basic designs are three wheeled (no longer made and, so, rare) and four wheeled. The four-wheel design affords reasonable stability and handling, but the three-wheeled ATV has a high center of gravity and is prone to rollover when turned sharply. Listed below are the four most common mechanisms.

- Vehicle rollover
- Fall-off of rider or passenger
- Forward deceleration of rider from vehicle impact with stationary object
- Impact of rider or passenger's head or extremities when passing too close to stationary objects (trees)

The injuries produced depend upon the mechanism and the part of the anatomy that is impacted. The most frequent injuries are fractures, about half of which are above and half below the diaphragm. The major bony injuries involve the clavicles, sternum, and ribs. Be very suspicious for head or spinal injury.

Personal Watercraft: The use of personal watercraft (such as the Jet Ski, Sea Doo, Wave Runner) has become popular in water recreational activities. Over a million PWCs are in operation in the United States. The U.S. Coast Guard reports that after a 400 percent increase in the number of reported injuries from PWCs between 1990 and 1997 (2,860–12,000), there has been a decline in reported injuries every year since (last report 2004). The number of reported PWC-related injuries, however, is thought to be inaccurate, because many are never reported to law enforcement agencies. The rate of emergency department–treated injuries related to PWC is about 8.5 times higher than the rate of that of motorboats. The death rate is about 3 times higher.

These watercraft are designed to be operated by the driver in a sitting, standing, or kneeling position, with one or more passengers located behind the driver in tandem. PWCs are able to obtain high speeds quickly, but have no braking mechanism. Like motorcycles, PWCs offer no protection to the driver or passengers. Most injuries are caused by PWC collisions, either with other watercraft or with fixed objects such as docks or tree stumps. PWC collisions produce injury patterns similar to those encountered with motorcycle–auto collisions. Rectal and vaginal trauma may occur when rear-seat passengers or the driver fall off backwards, impacting the water (buttocks first) at high speeds. The likelihood of drowning (even with the use of personal flotation devices) is always a danger. Remember, water is not soft when a body impacts with it at high speeds; therefore, you must assess and practice the same index of suspicion as with any high-energy event.

Snowmobiles: Snowmobiles are used both as recreational and utility vehicles. The snowmobile has a low clearance and a low center of gravity. The injuries common to this vehicle are similar to those that occur with the ATV. Turnovers are somewhat more common, and since the vehicle is usually heavier than an ATV, crush injuries are seen more frequently. Again, the injury pattern depends on the part of the anatomy that is directly involved. Be alert for possible coexisting hypothermia. A common injury with the snowmobile is the "hangman" or "clothes line" injury that results from running under wire fences. Be alert for occult cervical-spine injuries and potential airway compromise.

Pedestrian Injuries

The pedestrian struck by a car almost always suffers severe internal injuries as well as fractures. This is true even if the vehicle is traveling at low speed. The mass of the auto is so large that high speed is not necessary to impart high-energy transfer. When high speed is involved the results are disastrous.

There are two mechanisms of injury. The first is when the bumper of the auto strikes the body, and the second is when the body, accelerated by the transfer of forces, strikes the ground or some other object. An adult usually has bilateral lower leg or knee fractures plus whatever secondary injuries occur when the body strikes the hood of the car and then later the ground. Children are shorter, so the bumper is more likely to hit them in the pelvis or torso. They usually land on their heads in the secondary impact. When answering a call to an auto–pedestrian accident, be prepared for broken bones, internal injuries, and head injuries.

FALLS

The mechanism for falls is vertical deceleration. The types of injuries sustained depend on the following three factors, which you must identify and relay to medical direction.

- Distance of fall
- Anatomic area impacted
- Surface struck

The primary groups involved in vertical falls are adults and children under the age of 5 years. In children, the falls most commonly involve boys and occur mostly in the summer months in urban high-rise, multiple-occupant dwellings. Predisposing factors include poor supervision, defective railings, and the curiosity associated with that age group. Head injuries are common in falls by children, because the head is the heaviest part of the body and thus impacts first. Adult falls are generally occupational or due to the influence of alcohol or drugs. It is not uncommon for falls to occur during attempts to escape from fire or criminal activity. Generally, adults attempt to land on their feet; thus their falls are more controlled. In this landing form, the victim usually impacts initially on the feet and then falls backwards, landing on the buttocks and outstretched hands. Classically, this "lover's leap" fall may result in the following injuries (Figure 1-15).

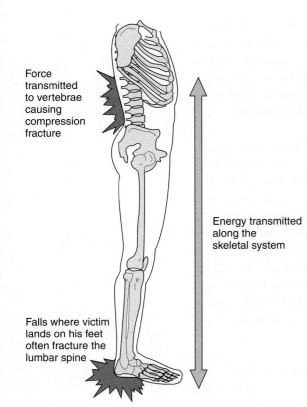

Force transmitted to vertebrae causing compression fracture

Energy transmitted along the skeletal system

Falls where victim lands on his feet often fracture the lumbar spine

FIGURE 1-15 Axial loading.

- Fractures of the feet or legs
- Hip and/or pelvic injuries
- Axial loading to the lumbar and cervical spine
- Vertical deceleration forces to the organs
- Colles fracture of the wrists

The greater the height, the greater is the potential for injury. However, serious injury can occur in a short-distance fall. Surface density (concrete versus sawdust) and irregularity (gym floor versus staircase) also influence the severity of injury. Relay information about distance fallen and surface struck to medical direction with other pertinent information.

PENETRATING INJURIES

Numerous objects are capable of producing penetrating injuries. These range from the industrial saw blade that breaks off at an extremely high rate of speed to the foreign body hurled by a lawn mower. Most high-velocity objects are capable of penetrating the thorax or abdomen. Common forms of penetrating wounds come from the knife and gun.

Knife-wound severity depends on the anatomic area penetrated, length of the blade, and angle of penetration (Figure 1-16). Remember, an upper abdominal stab wound may cause intrathoracic organ injury, and stab wounds below the fourth intercostal space may have penetrated the abdomen. The golden rule with any impaled object is to stabilize it in place. It will be removed at the hospital. Impaled objects in the cheek of the face and those blocking the airway are exceptions to this rule.

Most penetrating wounds inflicted by firearms are due to handguns, rifles, and shotguns. Important factors to obtain, if possible, are the type of weapon, its caliber, and the distance from which the weapon was fired. However, remember that you treat the patient and the wound, not the weapon.

Wound Ballistics

Because the kinetic energy (kinetic energy = $\frac{1}{2}$ mass × velocity^2) produced by a projectile is mostly dependent upon velocity, weapons are clas-

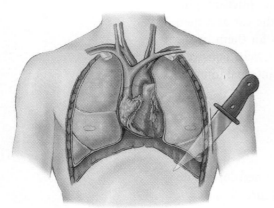

Stab wounds at nipple level or below frequently penetrate the abdomen.

FIGURE 1-16 Stab wounds.

sified as high or low velocity. Weapons with velocities less than 2,000 feet per second are considered low velocity and include essentially all handguns and some rifles. Injuries from these weapons are much less destructive than those sustained from high-velocity weapons, such as a military rifle. Low-velocity weapons are certainly capable of lethal injuries, depending on the body area struck. More civilians are killed by low-velocity bullets, because they are more often shot by low-velocity weapons. All wounds inflicted by high-velocity weapons carry the additional factor of hydrostatic pressure. This factor alone can increase the injury.

Factors that contribute to tissue damage include:

- *Missile size.* The larger the bullet, the more resistance and the larger the permanent tract.
- *Missile deformity.* Hollow point and soft nose flatten out on impact, resulting in the involvement of a larger surface.
- *Semijacket.* The jacket expands and adds to surface area.
- *Tumbling.* Tumbling of the missile causes a wider path of destruction.
- *Yaw.* The missile can oscillate vertically and horizontally (wobble) about its axis, resulting in a larger surface area presenting to the tissue.

The wounds consist of the following three parts.

- *Entry wound.* Usually smaller than the exit wound, it may have darkened, burned edges if the bullet is fired from very close range (Figure 1-17a).
- *Exit wound.* Not all entry wounds will have exit wounds, and on occasion there may be multiple exits due to fragmentation of bone and missile. Generally, the exit wound is larger and has ragged edges (Figure 1-17b).
- *Internal wound.* Low-velocity projectiles inflict damage primarily by damaging tissue that the missile contacts. High-velocity projectiles inflict damage by tissue contact and transfer of kinetic energy to surrounding tissues (Figure 1-18). Damage is related to the following:
  - Shock waves
  - Temporary cavity, which is 30 to 40 times the bullet's diameter and creates immense tissue pressures
  - Pulsation of the temporary cavity, which creates pressure changes in the adjacent tissue

Generally damage done is proportional to tissue density. Highly dense organs such as bone, muscle, and liver sustain more damage than less dense organs such as lungs. A

PEARLS
Basic Ballistics

Know the information offered here, but remember: Treat the patient, not the weapon.

- *Caliber*—the internal diameter of the barrel; this corresponds to the ammunition used for the particular weapon
- *Rifling*—a series of spiral grooves in the interior surface of the barrel of some weapons
- *Ammunition*—case, primer, powder, and bullet
- *Bullet construction*—usually solid lead alloy; may have a full or partial copper or steel jacket. The shape of the nose of the bullet may be rounded, flat, conical, or pointed. The bullet nose may also be soft or hollow (for expansion or fragmentation).

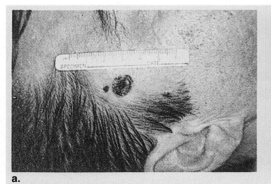
a.
ENTRANCE WOUND (Bullet —
Close Range)

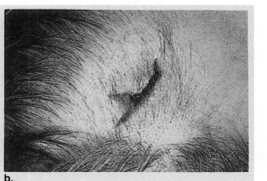
b.
EXIT WOUND (Bullet)

FIGURE 1-17 Comparison of (a) an entrance wound and (b) an exit wound.

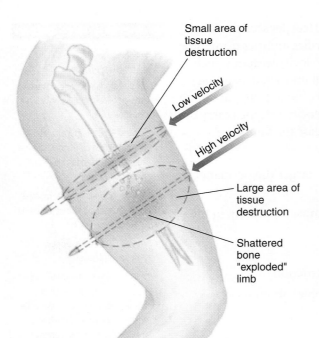

FIGURE 1-18a High-velocity versus low-velocity injury.

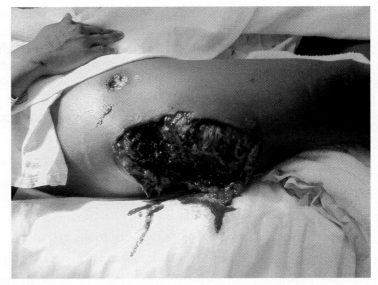

FIGURE 1-18b Example of a high-velocity wound of leg. *(Photo courtesy of Roy Alson, MD)*

key factor to remember is that once a bullet enters a body, its trajectory will not always be in a straight line. Any patient with a missile penetration of the head, thorax, or abdomen should be transported immediately. Personnel who have been shot while wearing a flak vest should be managed with caution; be alert for possible cardiac and other organ contusion.

In shotgun wounds, injury is determined by kinetic energy at impact, which is influenced by:

■ Powder charge
■ Size of pellets
■ Choke of muzzle
■ Distance to target

Velocity and kinetic energy dissipate rapidly as distance is traveled. At 40 yards, the velocity is one-half the initial muzzle velocity.

BLAST INJURIES

Blast injuries in this country occur primarily in industrial settings such as grain elevator and gas fume explosions. Because threat of terrorist activity is now both common and worldwide, blast injury management also must be added to ITLS training and knowledge.

The mechanism of injury by blast/explosion is due to three factors:

■ *Primary*—initial air blast
■ *Secondary*—patient being struck by material (shrapnel) propelled by the blast force
■ *Tertiary*—body being thrown and impacting on ground or other object

Now that terrorists are using explosives to disperse chemical, biological, or radiological material, some now classify injuries resulting from this as "quaternary injuries."

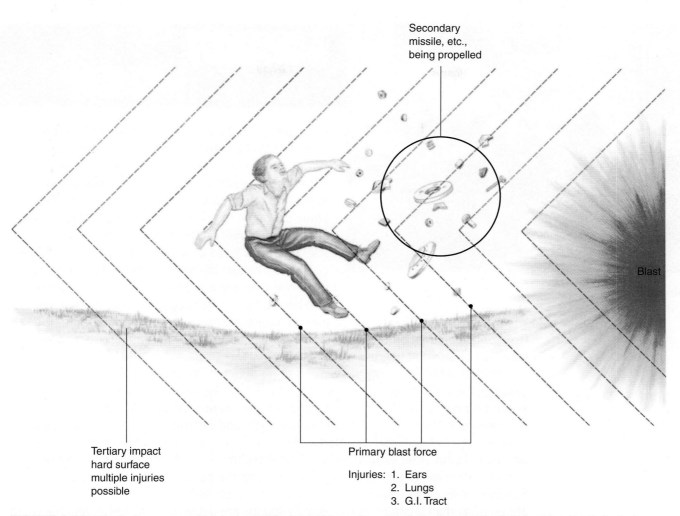

FIGURE 1-19a Explosions can cause injury with the initial blast, when the victim is struck by debris, or by the victim being thrown against the ground or other fixed objects by the blast.

Injuries due to the primary air blast are almost exclusive to the air-containing organs. The auditory system usually involves ruptured tympanic membranes. Lung injuries may include pneumothorax, parenchymal hemorrhage, and especially, alveolar rupture. Alveolar rupture may cause air embolus that may be manifested by bizarre central nervous system symptoms. Gastrointestinal tract injuries may vary from mild intestinal and stomach contusions to frank rupture. Always suspect lung injuries in a blast victim.

Injuries caused by the secondary factors may be penetrating or blunt. Fragments of shrapnel from an explosion may attain velocities of 14,000 feet per second. This is over 4 times the velocity of the most powerful high-velocity rifle bullets. A piece of shrapnel traveling at this velocity would impart more than 16 times the energy of a similarly sized high-velocity rifle bullet. Any shrapnel wound should be considered serious.

Tertiary injuries are much the same as when a person is ejected from an automobile (Figure 1-19).

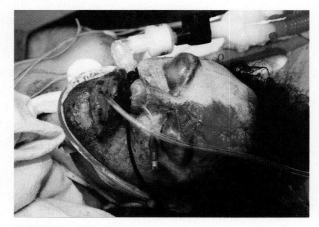

FIGURE 1-19b Tertiary injury from being thrown into a wall by the blast. *(Photo courtesy of Roy Alson, MD)*

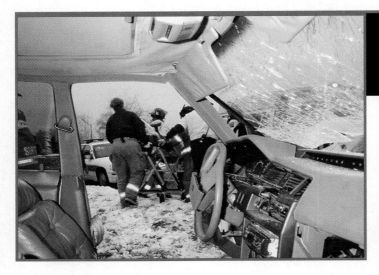

(Photo © Jeff Forster)

Dan, Joyce, and Buddy of the Emergency Transport Service (ETS) have been dispatched to a two-car collision in which one auto ran into the side of the other. They are informed that a rescue truck is on-scene and attempting to extricate one of the drivers. While driving to the scene they decide that Joyce will act as team leader on this case.

On arrival, Joyce gets the trauma box and cervical collars and begins the Scene Size-up. Dan gets the oxygen and airway equipment and Buddy gets the backboard. As she sizes up the scene, Joyce notes that the police are there and the scene is safe. The team dons personal protective equipment. They approach, each carrying some of the essential equipment needed at the scene.

Neither vehicle had any passengers other than the driver. The first car has front-end damage, the air bag deployed, and the driver is walking around with no complaints. The second car was struck in the driver's door with major intrusion into the passenger compartment. The driver is pinned in the vehicle and extrication requires removing the door in order to free him. He is alert and oriented, but complains of chest and abdominal pain. After extrication, Dan stabilizes the cervical spine and applies the nonrebreather oxygen mask while Joyce performs the assessment. Joyce's Rapid Trauma Survey reveals crepitation of the lower ribs on the left with a tender, distended abdomen and an unstable pelvis. Breath sounds are decreased on the left and the chest is dull to percussion. The patient is in shock. They quickly package him and immediately load and go.

Vital signs are pulse 140, respiration 28, BP 70/40. The patient states he has no allergies, takes no medications, has always been healthy, and last food was about 4 hours ago. While Dan starts two large-bore IVs and cautiously gives normal saline at a rate to maintain a BP of 80–90 systolic, Joyce calls on-line medical direction (OLMD) and reports that she is transporting a patient who is in shock. She suspects that the patient has rib fractures, a hemothorax, intra-abdominal injuries, and a fractured pelvis. OLMD agrees with her decision to limit IV fluids because of the hemothorax and tells her to transport the patient to the local level-one trauma center.

The trauma team is mobilized and waiting when they arrive. The patient is found to have a fractured pelvis, ruptured spleen, fractured left ribs, and a hemothorax. He requires surgery and multiple blood transfusions but eventually recovers and returns to work. The emergency physician credits prompt prehospital management for helping save the patient's life.

The mechanism of injury of a T-bone or lateral-impact collision is straight deceleration for the auto hitting the side of the other auto. For the auto that sustains the lateral impact, the mechanism depends on the height of the blow. A sports utility vehicle or large truck would strike the auto higher than a passenger car and so would more likely cause upper chest, shoulder, neck, and head injuries. A passenger car would strike lower and, depending on how low, would be more likely to cause pelvis fractures, intra-abdominal injuries, and rib and lower chest injuries. With major intrusion into the passenger compartment, expect these to be serious injuries. All patients in shock are load-and-go.

SUMMARY

Trauma is the most serious disease affecting young people. Being a rescuer is among the most important professions but requires great dedication and continuous training. Saving patients who have sustained severe trauma requires attention to detail and careful management of time. Teamwork is essential, as many actions must occur at the same time.

At the scene of an injury, there are certain important steps to perform before you begin care of the patient. Failure to perform a Scene Size-up will subject you and your patient to danger and may cause you to fail to anticipate serious injuries that your patient may have sustained. Take standard precautions and assess the scene for dangers first. Then determine the total number of patients and the need for additional rescuers or special equipment. If there are more patients than your team can manage, report to dispatch and initiate MCI protocols.

Identify the mechanism of injury and consider it as part of the overall management of the trauma patient. Ask yourself: What happened? What type of energy was applied? How much energy was transmitted? What part of the body was affected? If there is a MVC, consider the form of the crash and survey the vehicle's interior and exterior for damage.

Note that tractor accidents require careful stabilization of the machine to prevent a second injury to the patient. Falls require identification of distance fallen, surface struck, and position of the patient upon impact. Stab wounds require knowledge of the length of the instrument as well as the angle at which it entered the body. When evaluating a shooting victim, you need to know the weapon, caliber, and distance from which it fired.

Information about the high-energy event (e.g., falls, vehicle collision) is also important to the emergency physician. Be sure not only to record your findings but also to give a verbal report to the emergency department physician or trauma surgeon when you arrive. With this knowledge and a high index of suspicion, you can give your patient the greatest chance of survival.

BIBLIOGRAPHY

1. Almogy, G., Y. Mintz, et al. 2006. Suicide bombing attacks: Can external signs predict internal injuries? *Annals of Surgery* 243(4):541–46.

2. American College of Surgeons, Committee on Trauma. 2004. Appendix 3: Biomechanics of injury. In *Advanced Trauma Life Support Student Manual.* 7th ed. Chicago: American College of Surgeons.

3. Committee on Injury and Poison Prevention. 2000. American Academy of Pediatrics: Personal watercraft use by children and adolescents. *Pediatrics* 105(2): 452–53.

4. DeHaven, H. 2000. Mechanical analysis of survival in falls from heights of fifty to one hundred and fifty feet. *Injury Prevention* 6: 62–68.

5. McSwain, N. E. Jr. 1999. *Pre-hospital trauma life support.* 4th ed. St. Louis: Mosby, Inc. 1–33.

6. Newgard, C., K. Martens, E. Lyons. 2002. Crash scene photography in motor vehicle crashes without air bag deployment. *Academic Emergency Medicine* 9(9): 924–29.

7. Wightman, J., S. Gladish. 2001. Explosions and blast injuries. *Annals of Emergency Medicine,* 37(6): 664–78.

Assessment and Initial Management of the Trauma Patient

John E. Campbell, MD, FACEP

John T. Stevens, EMT-P

Leon Charpentier, EMT-P

OBJECTIVES

Upon completion of this chapter, you should be able to:

1. Outline the steps in trauma assessment and management.

2. Describe the ITLS Primary Survey.

3. Explain the Initial Assessment and how it relates to the Rapid Trauma Survey and the Focused Exam.

4. Describe when the Initial Assessment can be interrupted.

5. Describe when critical interventions should be made and where to make them.

6. Identify which patients have critical conditions and how they should be managed.

7. Describe the ITLS Secondary Survey.

8. Describe the ITLS Ongoing Exam.

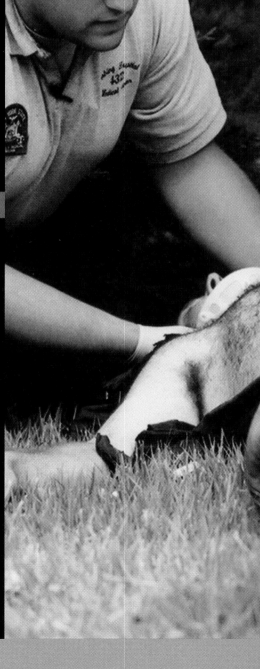

(© Craig Jackson/
In the Dark Photography)

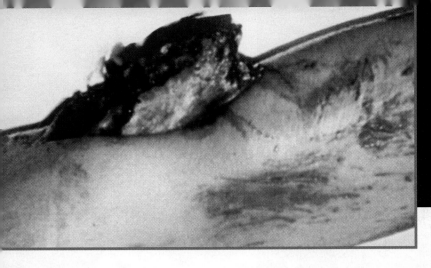

Dan, Joyce, and Buddy of the Emergency Transport System (ETS) have been called to the scene of a construction accident where a man fell from a scaffold onto a pile of lumber. Their Scene Size-up reveals that the scene is safe and there is only one victim. He has been pulled from the lumber pile, but appears to be pale and diaphoretic and has an obvious open fracture of his left lower leg. He is clutching a piece of wood that is sticking out of his left chest. *How would you approach this patient? What is the mechanism of injury? What type of assessment would you perform? What would you do first? Is this a load-and-go situation?* Keep these questions in mind as you read the chapter. Then, at the end of the chapter, find out how the rescuers completed this call.

INTRODUCTION

ITLS patient assessment (Primary Survey, Secondary Survey, and Ongoing Exam) is consistent with U.S. Department of Transportation guidelines. The ITLS Primary Survey is made up of the Scene Size-up, Initial Assessment (a very brief exam of the level of consciousness and the ABCs), and a Rapid Trauma Survey (a rapid head-to-toe exam) to determine if *immediately* life-threatening conditions exist and to identify those patients who should have immediate transport. The Primary Survey differs from the Secondary Survey in that the Secondary Survey is an evaluation for all injuries, not just life-threatening ones. The Ongoing Exam is meant to identify changes in the patient's condition.

The patient with the most minor-appearing injury will get a brief Initial Assessment before you concentrate on the minor injury. Critical patients will get a much more comprehensive exam, but in each case the exam will begin in the same way (Initial Assessment). The Scene Size-up will set the stage for how you will perform the rest of the ITLS Primary Survey.

If there is a dangerous generalized mechanism of injury (auto crash, fall from a height, etc.) or if the patient is unconscious, you should go from Initial Assessment directly to the Rapid Trauma Survey. You would then perform interventions, transport, Ongoing Exams, and possibly a Secondary Survey en route.

If there is a dangerous focused mechanism of injury suggesting an isolated injury (bullet wound of thigh, stab wound to the chest, etc.), you would perform the Initial Assessment but the Focused Exam would be limited to the area of injury. The full Rapid Trauma Survey is not required. You would then perform interventions, transport, Ongoing Exams, and possibly a Secondary Survey.

If there is no significant life threat in the mechanism of injury (e.g., shot off big toe) you would do the Initial Assessment and, if normal, go directly to a Focused Exam based on the patient's chief complaint. The Secondary Survey would not be necessary.

To make the most efficient use of time, ITLS prehospital assessment and management of the trauma patient is divided into three exams (Primary Survey, Secondary Survey, and Ongoing Exam), and each exam is made up of certain steps (Figure 2-1). These exams are the foundation on which prehospital trauma care is built.

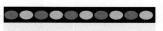

PEARLS
A Systematic Approach
Use the same systematic ITLS approach for each trauma patient.

PATIENT ASSESSMENT

ITLS Primary Survey

The ITLS Primary Survey includes an evaluation of the scene and preparation for patient assessment and management. It begins with the Scene Size-up and then, if the scene is safe to enter, moves on to the Initial Assessment and a Rapid Trauma Survey or Focused Exam.

Scene Size-up: On-scene trauma assessment begins with certain actions that are performed before you approach the patient. It cannot be stressed too much that failure to perform preliminary actions can jeopardize your life as well as the patient's. Perform the Scene Size-up as described in Chapter 1.

PEARLS
Safety
Do not approach the patient before doing a Scene Size-up. Foolish haste may subtract a rescuer and add a patient.

Once you begin your assessment of the critical patient, you may not have time to return to the vehicle for needed equipment. For this reason, you should always carry essential medical equipment with you to the patient's side. Anticipate that the following equipment may be needed for trauma patients.

- Personal protection equipment (See Chapters 1 and 22.)
- Long backboard with effective strapping and head motion-restriction device
- Appropriately sized rigid cervical extrication collar
- Airway kit (separate kits or separate sections for adult and pediatric patients)
  - Oxygen
  - Airway and intubation equipment
  - Bag-valve mask (BVM)
  - Suction
- Trauma box (separate boxes for adult and pediatric patients)
  - Dressings, bandages, and hemostatic agents to aid in bleeding control
  - Pleural decompression equipment
  - Blood pressure cuff
  - Stethoscope
  - Tourniquets

Once the scene is safe to enter, as team leader, you must focus on the rapid assessment of your patient. All decisions on treatment require that you have identified life-threatening conditions. Experience has shown that most mistakes occur because the team leader stops to perform an intervention and forgets to perform part of the assessment. If immediate interventions are needed, delegate them to your team members while you continue the assessment.

Remember, once you begin patient assessment in the ITLS Primary Survey, only three things should cause you to interrupt the completion of the assessment. You may interrupt the assessment sequence if the scene becomes unsafe, if you must treat an airway obstruction, or if you must treat cardiac arrest. (Respiratory arrest or dyspnea may be addressed by Rescuer 2 while you continue assessment of the patient.)

For critical patients, the goal should be to have on-scene times of 5 minutes or less. While interventions may be important, the only thing proven to increase survival of trauma patients is decreasing time to definitive care (trauma center).

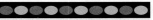

PEARLS
Interruptions
The team leader should delegate any intervention required during the ITLS Primary Survey and should not interrupt the completion of the survey except for airway obstruction, cardiac arrest, or scene danger.

ITLS Patient Assessment

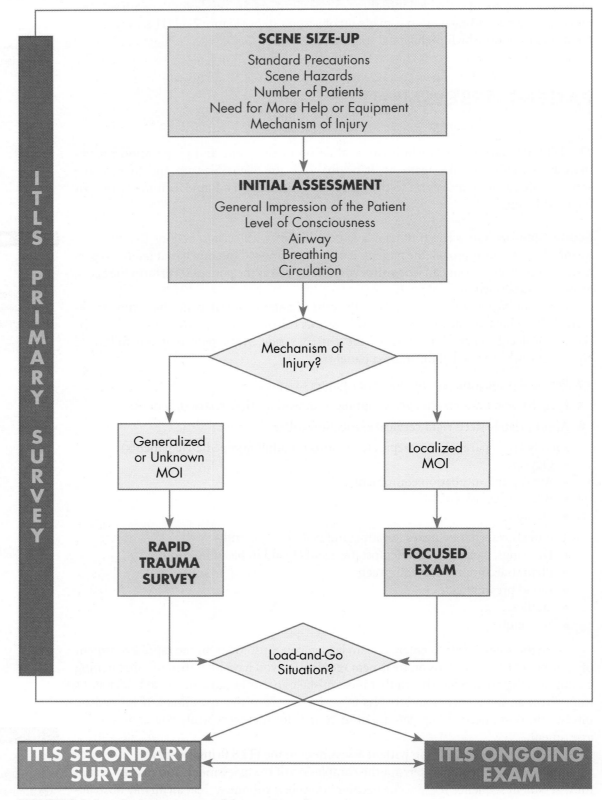

FIGURE 2-1 Steps in the assessment of the trauma patient.

Initial Assessment: The purpose of the Initial Assessment is to prioritize the patient and to determine the existence of immediately life-threatening conditions. The information gathered is used to make decisions about critical interventions and time of transport. Once you determine that the patient may be safely approached, assessment should proceed quickly and smoothly. (The Initial Assessment and Rapid Trauma Survey should take less than 2 minutes.) As you begin, direct Rescuer 2 (who should have the cervical collar and airway equipment) to stabilize the patient's neck (if needed) and to assume responsibility for the airway. Rescuer 3 will place the backboard and the trauma box beside the patient while you are proceeding with your exam. This team approach makes the most efficient use of time and allows you to rapidly perform the Initial Assessment without performing noninvasive airway interventions yourself, which can interrupt your thought process.

The Initial Assessment is made up of your general impression upon approaching the patient, an evaluation of the patient's level of consciousness (LOC), manual stabilization of the cervical spine (if needed), and an assessment of the patient's airway, breathing, and circulation (ABCs).

Form a General Impression of the Patient on Approach: You have already sized up the scene, determined the total number of patients, and initiated MCI protocols if there are more patients than your team can effectively handle (see Chapter 1 and Appendix I). As you approach, note the patient's approximate age, sex, weight, and general appearance. The old and the very young are at increased risk. Female patients may be pregnant. Observe the position of the patient, both body position and position in relation to surroundings. Note the patient's activity. (Is the patient aware of surroundings, anxious, obviously in distress, etc.?) Does the patient have any obvious major injuries or major bleeding? Your observation of the patient in relation to the scene and the mechanism of injury will help you prioritize the patient.

If there are multiple patients, rapidly triage them and begin evaluation of the most seriously injured patient first. (You may have to delegate a member of your team to assess other patients until help arrives.)

Evaluate Initial Level of Consciousness While Obtaining Cervical-Spine Stabilization: Assessment begins immediately, even if the patient is being extricated. As team leader, try to approach the patient from the front (face to face, so the patient does not turn the head to see you). If there is a mechanism of injury that suggests spinal injury, Rescuer 2 immediately and gently but firmly stabilizes the head and neck in a neutral position. Holding the head keeps the hands from being in the way when another team member applies a cervical collar later. As team leader you may need to initially stabilize the neck if there is not a second rescuer immediately available. If the head or neck is held in an angulated position and the patient complains of pain on any attempt to straighten it, you should stabilize it in the position found. The same is true of the unconscious patient whose neck is held to one side and does not move when you gently attempt to straighten it. The rescuer stabilizing the neck must not release it until he or she is relieved or a suitable motion-restriction device is applied.

The team leader should say to the patient, "My name is _____. We are here to help you. Can you tell me what happened?" The patient's reply gives immediate information about both the airway and the level of consciousness. If the patient responds appropriately to questioning, you can assume that the airway is open and the level of consciousness (LOC) is normal. If the response is not appropriate (the patient is unconscious or awake but confused), make a mental note of the LOC using the AVPU scale (Table 2-1). Anything below "A" (alert) should trigger a systematic search for the causes during the Rapid Trauma Survey.

■ **TABLE 2-1** *Levels of Mental Status (AVPU)*
A—Alert (awake and oriented)
V—Responds to Verbal stimuli (awake but confused, or unconscious but responds in some way to verbal stimuli)
P—Responds to Pain (unconscious but responds in some way to painful stimuli)
U—Unresponsive (no gag or cough reflex)

Assess the Airway: If the patient cannot speak or is unconscious, further evaluation of the airway should follow. Look, listen, and feel for movement of air. The team leader or Rescuer 2 should position the airway as needed. Because of the ever-present danger of spinal injury, avoid extending the neck to open the airway of a trauma patient. If the airway is obstructed (apnea, snoring, gurgling, stridor), use an appropriate method (reposition, sweep, suction) to open it immediately (Figure 2-2). Failure to quickly provide an open airway is one of the three reasons to interrupt the patient assessment part of the ITLS Primary Survey. If simple positioning and suctioning fail to provide an adequate airway, or if the patient has stridor, advanced airway techniques may be necessary immediately.

Assess Breathing: Look, listen, and feel for movement of air. If the patient is unconscious, place your ear over the patient's mouth so you can judge both the depth (tidal volume; see Chapter 4) and rate of ventilations. Look at the movement of the chest (or abdomen), listen to the sound of air movement, and feel both the movement of air on your cheek and the movement of the chest wall with your hand. Notice if the patient uses accessory muscles to breathe. If ventilation is inadequate (less than 8 per minute or too shallow), Rescuer 2 should begin to assist ventilation immediately, using his knees to restrict movement of the patient's neck and free his hands to apply oxygen or a bag-valve mask to assist ventilation (Figure 2-3). When assisting or providing ventilation, be sure that the patient gets an adequate ventilatory rate (one breath every 6 to 8 seconds) and an adequate volume (Table 2-2). Rescuers tend to ventilate too fast. If you monitor ventilation with capnography (recommended), you should maintain the pCO_2 at about 35–40. All patients who are breathing too fast should receive supplemental high-flow oxygen. As a general rule, all patients with multisystem trauma should receive supplemental high-flow oxygen.

Assess Circulation: As soon as you have ensured a patent airway and adequate ventilation, note the rate and quality of the pulses at the wrist (brachial in the infant). Checking the

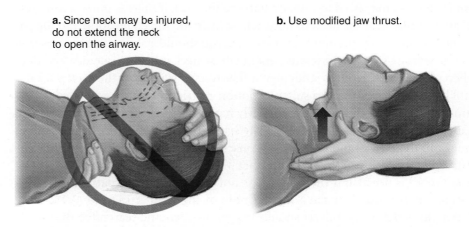

a. Since neck may be injured, do not extend the neck to open the airway.

b. Use modified jaw thrust.

FIGURE 2-2 Opening the airway using the modified jaw thrust. Maintain in-line stabilization while pushing up on the angles of the jaw with your thumbs.

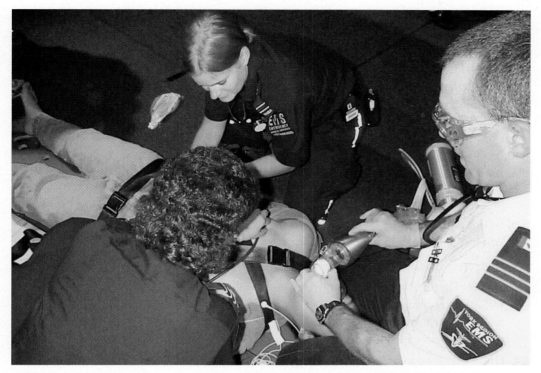

FIGURE 2-3 Using your knees to maintain stabilization of the neck will free your hands to assist ventilation. *(Photo courtesy of ITLS Ontario, Steve McNenly, Jennifer Lundgren, and Sheryl Jackson)*

TABLE 2-2 *Normal and Abnormal Respiratory Rates*

	Normal	Abnormal
Adult	10–20	<8 and >24
Small child	15–30	<15 and >35
Infant	25–50	<25 and >60

pulse in the neck is not necessary if the patient is awake and alert or has a palpable peripheral pulse. Quickly note whether the rate is too slow (<60 in an adult) or too fast (>120), and note also its quality (thready, bounding, weak, irregular). If pulses are absent at the neck, immediately start CPR (unless there is massive blunt trauma) and prepare for immediate transport. This is also one of the three reasons to interrupt assessment during the ITLS Primary Survey.

While at the wrist, note skin color, temperature, and condition (and capillary refill in an infant or small child). Pale, cool, clammy skin; thready radial pulse; and decreased LOC are the best early assessments of decreased perfusion (shock). Be sure the bleeding has been controlled (direct Rescuer 3 to do this). Most bleeding can be stopped by direct pressure or pressure dressings. Air splints or the pneumatic antishock garment (PASG) may be used to tamponade bleeding. Tourniquets have been discouraged in the past, but recent military experience has found that for bleeding not adequately controlled with pressure, an appropriate tourniquet should be used immediately. If a dressing becomes blood soaked, remove the dressing and redress once to be sure direct pressure is being placed on the bleeding area. Hemostatic agents such as QuickClot or Celox can be used in this situation. It is important to report excessive bleeding to the receiving physician. Do not use clamps to stop bleeders; this may cause injuries to other structures (nerves are present alongside arteries).

Rapid Trauma Survey or Focused Exam: The choice between the Rapid Trauma Survey and the Focused Exam depends on the mechanism of injury and/or the results of the Initial Assessment. If there is a dangerous generalized mechanism of injury (such as an auto crash or fall from a height) or if the patient is unconscious, perform the Rapid Trauma Survey. If there is a dangerous focused mechanism of injury suggesting an isolated injury (bullet wound of thigh or stab wound to the chest, for example), you may perform the Focused Exam, which is limited to the area of injury. If there is no significant mechanism of injury (e.g., dropped a rock on a toe) and the Initial Assessment is normal (alert with no loss of consciousness, normal breathing, radial pulse less than 120, and no complaint of dyspnea, chest, abdominal, or pelvic pain), you may move directly to the Focused Exam based on the patient's chief complaint.

If you identify a priority (high-risk) patient, you need to find the cause of the abnormal findings and identify if this is a load-and-go patient.

You have identified a priority patient if you find any of the following:

■ Dangerous mechanism of injury

■ History that reveals:
  • Loss of consciousness
  • Difficulty breathing
  • Severe pain of head, neck, or torso

■ High-risk group (such as very young, very old, chronically ill)
  • Altered mental status
  • Difficulty breathing
  • Abnormal perfusion
  • Any abnormality revealed during the Initial Assessment

Rapid Trauma Survey: The Rapid Trauma Survey is a brief exam done to find all life-threats (Figure 2-4). (A more thorough assessment—the ITLS Secondary Survey—will follow later if time permits.) To begin the Rapid Trauma Survey, briefly assess (look and feel) the head and neck for injuries and see if the neck veins are flat or distended and the trachea is in the midline. A rigid cervical extrication collar may be applied at this time. Note: If the team leader elected to stabilize the neck, this duty should be transferred to another rescuer at this time.

Now expose and look, feel, and listen to the chest. Look for both asymmetrical and paradoxical movement. Note if the ribs rise with respiration or if there is only diaphragmatic breathing. Look for signs of blunt trauma or open wounds. Feel for tenderness, instability, and crepitation (TIC). Then listen to see if breath sounds are present and equal bilaterally. Listen with the stethoscope over the lateral chest about the fourth intercostal space in the midaxillary line on both sides. If breath sounds are not equal (decreased or absent on one side), percuss the chest to determine whether the patient is just splinting from pain or if a pneumothorax or a hemothorax is present. If abnormalities are found during the chest exam (open chest wound, flail chest, tension pneumothorax, hemothorax), delegate the appropriate intervention (seal open wound, stabilize flail, decompress severe tension pneumothorax). Very briefly notice the heart sounds so you will have a baseline for changes such as development of muffled heart sounds.

Rapidly expose and look at the abdomen (distension, contusions, penetrating wounds), and gently palpate the abdomen for tenderness, guarding, and rigidity.

Check the pelvis. Look for deformity or penetrating wounds. Feel for tenderness, instability, and crepitation by gently pressing down on the symphysis and gently squeezing in on the iliac crests. Note that tenderness is not the same thing as being unstable. The pelvis may be tender and yet stable. If the pelvis is unstable, you can feel the pelvic ring collapse as you apply pressure. If the pelvis is unstable, do not check again!

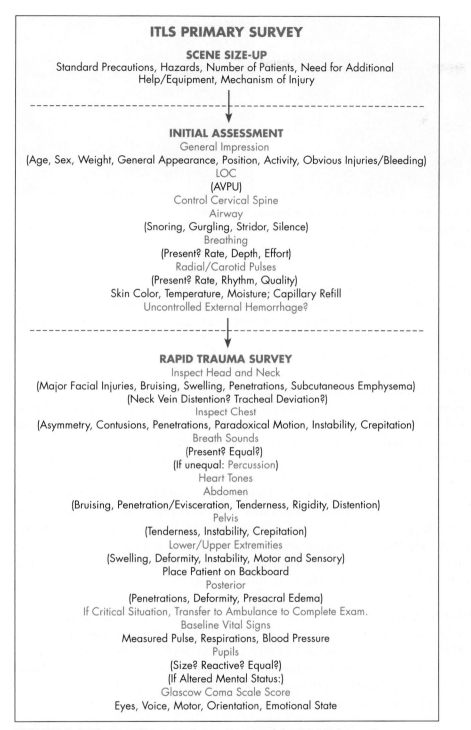

ITLS PRIMARY SURVEY

SCENE SIZE-UP
Standard Precautions, Hazards, Number of Patients, Need for Additional
Help/Equipment, Mechanism of Injury

INITIAL ASSESSMENT
General Impression
(Age, Sex, Weight, General Appearance, Position, Activity, Obvious Injuries/Bleeding)
LOC
(AVPU)
Control Cervical Spine
Airway
(Snoring, Gurgling, Stridor, Silence)
Breathing
(Present? Rate, Depth, Effort)
Radial/Carotid Pulses
(Present? Rate, Rhythm, Quality)
Skin Color, Temperature, Moisture; Capillary Refill
Uncontrolled External Hemorrhage?

RAPID TRAUMA SURVEY
Inspect Head and Neck
(Major Facial Injuries, Bruising, Swelling, Penetrations, Subcutaneous Emphysema)
(Neck Vein Distention? Tracheal Deviation?)
Inspect Chest
(Asymmetry, Contusions, Penetrations, Paradoxical Motion, Instability, Crepitation)
Breath Sounds
(Present? Equal?)
(If unequal: Percussion)
Heart Tones
Abdomen
(Bruising, Penetration/Evisceration, Tenderness, Rigidity, Distention)
Pelvis
(Tenderness, Instability, Crepitation)
Lower/Upper Extremities
(Swelling, Deformity, Instability, Motor and Sensory)
Place Patient on Backboard
Posterior
(Penetrations, Deformity, Presacral Edema)
If Critical Situation, Transfer to Ambulance to Complete Exam.
Baseline Vital Signs
Measured Pulse, Respirations, Blood Pressure
Pupils
(Size? Reactive? Equal?)
(If Altered Mental Status:)
Glascow Coma Scale Score
Eyes, Voice, Motor, Orientation, Emotional State

FIGURE 2-4 The Rapid Trauma Survey as part of the ITLS Primary Survey.

Check the extremities. Assess both upper legs, looking for deformity and feeling for TIC. Remember that bilateral femur fractures can produce enough internal blood loss to be life threatening. Scan for obvious wounds or deformities of the arms and lower legs. Note whether the patient can move fingers and toes before transferring to the backboard.

At this point, transfer the patient to a long backboard, checking the posterior of the patient as you do this. If the patient has an unstable pelvis or bilateral femur fractures, to prevent further injuries, use a scoop stretcher (Figure 2-5) to transfer the patient to a long backboard. A scientific study has shown that at least one brand of scoop stretcher

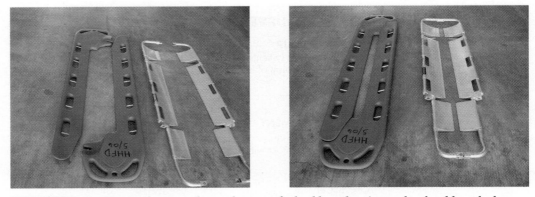

FIGURE 2-5 Scoop stretchers may be used to transfer backboard patients who should not be log rolled. The newer, more rigid scoop stretchers (as shown) can replace standard backboards. *(Photos courtesy of Leon Carpentier, EMT-P)*

(Ferno) provides stabilization equal or superior to a rigid backboard and you may simply use it instead of a backboard (see Bibliography). Remember that if you use a scoop stretcher, you are still responsible to do your best to evaluate the posterior side of the patient.

You now obtain baseline vital signs (blood pressure, pulse, and respiratory rate) and the rest of the SAMPLE history (see below). If a critical situation is present (see Transport Decision below), transport now and obtain the vital signs during transport.

If the patient has an altered mental status, do a brief neurological exam to identify possible increased intracranial pressure (ICP). It is critical to identify this condition (see Chapter 10) as it will have important implications with respect to the rate you assist ventilation and your aggressiveness in treating shock. This exam should include the pupils, Glasgow Coma Scale (GCS) score, and signs of cerebral herniation (see Chapter 10). Also look for medical identification devices. Head injury, shock, and hypoxia are not the only things that cause altered mental status; also think about nontraumatic causes such as hypoglycemia and drug or alcohol overdose. All patients with altered mental status should have a finger-stick glucose performed as soon as they are placed in the ambulance. Because altered mental status is one of the criteria for immediate transport (see next page), this brief neurological exam is always performed during transport.

SAMPLE History: At the same time as you are performing the patient assessment part of the ITLS Primary Survey (Initial Assessment and Rapid Trauma Survey or Focused Exam), you or one of the other rescuers should obtain a SAMPLE history (Table 2-3). This is especially important if you must gather information from bystanders, since they will not be going with you when you transport the patient. Remember, prehospital providers are the only ones who get to see the scene and also may be the only ones who get to take a history,

TABLE 2-3 *SAMPLE History*
S —Symptoms
A —Allergies
M—Medications
P —Past medical history (Other illnesses?)
L —Last oral intake (When was the last time there was any solid or liquid intake?)
E —Events preceding the incident (Why did it happen?)

since many patients who are initially alert lose consciousness before arriving at the hospital. You are not only making interventions to deliver a living patient to the hospital, you also must be the detective who figures out what happened and why. Pay special attention to the patient's complaints (symptoms) and events prior to the incident (the "S" and "E" of the SAMPLE history). A more detailed history may be taken later during the ITLS Secondary Survey. The patient's symptoms can suggest other injuries, and this will affect further examination. It is important to know as much about the mechanism as possible. (Was she restrained? How far did she fall? What caused her to fall?) Look for clues to serious injury such as history of loss of consciousness, shortness of breath, or pain in the neck, back, chest, abdomen, or pelvis.

Critical Interventions and Transport Decision: When you have completed the Initial Assessment and Rapid Trauma Survey or Focused Exam, enough information is available to decide if a critical situation is present. Patients with critical trauma situations are transported immediately. Most treatment interventions will be done during transport.

If your patient has any of the following critical injuries or conditions, transport immediately.

- *Initial Assessment reveals:*
  - Altered mental status
  - Abnormal respiration
  - Abnormal circulation (shock or uncontrolled bleeding)
- *Signs discovered during the Rapid Trauma Survey of conditions that rapidly lead to shock:*
  - Abnormal chest exam (flail chest, open wound, tension pneumothorax, hemothorax)
  - Tender, distended abdomen
  - Pelvic instability
  - Bilateral femur fractures
- *Significant mechanism of injury and/or poor general health of patient.* As you consider mechanisms, age, general appearance, chronic illnesses, and so on, you may decide that the patient is at higher risk than the ITLS Primary Survey alone would suggest. These higher risk patients should go to a trauma center even though they might not meet other criteria to go there. Remember that there are more considerations than just the physical exam of the patient.

If the patient has one of the critical conditions listed above, after the Rapid Trauma Survey or Focused Exam, immediately load her into an ambulance, and transport rapidly to the nearest appropriate emergency facility. When in doubt, transport early.

The following procedures are done at the scene, and most of them can be delegated to team members to perform while you continue the ITLS Primary Survey.

- Manage the airway.
- Assist ventilation.
- Administer oxygen.
- Begin CPR.
- Control major external bleeding.
- Seal sucking chest wounds.
- Stabilize flail chest.
- Decompress tension pneumothorax.
- Stabilize impaled objects.
- Complete packaging of the patient.

PEARLS
On-Scene Time
Critical trauma patients need definitive care in the operating room. Limit on-scene time. Survival of the critical trauma patient is time dependent. Most interventions should be performed in the ambulance during transport to an appropriate facility.

Procedures that are not life saving, such as splinting, bandaging, insertion of IV lines, or even emergency endotracheal intubation, must not hold up transport of the critical patient. At this point, the ITLS Primary Survey is over and the team leader may help the other rescuers with patient care. Be sure to call medical direction early so that the hospital is prepared for the patient's arrival.

Contacting Medical Direction: When you have a critical patient, it is extremely important to contact medical direction as early as possible. It takes time to get the appropriate surgeon and the operating room team in place, and the critical patient has no time to wait. Always notify the receiving facility of your estimated time of arrival (ETA), the condition of the patient, and any special needs on arrival (see Appendix B).

ITLS Secondary Survey

The ITLS Secondary Survey is a more comprehensive exam to pick up additional injuries that might have been missed in the brief ITLS Primary Survey. This assessment also establishes the baseline from which treatment decisions will eventually be made. It is important to record the information discovered in this assessment. Whether or not to perform a Secondary Survey as well as when to perform one depends on the situation.

- Critical patients should have this assessment done during transport rather than on scene.
- If there is a short transport and you must perform interventions, you may not have time to do the Secondary Survey.
- If the Primary Survey does not reveal a critical condition, the Secondary Survey may be performed on scene.

When you perform the Secondary Survey, routinely repeat the Initial Assessment. You can do this as you check the vital signs. Even though the patient appears to be stable, if there is a dangerous mechanism or other dangers (such as age, poor general health, death of another passenger in the same auto), consider early transport. "Stable" patients may become unstable quite rapidly. Stable patients with no dangerous mechanism of injury (e.g., dropped rock on toe) do not require a Secondary Survey.

You should have obtained most of the pertinent history during the ITLS Primary Survey, but now you can obtain further information if needed. You should perform your Secondary Survey while you are obtaining the rest of the SAMPLE history (if the patient is conscious).

PROCEDURE
❖ Performing a Secondary Survey

The exam should contain the following elements (Figure 2-6).

1. Repeat the Initial Assessment.
2. Record vital signs again. Record pulse, respiration, and blood pressure. Remember, the pulse pressure is as important as the systolic pressure. Many people now consider the pulse oximetry reading one of the vital signs. It is a good tool but you must know its limitations (see Chapters 4 and 5).
3. Consider using monitors (cardiac, pulse oximeter, CO_2). These are usually applied during transport.

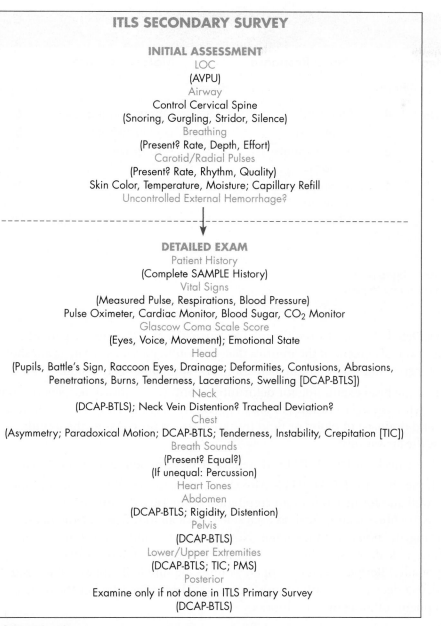

ITLS SECONDARY SURVEY

INITIAL ASSESSMENT
LOC
(AVPU)
Airway
Control Cervical Spine
(Snoring, Gurgling, Stridor, Silence)
Breathing
(Present? Rate, Depth, Effort)
Carotid/Radial Pulses
(Present? Rate, Rhythm, Quality)
Skin Color, Temperature, Moisture; Capillary Refill
Uncontrolled External Hemorrhage?

- -

DETAILED EXAM
Patient History
(Complete SAMPLE History)
Vital Signs
(Measured Pulse, Respirations, Blood Pressure)
Pulse Oximeter, Cardiac Monitor, Blood Sugar, CO_2 Monitor
Glasgow Coma Scale Score
(Eyes, Voice, Movement); Emotional State
Head
(Pupils, Battle's Sign, Raccoon Eyes, Drainage; Deformities, Contusions, Abrasions,
Penetrations, Burns, Tenderness, Lacerations, Swelling [DCAP-BTLS])
Neck
(DCAP-BTLS); Neck Vein Distention? Tracheal Deviation?
Chest
(Asymmetry; Paradoxical Motion; DCAP-BTLS; Tenderness, Instability, Crepitation [TIC])
Breath Sounds
(Present? Equal?)
(If unequal: Percussion)
Heart Tones
Abdomen
(DCAP-BTLS; Rigidity, Distention)
Pelvis
(DCAP-BTLS)
Lower/Upper Extremities
(DCAP-BTLS; TIC; PMS)
Posterior
Examine only if not done in ITLS Primary Survey
(DCAP-BTLS)

FIGURE 2-6 ITLS Secondary Survey for the stable patient.

4. Do a neurological exam. It gives important baseline information that is used in later treatment decisions. This exam should include the following:

   a. *Level of consciousness:* If the patient is conscious, describe her orientation and emotional status. If she has an altered mental status, record her level of coma (for Glasgow Coma Scale score, see Table 2-4). If there is altered mental status, check finger-stick blood glucose and check the oxygen saturation level. If there is any chance of narcotic overdose, give 2 mg of naloxone IV.

   b. *Pupils:* Note size and whether they are equal or unequal. Do they respond to light?

   c. *Motor:* Can the patient move fingers and toes?

   d. *Sensation:* Can she feel you when you touch her fingers and toes? Does the unconscious patient respond when you pinch her fingers and toes?

TABLE 2-4 *Glasgow Coma Scale*

Eye Opening	Points	Verbal Response	Points	Motor Response	Points
Spontaneous	4	Oriented	5	Obeys commands	6
To voice	3	Confused	4	Localizes pain	5
To pain	2	Inappropriate words	3	Withdraws	4
None	1	Incomprehensible sounds	2	Abnormal flexion	3*
		Silent	1	Abnormal extension	2**
				No movement	1

*Decorticate posturing to pain
**Decerebrate posturing to pain

5. Perform a Detailed (head-to-toe) Exam. Pay particular attention to the patient's complaints and also recheck the injuries that you found previously. The exam should consist of inspection, auscultation, palpation, and sometimes percussion.

   a. Begin at the head examining for deformities, contusions, abrasions, penetrations, burns, tenderness, lacerations, or swelling (DCAP-BTLS), raccoon eyes, Battle's sign, and drainage of blood or fluid from the ears or nose. Assess the mouth. Assess the airway again.

   b. Check the neck for DCAP-BTLS, distended neck veins, and deviated trachea.

   c. Check the chest for DCAP-BTLS. Also check for paradoxical movement of the chest wall and for instability and crepitation of the ribs. Be sure that breath sounds are present and equal on each side (check all four fields). Note rales, wheezing, or "noisy" breath sounds. Notice if heart sounds are as loud as before. (A noticeable decrease in heart sounds may be an early sign of cardiac tamponade.) Recheck seals over open wounds. Be sure flails are well stabilized. If you detect decreased breath sounds, percuss to determine whether the patient has a pneumothorax or hemothorax.

   d. Perform an abdominal exam. Look for signs of blunt or penetrating trauma. Feel all four quadrants for tenderness or rigidity. Do not waste time listening for bowel sounds; it gives you no useful information. If the abdomen is painful to gentle pressure during examination, you can expect the patient to be bleeding internally. If the abdomen is both distended and painful, you can expect hemorrhagic shock to occur very quickly.

   e. Assess pelvis and extremities (unstable pelvis noted in Rapid Trauma Survey is not rechecked). Check for DCAP-BTLS. Be sure to check and record pulse, motor function, and sensation (PMS) on all fractures. Do this before and after straightening any fracture. Angulated fractures of the upper extremities are usually best splinted as found. Most fractures of the lower extremities are gently straightened and then stabilized using traction splints or air splints. Critical patients have all splints applied during transport.

   Transport immediately if the ITLS Secondary Survey reveals the development of any of the critical trauma situations. After you finish the Secondary Survey, you should finish bandaging and splinting.

ITLS Ongoing Exam

Ongoing assessment and management includes the critical procedures performed on scene and during transport and communication with medical direction. The ITLS Ongoing Exam is an abbreviated exam to assess for changes in the patient's condition. In contrast to the ITLS Secondary Survey that is performed only once, the Ongoing Exam may be performed multiple times during a long transport. In critical cases with short transport times, there may not be time to perform a Secondary Survey; the Ongoing Exam may take its place. It should be performed and recorded no less than every 5 minutes for critical patients and every 15 minutes for stable patients. The Ongoing Exam also should be performed:

- Each time the patient is moved.
- Each time an intervention is performed.
- Any time the patient's condition worsens.

This exam is meant to find any changes in the patient's condition, so concentrate on reassessing only those things that may change. For example, if you have applied a traction splint, reassess the limb for decreased pain and for the presence of distal pulses, motor function, and sensation (PMS). On the other hand, if you decompress a chest, you must reassess everything in the Initial Assessment and Rapid Trauma Survey down through the abdominal exam.

PROCEDURE

Performing an Ongoing Exam

The ITLS Ongoing Exam should be performed in the following order:

1. Ask the patient if there have been any changes in how she feels.
2. Reassess mental status (LOC and pupils, recheck GCS if the patient has an altered mental status).
3. Reassess the ABCs.
   a. Reassess the airway.
      (1) Recheck patency.
      (2) If this is a burn patient, assess for signs of inhalation injury.
   b. Reassess breathing and circulation.
      (1) Recheck vital signs.
      (2) Note skin color, condition, and temperature.
      (3) Check the neck for jugular venous distention (JVD) and tracheal deviation. (If a cervical collar has been applied, remove the front to examine the neck.)
      (4) Recheck the chest. Notice the quality of breath sounds. If breath sounds are unequal, evaluate for splinting, pneumothorax, and hemothorax. Listen to the heart to see if the sounds have become muffled.
4. Reassess the abdomen (if mechanism suggests possible injury). Note the development of tenderness, distention, or rigidity.
5. Check each of the identified injuries (lacerations for bleeding, PMS distal to all injured extremities, flails, pneumothorax, open chest wounds, and so on).
6. Check interventions.
   a. Check ET tube for patency and position.
   b. Check oxygen for flow rate.
   c. Check IVs for patency and rate of fluid.

   d. Check seals on sucking chest wounds.

   e. Check patency of tension pneumothorax decompression needle.

   f. Check splints and dressings.

   g. Check impaled objects to be sure they are well stabilized.

   h. Check body position of pregnant patients.

   i. Check cardiac monitor, capnograph, and pulse oximeter.

Accurately record what you see and what you do. Record changes in the patient's condition during transport. Record the time that you perform each intervention. Extenuating circumstances or significant details should be recorded in the comments or remarks section of the written report (review documentation in Appendix C).

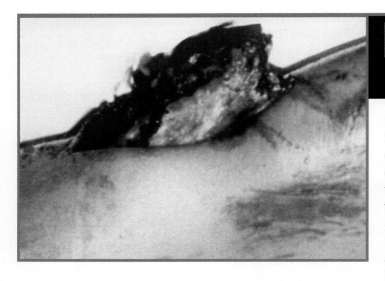

Case Study
continued

Dan, Joyce, and Buddy of the Emergency Transport System (ETS) have been called to the scene of a construction accident where a man fell from a scaffold onto a pile of lumber. Their Scene Size-up revealed that the scene was safe to enter. There they found their patient who is awake and appears to be about 50 years old (high-risk group). The general impression is poor, because the patient is pale and diaphoretic and appears to be having some trouble breathing. He is clutching a 2-foot piece of wood that is protruding from his left chest. In addition, the bone can be seen in an open wound of his left lower leg. Buddy is acting as team leader on this call. The team dons personal protective equipment, gathers the essential equipment, and approaches the patient.

Buddy begins his Initial Assessment by introducing the team. At the same time, Joyce stabilizes the patient's neck by holding his head with her knees and prepares to apply a nonrebreather oxygen mask. Dan places the long backboard beside the patient and checks the pulse in his left foot before splinting the lower leg. When questioned about what happened, the patient states he was building a concrete wall and was on a scaffold about 10 feet high. He was lifting a concrete block when he felt a "fluttering" in his chest and the next thing he knew his friends were bending over him asking him what happened. His friends state he was unconscious for about 2 to 3 minutes.

Buddy notes the patient has a good airway but his breathing is rapid and shallow. He has a rapid, thready pulse at the wrist. Dan has applied a compression dressing to the open wound on the left lower leg and is applying a splint at this time. There is no bleeding now. Because of the mechanism of injury, Buddy chooses to perform a Rapid Trauma Survey. He has already determined that this is a priority patient because of the abnormal Initial Assessment and this is also a load-and-go situation because of the loss of consciousness and the respiratory difficulty.

Brief exam of the head and face reveals no evidence of head trauma and Joyce notes that the pupils are 4 mm and react equally. The neck veins are flat and the trachea is midline. There is no tenderness or deformity of the neck. At this time Buddy and Joyce choose the correct-size rigid cervical collar and apply it while maintaining motion restriction of the cervical spine in a neutral position. Buddy notes the 2-inch-wide piece of wood enters from the front of the left chest but does not protrude from the back. There is no paradoxical movement of the chest. The breath sounds are markedly decreased on the left and the left chest is dull to percussion. The heart sounds are good but slightly irregular. The abdomen is negative for DCAP-BTLS and is soft and nontender. The pelvis is stable and nontender. Exam of the extremities is normal except for the left lower leg, which has an open fracture that has been splinted and dressed. The patient is able to move his fingers and toes and has sensation in all extremities. Because of the history of loss of consciousness, a brief neurological exam is done. It reveals normal level of consciousness with good PMS in all extremities. The Glasgow Coma Scale score is 15.

After stabilizing the impaled piece of wood, they decide not to log roll the patient, but to carefully strap him onto a scoop stretcher. He is then immediately moved to the ambulance and transported. Dan drives while Buddy and Joyce provide patient care. While Buddy obtains the rest of the SAMPLE history and obtains baseline vital signs, Joyce starts two large-bore IVs, applies a pulse oximeter, attaches a cardiac monitor, performs a 12-lead EKG, and performs a rapid blood-glucose check. The patient states that he hurts in his chest and left lower leg and feels short of breath. He has no allergies. His past medical history is positive for hypertension but he has never had any heart disease or palpitations in the past. He takes one aspirin tablet each day (and has taken his dose today) and medication for hypertension but is not sure of the name. His last oral intake was breakfast. It is now 11:00 AM.

The vital signs are blood pressure 70/40, pulse 130 and irregular, respiratory rate 30 and shallow. The pulse oximeter reading is 92 percent on 100 percent oxygen, the blood glucose is normal, and the 12-lead EKG shows an acute injury pattern with frequent premature ventricular contractions.

Buddy notifies medical direction that he is transporting a patient who had syncope after cardiac palpitations and fell about 10 feet, sustaining a penetrating wound of his left chest and an open fracture of his left lower leg. He also notifies medical direction that the patient's EKG shows an acute injury pattern. Buddy is ordered to give cautious small fluid boluses to try to raise the blood pressure to no higher than 90–100 systolic, while watching carefully for signs of congestive heart failure.

The trauma team and cardiologist are waiting upon their arrival and the patient is taken to surgery where the impaled wood is removed (no cardiac damage from the wood) and the open fracture is irrigated and repaired. A balloon angioplasty and stent insertion is performed and the patient receives three units of blood. After a stormy course he eventually recovers.

Case Study Wrap-up

This is a complex case in which a medical event (acute myocardial infarction with arrhythmia) causes syncope, which in turn causes serious traumatic injury. If the team had not carefully performed every step in the ITLS Primary Survey, they would have missed the cardiac problem, with potentially disastrous results.

SUMMARY

Patient assessment is key to trauma care. The interventions required are not difficult, but their timing often is critical. If you know what questions to ask and how to perform the exam, you will know when to perform the life-saving interventions. This chapter has described a rapid, orderly, and thorough examination of the trauma patient with examination and treatment priorities always in mind. The continuous practice of approaching the patient in the way described here will allow you to concentrate on the patient, rather than on what to do next. Optimum speed is achieved by teamwork. Teamwork is achieved by practice. You should plan regular exercises in patient evaluation to perfect each team member's role.

BIBLIOGRAPHY

1. Alam, H. B., et al. 2005. Hemorrhage control in the battlefield: Role of new hemostatic agents. *Military Medicine* 170: 63–69.
2. Krell, J. M., et al. 2006. Comparison of the Ferno scoop stretcher with the long backboard for spinal immobilization. *Prehospital Emergency Care* 10: 46–51.

Patient Assessment Skills

Donna Hastings, EMT-P

OBJECTIVES

Upon completion of this chapter, you should be able to:

ITLS Primary Survey

1. Correctly perform the ITLS Primary Survey.

2. Identify within 2 minutes which patients require load and go.

3. Describe when to perform critical interventions.

ITLS Secondary Survey and ITLS Ongoing Exam

4. Correctly perform the Secondary Survey.

5. Correctly perform the Ongoing (reassessment) Exam.

6. Describe when to perform critical interventions.

7. Demonstrate proper communications with medical direction.

Assessment and Management of the Trauma Patient

8. Demonstrate the proper sequence of rapid assessment and the management of the multiple-trauma patient.

(© Craig Jackson/
In the Dark Photography)

PEARLS
ITLS Primary Survey

- Do not approach the patient until you have done a Scene Size-up.

- Do not interrupt the ITLS Primary Survey except for airway obstruction, cardiac arrest, or if the scene becomes too dangerous. Team members may perform other critical interventions while you complete the Survey.

- Give ventilation instructions as soon as you assess airway and breathing.

- Prophylactic hyperventilation is not recommended for patients with decreased LOC. Use it only for head-injury patients who show signs of the cerebral herniation syndrome.

- Assist ventilations in anyone who is hypoventilating (less than 8 breaths per minute).

- Give oxygen to all multiple-trauma patients. If in doubt, give oxygen.

- Remember that unconscious patients with no gag reflex cannot protect their airways.

- Endotracheal tubes are the best method to protect the airway and ventilate the adult patient.

- Transfer the patient to the backboard as soon as the ITLS Primary Survey is completed.

- When the ITLS Primary Survey is completed, decide if the patient is critical or stable.

- Call medical direction early if you have a critical patient. (Other physicians may have to be called from home to treat the patient.)

- If the patient has a critical trauma situation, load him into the ambulance and transport. (Transport pregnant patients with the backboard tilted slightly to the left. Do not let them roll over onto the floor.)

(continued on page 48)

PROCEDURE

Short written scenarios will be used along with a model (to act as the patient). You will divide into teams to practice performing the Initial Assessment, critical interventions, and transport decision. Each member of the team must practice being team leader at least once. The Critical Information represents the answers you should be seeking at each step of the survey. The Treatment Decision Tree at the end of the chapter represents the actions that should be taken (personally or delegated) in response to your assessment.

❂ ITLS Primary Survey—Critical Information

If you ask the right questions, you will get the information you need to make the critical decisions necessary in the management of your patient. The following questions are presented in the order in which you should ask yourself as you perform patient assessment. This is the minimum information that you will need as you perform each step (Figure 3-1).

Scene Size-up

- Have I taken standard precautions?
- Do I see, hear, smell, or sense anything dangerous?
- Are there any other patients?
- Are additional personnel or resources needed?
- Do we need special equipment?
- What is the mechanism of injury here?
- Is it generalized or focused?
- Is it potentially life-threatening?

Initial Assessment

General Impression

- What is my general impression of the patient as I approach?

Level of Consciousness (AVPU)

- Introduce yourself and say: "We are here to help you. Can you tell us what happened?"

Airway

- Is the airway open and clear?

Breathing

- Is the patient breathing?
- What is the rate and quality of respiration?

Ventilation Instructions

- Order oxygen for any patient with abnormal respiration, altered mental status, shock, or major injuries.
- Delegate assisted ventilation if the patient is hypoventilating (less than 8 breaths per minute) or if there is inadequate movement of air.
- Hyperventilate only those head-injury patients who are unresponsive and show signs of cerebral herniation (see Chapter 10).

ITLS Patient Assessment

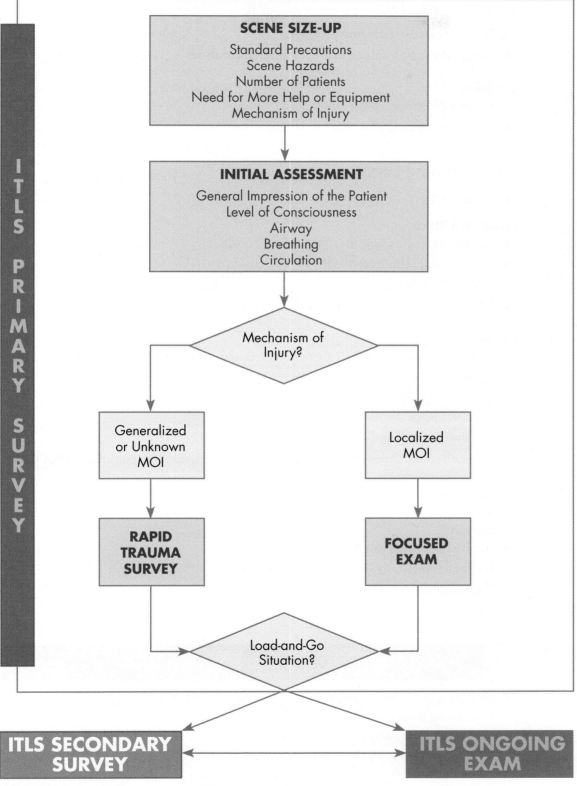

FIGURE 3-1 Steps in the assessment of the trauma patient.

Circulation
- What is the rate and quality of the pulse at the wrist (and at the neck, if not palpable at the wrist)?
- Is major external bleeding present?
- What are the skin color, condition, and temperature?

Decision
- Is this a critical situation (Table 3-1)?
- Are there interventions that I must make now?

Rapid Trauma Survey

(See Figure 3-2.)

Head and Neck
- Are there obvious wounds of the head or neck?
- Are the neck veins distended?
- Does the trachea look and feel midline or deviated?
- Is there deformity or tenderness of the neck?

Chest
- Is the chest symmetrical? Is there paradoxical movement? Is there any obvious blunt or penetrating trauma?
- Are there any open wounds?
- Is there TIC of the ribs?
- Are the breath sounds present and equal?
- If breath sounds are not equal, is the chest hyperresonant (pneumothorax) or dull (hemothorax)?
- Are heart sounds normal or decreased?

Abdomen
- Are there obvious wounds?
- Is the abdomen soft, rigid, or distended?
- Is there tenderness?

◪ TABLE 3-1 *Critical Trauma Situations*
Critical trauma situations are characterized by any of the following: • Decreased level of consciousness • Difficulty with airway or breathing • Shock or uncontrolled bleeding • Tender abdomen • Unstable pelvis • Bilateral femur fractures • High-risk group

ITLS PRIMARY SURVEY

SCENE SIZE-UP
Standard Precautions, Hazards, Number of Patients, Need for Additional
Help/Equipment, Mechanism of Injury

- → -

INITIAL ASSESSMENT
General Impression
(Age, Sex, Weight, General Appearance, Position, Activity, Obvious Injuries/Bleeding)
LOC
(AVPU)
Control Cervical Spine
Airway
(Snoring, Gurgling, Stridor, Silence)
Breathing
(Present? Rate, Depth, Effort)
Radial/Carotid Pulses
(Present? Rate, Rhythm, Quality)
Skin Color, Temperature, Moisture; Capillary Refill
Uncontrolled External Hemorrhage?

- → -

RAPID TRAUMA SURVEY
Inspect Head and Neck
(Major Facial Injuries, Bruising, Swelling, Penetrations, Subcutaneous Emphysema)
(Neck Vein Distention? Tracheal Deviation?)
Inspect Chest
(Asymmetry, Contusions, Penetrations, Paradoxical Motion, Instability, Crepitation)
Breath Sounds
(Present? Equal?)
(If unequal: Percussion)
Heart Tones
Abdomen
(Bruising, Penetration/Evisceration, Tenderness, Rigidity, Distention)
Pelvis
(Tenderness, Instability, Crepitation)
Lower/Upper Extremities
(Swelling, Deformity, Instability, Motor and Sensory)
Place Patient on Backboard
Posterior
(Penetrations, Deformity, Presacral Edema)
If Critical Situation, Transfer to Ambulance to Complete Exam.
Baseline Vital Signs
Measured Pulse, Respirations, Blood Pressure
Pupils
(Size? Reactive? Equal?)
(If Altered Mental Status:)
Glasgow Coma Scale Score
Eyes, Voice, Motor, Orientation, Emotional State

FIGURE 3-2 The Rapid Trauma Survey as part of the ITLS Primary Survey.

Pelvis
- Are there obvious wounds or deformity?
- Is there TIC?

Upper Legs
- Are there obvious wounds, swelling, or deformity?
- Is there TIC?

Lower Legs and Arms

- Are there obvious wounds, swelling, or deformity?
- Is there TIC?
- Can the patient feel/move fingers and toes?

Posterior

This exam is performed during transfer to the backboard.

- Is there any deformity, contusions, abrasions, penetrations, burns, tenderness, lacerations, or swelling (DCAP-BTLS) of the patient's posterior side?

Decision

- Is there a critical situation?
- Are there interventions that I must make now?

History

- What is the SAMPLE history (may have been obtained during the exam)?

Baseline Vital Signs

- Are the vital signs abnormal?

Disability

Perform this exam now if there is altered mental status. Otherwise, postpone this exam until you perform the ITLS Secondary Survey.

- Are the pupils equal and reactive?
- What is the Glasgow Coma Scale score?
- Are there signs of cerebral herniation (unconscious, dilated pupil(s), hypertension, bradycardia, posturing)?
- Does the patient have a medical identification device?

PROCEDURE

Short written scenarios will be used along with a model (to act as the patient). You will divide into teams to practice performing the ITLS Secondary Survey. Each member of the team must practice being team leader at least once. The Critical Information represents the answers you should be seeking at each step of the exam.

❄ ITLS Secondary Survey—Critical Information

As a general rule, you should repeat the Initial Assessment before you begin the ITLS Secondary Survey. You can do this as you check the vital signs. If you ask the right questions, you will get the information you need to make the critical decisions necessary in the management of your patient. The following questions are presented in the order in which you should ask yourself as you perform the Secondary Survey. This is the minimum information that you will need as you perform each step of the exam (Figure 3-3).

SAMPLE History

Complete the SAMPLE history now if you have not already done so.

- What is the patient's history?

PEARLS
ITLS Secondary Survey

- Critical patients get an ITLS Secondary Survey en route to the hospital if time permits.
- Stable patients may get an ITLS Secondary Survey at the scene (on the backboard).
- Transport immediately if your Detailed Exam reveals any of the critical trauma situations.
- Critical patients should not have traction splints applied at the scene. They take too long.

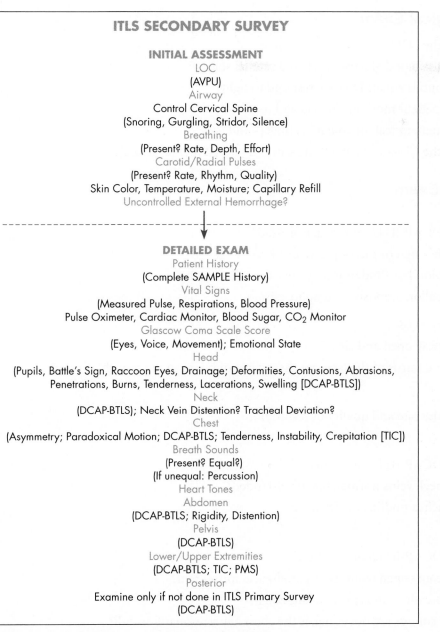

ITLS SECONDARY SURVEY

INITIAL ASSESSMENT
LOC
(AVPU)
Airway
Control Cervical Spine
(Snoring, Gurgling, Stridor, Silence)
Breathing
(Present? Rate, Depth, Effort)
Carotid/Radial Pulses
(Present? Rate, Rhythm, Quality)
Skin Color, Temperature, Moisture; Capillary Refill
Uncontrolled External Hemorrhage?

DETAILED EXAM
Patient History
(Complete SAMPLE History)
Vital Signs
(Measured Pulse, Respirations, Blood Pressure)
Pulse Oximeter, Cardiac Monitor, Blood Sugar, CO_2 Monitor
Glasgow Coma Scale Score
(Eyes, Voice, Movement); Emotional State
Head
(Pupils, Battle's Sign, Raccoon Eyes, Drainage; Deformities, Contusions, Abrasions,
Penetrations, Burns, Tenderness, Lacerations, Swelling [DCAP-BTLS])
Neck
(DCAP-BTLS); Neck Vein Distention? Tracheal Deviation?
Chest
(Asymmetry; Paradoxical Motion; DCAP-BTLS; Tenderness, Instability, Crepitation [TIC])
Breath Sounds
(Present? Equal?)
(If unequal: Percussion)
Heart Tones
Abdomen
(DCAP-BTLS; Rigidity, Distention)
Pelvis
(DCAP-BTLS)
Lower/Upper Extremities
(DCAP-BTLS; TIC; PMS)
Posterior
Examine only if not done in ITLS Primary Survey
(DCAP-BTLS)

FIGURE 3-3 The ITLS Secondary Survey for a stable patient.

Vital Signs and Repeat Initial Assessment

▪ What are the vital signs?
▪ Airway
  • Is the airway open and clear?
  • Is the sound of breathing normal (snoring, gurgling, stridor)?
▪ Breathing
  • What is the quality of respirations?
▪ Circulation
  • What is the rate and quality of the pulse?
  • What are the skin color, condition, and temperature (capillary refill in children)?
  • Is all external bleeding still controlled?

Neurological Exam

- What is the LOC?
- What is the blood glucose (if altered mental status)?
- Are the pupils equal? Do they respond to light?
- Can the patient move his fingers and toes?
- Can the patient feel me touch his fingers and toes?
- What is the Glasgow Coma Scale score (if altered mental status)?

Detailed Exam

Head

- Is there DCAP-BTLS of the face or head?
- Are Battle's sign or raccoon eyes present?
- Is there blood or fluid draining from the ears or nose?
- Is there pallor, cyanosis, or diaphoresis?

Airway

- Is the airway open and clear?
- If there are burns of the face, are there signs of burns in the mouth or nose?

Breathing

- What is the rate and quality of respiration?

Neck

- Is there DCAP-BTLS of the neck?
- Are the neck veins normal, flat, or distended?
- Is the trachea midline or deviated?

Chest

- Is there DCAP-BTLS of the chest?
- Are there any open wounds or paradoxical movement?
- Are the breath sounds present and equal?
- If breath sounds are not equal, is the chest hyperresonant or dull?
- Are heart sounds normal or decreased?
- If patient is intubated, is the endotracheal tube still in good position?

Abdomen

- Is there DCAP-BTLS of the abdomen?
- Is the abdomen soft, rigid, or distended?

Pelvis

If the pelvis has already been examined during the ITLS Primary Survey, no further exam should be done.

Lower Extremities

- Is there DCAP-BTLS of the legs?
- Is there normal PMS?
- Is range of motion normal? (optional)

Upper Extremities

- Is there DCAP-BTLS of the arms?
- Is there normal PMS?
- Is range of motion normal? (optional)

PROCEDURE

Short written trauma scenarios will be used along with a model (to act as the patient). You will divide into teams to practice performing the ITLS Ongoing Exam, making critical decisions and interventions. Each member of the team must practice being team leader at least once. The Critical Information represents the answers you should be seeking at each step of the exam.

⚕ ITLS Ongoing Exam—Critical Information

The following questions are presented in the order in which you should ask yourself as you perform the Ongoing (reassessment) Exam. This is the minimum information that you will need as you perform each step of the exam.

Subjective Changes

- Are you feeling better or worse now?

Mental Status

- What is the LOC?
- What is pupillary size? Are they equal? Do they react to light?
- If altered mental status, what is the Glasgow Coma Scale score now?

Reassess ABCs

- Airway
  - Is the airway open and clear?
  - If there are burns of the face, are there signs of inhalation injury?

- Breathing and circulation
  - What is the rate and quality of respiration?
  - What is the rate and quality of the pulse?
  - What is the blood pressure?
  - What are the skin color, condition, and temperature (capillary refill in children)?

- Neck
  - Is the trachea midline or deviated?
  - Are the neck veins normal, flat, or distended?
  - Is there increased swelling of the neck?

- Chest
  - Are the breath sounds present and equal?
  - If breath sounds are unequal, is the chest hyperresonant or dull?
  - Are heart sounds still normal or have they become muffled?

- Abdomen (if mechanism suggests possible injury)
  - Is there any tenderness?
  - Is the abdomen soft, rigid, or distended?

- Assessment of identified injuries
  - Have there been any changes in the condition of any of the injuries that I have found?

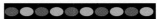

PEARLS
ITLS Ongoing Exam

- Repeat the ITLS Ongoing Exam:
  - If the patient's condition changes
  - If you make an intervention
  - If you move the patient (scene to ambulance, ambulance to hospital emergency department)
- Remain calm and think. Your knowledge, training, and concern are the most important tools you carry.

■ Check interventions. (Ask the appropriate question for your patient.)
  • Is the endotracheal tube still patent and in the correct position?
  • Is the oxygen rate correct?
  • Is the oxygen tubing connected?
  • Are the IVs running at the correct rate?
  • Is the open chest wound still sealed?
  • Is the decompression needle still working?
  • Are any of the dressings blood soaked?
  • Are the splints in good position?
  • Is the impaled object still well stabilized?
  • Is the pregnant patient tilted 20 to 30 degrees to the patient's left?
  • Is the cardiac monitor attached and working?
  • Is the pulse oximeter attached and working?
  • If intubated, is the capnograph attached and working?

PROCEDURE

❇ **Patient Assessment and Management**

Short written trauma scenarios will be used along with a model (to act as the patient). You will be divided into teams to practice the management of simulated trauma situations using the principles and techniques taught in the course. You will be evaluated in the same manner on the second day of the course. You will be expected to use all the principles and techniques taught in this course while managing these simulated patients. To familiarize yourself with the evaluation procedure, you will be given a copy of a scenario and a grade sheet. Review Chapter 2 and the previous surveys in this chapter.

Ground Rules for Teaching and Evaluation

1. You will be allowed to stay together in three-member groups (different-sized groups are optional) throughout the practice and evaluation stations.

2. You will have three practice scenarios. This allows each member of the team to be team leader once.

3. You will be evaluated as team leader once.

4. You will assist as a member of the rescue team during two scenarios in which another member of your team is being evaluated as team leader. You may assist, but the team leader must do all assessments. This gives you a total of six scenarios from which to learn: three practices, one evaluation, and two assists while others are evaluated.

5. Wait outside the door until the instructor comes out and gives you your scenario.

6. You will be allowed to look over your equipment before you start your exam.

7. Be sure to ask about scene safety if not provided in the scenario.

8. Be sure to apply your personal protective gear.

9. If you have a live model for a patient, you must talk to that person just as you would a real patient. It is best to explain what you are doing as you examine the patient. Be confident and reassuring.

10. You must ask your instructor for things you cannot find out from your patient. Examples are blood pressure, pulse, and breath sounds.

11. Wounds and fractures must be dressed or splinted just as if they were real. Procedures must be done correctly (such as blood pressure, log-rolling, strapping, and splinting).

12. If you need a piece of equipment that is not available, ask your instructors. They may allow you to simulate the equipment.

13. During practice and evaluation, you may be allowed to go (or may be directed) to any station, but you cannot go to the same station twice.

14. You will be graded on the following:

    a. Assessment of the scene

    b. Assessment of the patient

    c. Management of the patient

    d. Efficient use of time

    e. Leadership

    f. Judgment

    g. Problem-solving ability

    h. Patient interaction

15. When you finish your testing scenario, there is to be no discussion of the case. If you have any questions, they will be answered after the faculty meeting at the end of the course.

TRAUMA ASSESSMENT—*Treatment Decision Tree*

Initial Assessment	Action
SCENE SIZE-UP	
Safety	Put on gloves, protective clothing. Remove hazards or patient from hazards.
Number of patients	Call for help if needed.
Extrication needed	Call for special equipment if needed.
Mechanisms of injury	Suspect appropriate injuries (e.g., cervical spine).
GENERAL IMPRESSION	Begin to establish priorities.
Age, sex, weight	
Position (in surroundings, body position/posture)	
Activity	
LEVEL OF CONSCIOUSNESS	
Alert/responsive to voice	Maintain cervical-spine motion restriction.
Unresponsive to voice	Modified jaw thrust prn.
AIRWAY	
Snoring	Modified jaw thrust.
Gurgling	Suction.
Stridor	Intubate.
Silence	Attempt to ventilate. If unsuccessful: — Reposition; extricate immediately. — Visualize. — Suction. — Consider Heimlich maneuver. — Intubate. — Consider translaryngeal jet ventilation.

BREATHING

Absent.	Ventilate twice (check pulse before continuing ventilation at 8–10 + oxygen).
< 8.	Assist ventilation at 8–10 + oxygen.
Low tidal volume	Assist ventilation.
Labored.	Oxygen by nonrebreather at 15 liters/minute
Normal or rapid	Consider oxygen.

RADIAL PULSE

Absent.	Check carotid pulse (see below). Note late shock.
Present	Note rate and quality.
Bradycardia.	Consider spinal shock, head injury.
Tachycardia	Attempt to calm to reduce rate; consider shock.

CAROTID PULSE . . . . Done if no radial pulse.

Absent.	CPR + BVM + oxygen, load and go. Quick look and defibrillate as appropriate. Monitor.
Present	Note rate and quality.
Bradycardia.	Consider spinal shock, head injury.
Tachycardia	Consider shock.

SKIN . . . . Color and condition.

Pale, cool, clammy	Consider shock.
Cyanosis	Reconsider intubation/ventilation; check oxygen.

MAJOR BLEEDING . . . . Direct pressure, pressure dressing.

Rapid Trauma Survey	Action

HEAD

Major facial injuries.	Consider intubation.

NECK

Swelling, bruising, retracting	Consider intubation.
Neck vein distention.	Consider tamponade, tension pneumothorax.
Tracheal deviation.	Consider tension pneumothorax.
Deformity, tenderness.	**APPLY CERVICAL COLLAR NOW.**

CHEST . . . . Inspect and palpate.

Symmetrical, stable	Continue exam.
Bruises, crepitation.	Consider early cardiac monitoring.
Penetrating wounds	Occlusive dressing.
Paradoxical motion.	Stabilize flail; consider early intubation.

BREATH SOUNDS

Present and equal.	Continue exam.
Unequal.	Percuss chest to determine pneumothorax versus hemothorax.
With decreased LOC, absent radial pulses, cyanosis, JVD, possible tracheal deviation.	Consider needle decompression.

HEART TONES . . . . Note for comparison later.

   Muffled with JVD and bilateral breath sounds . . . Consider pericardial tamponade.

ABDOMEN, PELVIS, UPPER LEGS

   If tender abdomen, unstable pelvis, or bilateral
      femur fractures . . . . Expect development of shock.

MOVEMENT/SENSATION IN EXTREMITIES

   Present . . . . Record.

   Decreased or absent. . . . . Suspect spinal injury.

POSTERIOR

   Injuries identified. . . . . Appropriate management of identified injuries. Transfer
      to backboard.

      **TRANSPORT IMMEDIATELY IF CRITICAL TRAUMA
      SITUATION PRESENT.**

SAMPLE HISTORY . . . . Record.

VITAL SIGNS . . . . Measure and record pulse, respirations. Auscultate and
      record blood pressure.

   Systolic < 90 with signs of shock . . . . Consider IV fluid therapy en route.

   Systolic < 80 . . . . IV fluid therapy en route.

   Systolic < 60 . . . . IV fluid therapy en route.

   Pulse pressure > 60 with decreased LOC   Consider increased intracerebral pressure. Maintain
      systolic blood pressure of 110–120.

Neurological Exam	To Be Done If Altered Mental Status

PUPILS

   Unequal. . . . . Suspect head injury unless patient is alert, then suspect
      eye injury. Give 100% oxygen.

   Unequal or dilated and fixed with GCS ≤ 8 . . . . . . Give 100% oxygen; do not let patient get hypotensive.
      (Target systolic BP of 110–120.) Intubation and
      hyperventilation (20 breaths per minute) are indicated.
      (Unequal pupils or dilated and fixed pupils and GSC 8 or
      less are suggestive of cerebral herniation.)

   Pinpoint (with respiratory rate < 8). . . . . Consider naloxone.

   Dilated/reactive (with GCS ≤ 8) . . . . Give 100% oxygen; consider intubation.

GLASGOW COMA SCALE score (for decreased
   LOC) ≤ 8 . . . . Give 100% oxygen. Don't let patient get hypotensive
      (target systolic BP of 110–120). Intubation en route is
      indicated.

      Consider hyperventilation only if patient shows signs of
      cerebral herniation:

      — GCS ≤ 8 with extensor posturing

      — GCS ≤ 8 with pupillary asymmetry or nonreactivity

      — GCS ≤ 8 with a subsequent drop of more than 2 points

ALL PATIENTS WITH DECREASED LOC . . . . Check for medical identification devices. Do blood-glucose
      check.

Initial Airway Management

Kirk Magee, MD, MSc, FRCPC

Ronald D. Stewart, OC, BA, BSc, MD, FRCPC

John E. Campbell, MD, FACEP

OBJECTIVES

Upon completion of this chapter, you should be able to:

1. Describe the anatomy and physiology of the respiratory system.
2. Explain the importance of observation as it relates to airway control.
3. Describe methods to deliver supplemental oxygen to the trauma patient.
4. Briefly describe the indications, contraindications, advantages, and disadvantages of the following airway adjuncts:
   a. Nasopharyngeal airways
   b. Oropharyngeal airways
   c. Bag-valve masks
   d. Flow-restricted, oxygen-powered ventilation devices
   e. Blind insertion airway devices
   f. Endotracheal intubation
5. Describe the predictors of difficult mask ventilation and endotracheal intubation.
6. Describe the Sellick maneuver.
7. Describe the essential components of an airway kit.

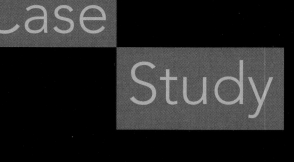
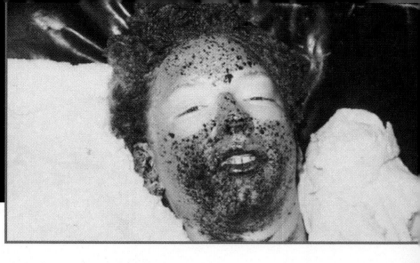

Dan, Joyce, and Buddy of the Emergency Transport System (ETS) have been called to the scene of a house fire. Their Scene Size-up reveals that the fire service is present, the scene is safe, and there is only one victim, a young woman. She had been asleep in a back bedroom where the firefighters found her and pulled her out of a window. She is covered in soot and is coughing. *How would you approach this patient? What is the mechanism of injury? What type of assessment would you perform? What would you do first? Is this a load-and-go situation?* Keep these questions in mind as you read the chapter. Then, at the end of the chapter, find out how the rescuers completed this call.

INTRODUCTION

Of all the tasks expected of field teams caring for the trauma patient, none is more important than that of airway control. Maintaining an open airway and adequate ventilation in the trauma patient can be a challenge in any setting, but it can be almost impossible in the adverse environment of the field with its poor lighting, the chaos that often surrounds the event, the position of the patient, and perhaps hostile onlookers.

Airway control is a task that you must master, because it frequently cannot wait until you get to the hospital. Patients who are cyanotic, underventilated, or both, are in need of immediate help—help that only you can give them in the initial stages of their care. It falls to you, then, to be familiar with the basic structure and function of the airway, to be versed in how to achieve and maintain an open airway, and to know how to oxygenate and ventilate a patient.

Because of the unpredictable nature of the field environment, you will be called on to manage patient airways in almost every conceivable situation: in wrecked cars, dangling above rivers, in the middle of a shopping center, or at the side of a busy highway. You therefore need *options* and alternatives from which to choose. What will help one patient may not work for another. One patient may require a simple jaw thrust to open an airway, while another may require a surgical procedure to prevent impending death.

Whatever the methods required, you must always start with the basics. It is of little value—and in some cases it may be downright dangerous—to apply "advanced" techniques of airway control before beginning basic maneuvers. The discussion of airway control in the trauma patient will be rooted in several fundamental truths: Air should go in and out, oxygen is good, and blue is bad. Everything else follows from this.

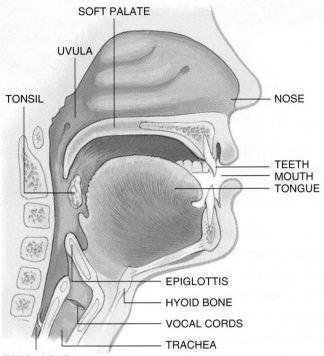

FIGURE 4-1 Anatomy of the upper airway. Note that the tongue, hyoid bone, and epiglottis are attached to the mandible by a series of ligaments. Lifting forward on the jaw will therefore displace all these structures anteriorly.

ANATOMY AND PHYSIOLOGY

The airway begins at the tip of the nose and the lips and ends at the *alveolocapillary membrane*, through which gas exchange takes place between the air sacs of the lung (the *alveoli*) and the lung's capillary network. The airway consists of chambers and pipes, which conduct air with its 21 percent oxygen content to the alveoli and carry away the waste *carbon dioxide* that diffuses from the blood into the alveoli.

Nasopharynx

The beginning of the respiratory tract (the nasal cavity and oropharynx) is lined with moist mucous membranes (Figure 4-1). This lining is delicate and highly vascular. It deserves all the respect that you can give it, and that means preventing undue trauma by using liberally lubricated tubes and avoiding unnecessary poking about. The *nasal cavity* is divided by a very vascular midline *septum*, and on the lateral walls of the nose are "shelves" called the *turbinates*. These projections can get in the way when tubes or other devices need to be inserted into the nostrils. Carefully sliding a well-lubricated tube's bevel along the floor or the septum of the nasal cavity will usually prevent traumatizing the turbinates.

Oropharynx

The teeth are the first obstruction we meet in the oral part of the airway. They may be more obstructive in some patients than in others. In any case, the same general principle always applies: *Patients should have the same number and condition of teeth at the end of an airway procedure as they had at the beginning.*

The tongue is mostly a large chunk of muscle and represents the next potential obstruction. These muscles are attached to the jaw anteriorly and through a series of muscles and ligaments to the *hyoid bone*, a wishbone-like structure just under the chin from which the cartilage skeleton (the larynx) of the upper airway is suspended. The *epiglottis* is also connected to the hyoid, so elevating the hyoid will lift the epiglottis upward and open the airway further.

Hypopharynx

The epiglottis is one of the main anatomic landmarks in the airway. You must be familiar with it and be able to identify it by sight and by touch. It looks like a floppy piece of cartilage covered by mucosa—which is exactly what it is—and it feels like the tragus, the cartilage at the opening of the ear canal. The epiglottis is attached to the hyoid and thence to the mandible by a series of ligaments and muscles. In the unconscious patient, the tongue can produce some airway obstruction by falling back against the soft palate and even the posterior pharyngeal wall. However, it is the epiglottis that will produce complete airway obstruction in the supine unconscious patient whose jaw is relaxed and whose head and neck are in the neutral position. In such patients the epiglottis will fall down against the glottic opening and prevent ventilation.

It is essential to understand this crucial fact in the management of the airway. To ensure an open (patent) airway in an unconscious supine patient, you can displace the hyoid anteriorly by lifting forward on the jaw (chin lift, jaw thrust) or by pulling on the tongue. This will lift the tongue out of the way and keep the epiglottis elevated and away from the posterior pharyngeal wall and glottic opening (Figure 4-2). Both nasotracheal and orotracheal intubation require elevation of the epiglottis by a laryngoscope or the fingers, by pulling on the tongue or by lifting forward on the jaw.

Larynx

On either side of the epiglottis is a recess called the *pyriform fossa*. An endotracheal tube can "catch up" in either one. Pyriform fossa placement of an endotracheal tube can be identified easily by "tenting" of the skin on either side of the superior aspect of the *laryngeal prominence* (Adam's apple) or by transillumination if a lighted stylet (or "lightwand") is being used to intubate.

The vocal cords are protected by the *thyroid cartilage*, a boxlike structure shaped like a "C," with the open part of the "C" representing its posterior wall, which is covered with muscle. In some patients, the cords can close entirely in *laryngospasm*, producing complete airway obstruction. The thyroid cartilage can easily be seen in most people on the anterior surface of the neck as the laryngeal prominence.

Inferior to the thyroid cartilage is another part of the larynx, the *cricoid*, a cartilage shaped like a signet ring with the ring in front and the signet behind. It can be palpated as a small bump on the anterior surface of the neck inferior to the laryngeal prominence. The esophagus is just behind the posterior wall of the cricoid cartilage. Pressure on the cricoid at the front of the neck will close off the esophagus to pressures as high as 100 cm H_2O. This maneuver (the *Sellick maneuver*, Figure 4-3) can be used to reduce the risk of gastric regurgitation during the process of intubation and to prevent insufflation of air into the stomach during positive pressure ventilation by mouth-to-mouth, bag-valve mask, or flow-restricted oxygen-powered ventilator. If there is any danger of cervical-spine injury, you must carefully support and stabilize the neck while performing the Sellick maneuver.

Connecting the inferior border of the thyroid cartilage with the superior aspect of the cricoid is the *cricothyroid membrane*, a very important landmark through which you can gain direct access to the airway below the cords. You can palpate the cricothyroid membrane on most patients by finding the most prominent part of the thyroid cartilage and then sliding your index finger down until you feel a second "bump" just before your finger palpates the last depression before the *sternal notch*. That second bump is the *cricoid cartilage*, and at the upper edge of this is the *cricothyroid membrane* (Figure 4-4). In some patients, especially those with a thick neck, you may find the cricoid cartilage more easily by going from the sternal notch upward until you feel the first prominent cartilage "bump." Just over the "top" of this bump is the cricothyroid membrane. The sternal notch is an important landmark as well because it is the point at which the cuff of a properly placed endotracheal tube should lie (Figure 4-5). The sternal notch is readily palpated at the junction of the clavicles with the upper edge of the sternum.

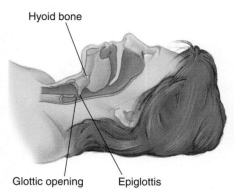

FIGURE 4-2a The epiglottis is attached to the hyoid and then to the mandible. When the mandible is relaxed and falls back, the tongue falls upward and against the soft palate and the posterior pharyngeal wall, while the epiglottis falls over the glottic opening.

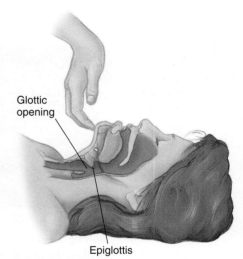

FIGURE 4-2b Extension of the head and lifting the chin will pull the tongue and the epiglottis upward and forward, exposing the glottic opening and ensuring the patent airway. In the trauma patient, only the jaw, or chin and jaw, should be displaced forward, while the head and neck should be kept in alignment.

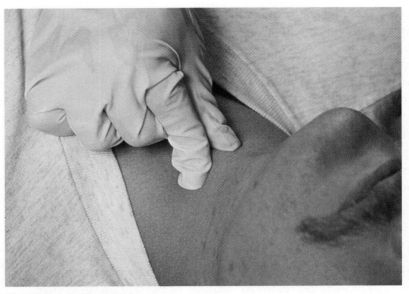

FIGURE 4-3 The Sellick maneuver.

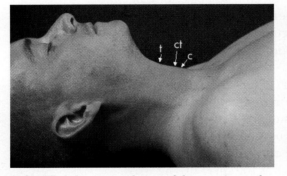

FIGURE 4-4a External view of the anterior neck, showing the surface landmarks for the thyroid cartilage (laryngeal) prominence, the cricothyroid membrane, and the cricoid cartilage.

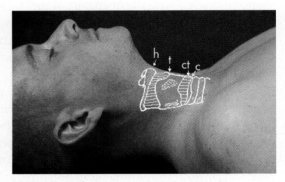

FIGURE 4-4b Cutaway view showing the important landmarks of the larynx and upper airway: hyoid, thyroid cartilage, cricothyroid membrane, and cricoid cartilage.

Trachea and Bronchi

The *tracheal rings* (C-shaped cartilaginous supports for the trachea) continue beyond the cricoid cartilage, and the trachea soon divides into the left and right *mainstem bronchi*. The point at which the trachea divides is called the *carina*. It is important to note that the right mainstem bronchus takes off at an angle that is slightly more in line with the trachea. As a result, tubes or other foreign bodies usually end up in the right mainstem bronchus. One of the goals of a properly performed endotracheal intubation is to avoid a right (or left) mainstem bronchus intubation.

You should know how far some of these major anatomic landmarks are from the teeth. Not only will a knowledge of these help you place an endotracheal tube at the correct level, but also by remembering only three numbers you will be able to detect a tube that is too far into the airway or not in far enough. The three numbers to remember are **15, 20,** and **25.** The first number, *15,* is the distance (in centimeters) from the teeth to the vocal cords of the average adult; *20* (5 cm farther down the airway) is the sternal notch; and 5 cm far-

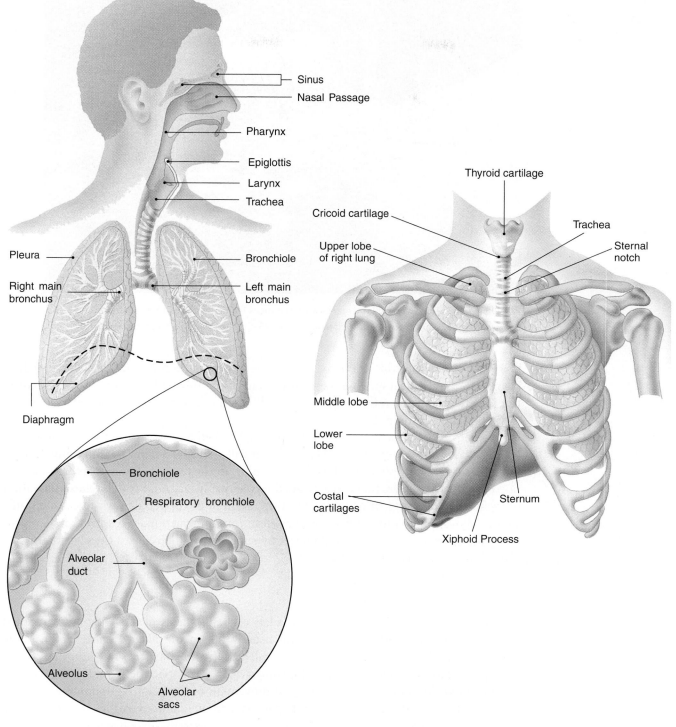

ALVEOLAR SACS

FIGURE 4-5 The respiratory system. Notice the sternal notch, at which point the clavicles join the sternum. It marks the position of the tip of a well-placed endotracheal tube.

ther again at *25* is the carina (Figure 4-6). These are average distances and can vary by several centimeters. Extension or flexion of the head of an intubated patient will move the endotracheal tube up or down as much as 2 to 2.5 cm. Tubes can easily become dislodged, and detection of misplacement can be difficult unless you are monitoring oxygen saturation and expired CO_2. Taping the head down or guarding against movement will not only

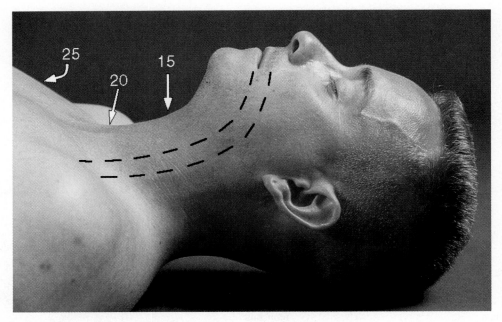

FIGURE 4-6 Major airway landmarks and distances from the teeth: 15 = 15 cm from teeth to cords, 20 = 20 cm from teeth to sternal notch, 25 = 25 cm from teeth to carina.

lessen the risk of tube displacement (even more important in children) but will also reduce trauma to the tracheal mucosa. Less movement of the tube will result in less stimulation to the patient's airway reflexes and may result in a more stable cardiovascular system and intracranial pressure in the patient.

To help protect the airway from becoming blocked and to reduce the risk of aspiration, the body has developed brisk reflexes that will attempt to expel any offending foreign material from the oropharynx, the glottic opening, or the trachea. These areas are well supplied by sensitive nerves that can activate the swallowing, gag, and cough reflex. Activation of swallowing, gagging, or coughing by stimulation of the upper airway can cause significant cardiovascular stimulation as well as elevation in intracranial pressure. You can protect patients from such unwanted effects by suppressing the reflexes through the use of topical lidocaine (see Chapter 5).

The Lungs

The *lungs* are the organs through which gas exchange takes place. They are contained within a "cage" formed by the ribs, and usually fill up the *pleural space*, which is the *potential space* between the internal chest wall and the lung surface. The lungs have only one opening to the outside, the *glottic opening*, which is the space between the vocal cords. Expansion of the chest wall (the cage) and movement of the diaphragm downward cause the lungs to expand (since the pleural space is airtight), and air rushes in through the *glottis*. The air travels down the smaller and smaller tubes to the alveoli, where gas exchange (respiration) takes place.

THE PATENT AIRWAY

One of the first maneuvers essential to caring for a patient is ensuring a *patent* or *open airway*. Without this, all other care is of little use. This must be done quickly, because patients cannot tolerate hypoxia for more than a few minutes. The effect of hypoxia and inadequate ventilation on an unconscious injured patient can be devastating, and if these are compounded by the absence of adequate perfusion, the patient is in even more difficult straits. Patients suffering from head trauma not only may have hypoxic brain damage from airway compromise but may also build up high levels of carbon dioxide that can increase blood flow to the injured brain, causing swelling and increased intracranial pressure.

Ensuring an open airway in a patient can be a major challenge in the prehospital setting. Not only can trauma disrupt the anatomy of the face and airway, but it can also result in bleeding, which can lead to airflow obstruction and obscure airway landmarks. Add to this the risk of cervical-spine injury, and the challenge is readily apparent. You must also remember that some airway maneuvers, including suction and insertion of nasopharyngeal and oropharyngeal airways, may stimulate a patient's protective reflexes and increase the likelihood of vomiting and aspiration, cardiovascular stimulation, and increased intracranial pressure.

The first step in providing a patent airway in the unconscious patient is to ensure that the tongue and epiglottis are lifted forward and maintained in that position. This is done by either the modified jaw thrust (Figure 4-7a) or the jaw lift (Figure 4-7b). Either of these maneuvers will prevent the tongue from falling backward against the soft palate or posterior pharyngeal wall. Either will pull forward on the hyoid, lifting the epiglottis up out of the way. These are essential maneuvers for both basic and advanced airway procedures. Done properly, they will open the airway without tilting the head backward or moving the neck.

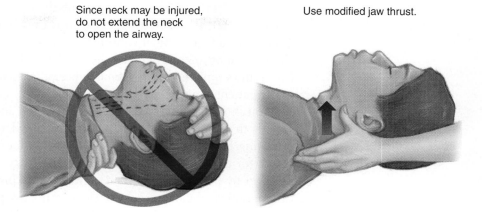

Since neck may be injured, do not extend the neck to open the airway.

Use modified jaw thrust.

FIGURE 4-7a Opening the airway using a modified jaw thrust. Maintain in-line stabilization while pushing up on the angle of the jaw with your thumbs.

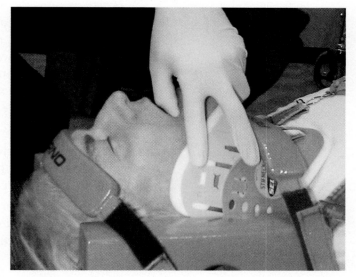

FIGURE 4-7b Jaw lift. *(Photo courtesy of Buddy Denson, EMT-P)*

Constant vigilance and care are required to maintain a patent airway in your patient. Following are essentials for this task:

- Continual observation of the patient in order to anticipate problems
- An adequate suction device with large-bore tubing and attachment
- Airway adjuncts

Observation

The patient who is injured is at risk of airway compromise even if completely conscious and awake. This is partially due to the fact that many patients have full stomachs, are anxious, and are prone to vomiting. Some patients will also be bleeding into their oropharynx and thus swallowing blood. In view of these facts, you should constantly observe your patient for airway problems following injury. One team member must be responsible for both airway control and adequate ventilation for any patient who might be at risk of airway compromise.

The general appearance of a patient, the respiratory rate, and any complaints must be noted and addressed. In a patient who is breathing spontaneously, you must check frequently for adequate tidal volume by feeling over the mouth and nose and by observing chest wall movements. Bare the chest—at least below the breasts—is a good rule to follow. Check the supplemental oxygen line periodically to ensure that oxygen is being delivered to the patient at a given flow rate or percentage.

You should always immediately clear blood and secretions. You must also be alert for sounds that indicate trouble. Be alert for this danger sign: *Noisy breathing is obstructed breathing.* If the patient has an endotracheal tube in place, monitor lung compliance and search for the cause of any change in compliance. If possible, monitor endotracheal tube position by pulse oximetry and continuous expiratory CO_2 monitoring. (For more on capnography, see Chapter 5.) Consider combative patients to be hypoxic until a systematic and rapid evaluation rules it out. Use of waveform capnography is strongly recommended in all intubated patients and use of pulse oximetry is recommended in all trauma patients (see Chapter 5).

Suction

All patients who are injured and who have cervical motion-restriction devices in place should be considered at high risk for airway compromise. In addition, one of the greatest threats to the patent airway is that of vomiting and aspiration, particularly in patients who have recently eaten a large meal washed down with large quantities of alcohol. As a result, portable suction devices should be considered basic equipment for field trauma care. A portable suction device should have the following characteristics (Figure 4-8).

■ It can be carried in an airway kit with an oxygen cylinder and other airway equipment. It should not be separated or stored remote from oxygen; otherwise, it represents an "extra" piece of equipment requiring extra hands.

■ It can be hand powered or battery powered rather than oxygen driven. Hand powered is preferred. You should always have a hand-powered suction as a backup if you use a battery-powered suction.

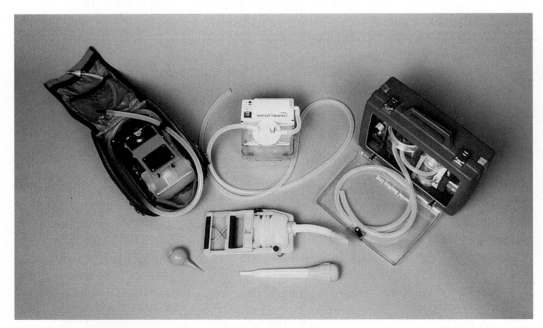

FIGURE 4-8 Examples of suction apparatus.

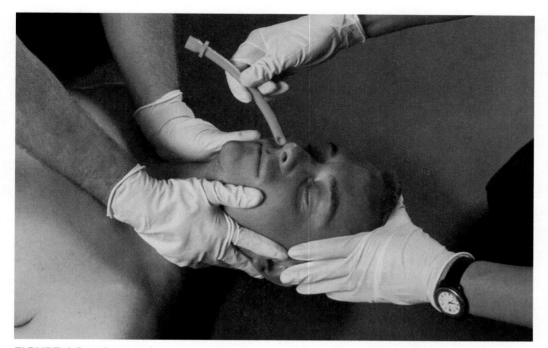

FIGURE 4-9a The nasopharyngeal airway is inserted with the bevel slid along the septum or floor of the nasal cavity.

■ It can generate sufficient suction and volume displacement to remove pieces of food, blood clots, and thick secretions from the oropharynx.

■ It has tubing of sufficient diameter (0.8–1 cm) to handle whatever is suctioned from the patient.

Suction tips should be of large bore, such as the rigid "tonsil-tip" suckers that can handle most clots and bleeding. In some cases the suction tubing itself can be used to withdraw large amounts of blood or gastric contents. A 6-mm endotracheal tube can be used with a connector as a suction tip. The tube's side hole removes the necessity for a proximal control valve to interrupt suction. Usually Rescuer 2 (see Chapter 2) assumes responsibility for the airway. As the VO (vomit officer), Rescuer 2 must be constantly alert to prevent the patient from aspirating.

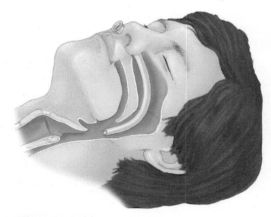

FIGURE 4-9b The nasopharyngeal airway rests between the tongue and the posterior pharyngeal wall.

Airway Adjuncts

Equipment to help ensure a patent airway will include various nasopharyngeal (NPA), oropharyngeal (OPA), blind insertion airway devices (BIAD), and endotracheal airways. Insertion of these devices must be reserved for patients whose protective reflexes are sufficiently depressed to tolerate them. Care must be taken not to provoke vomiting or gagging, since both occurrences are bad for these patients.

Nasopharyngeal Airways: Nasopharyngeal airways (NPAs) should be soft and of appropriate length. They are designed to prevent the tongue and epiglottis from falling against the posterior pharyngeal wall (see Chapter 5 for insertion technique). In a pinch, a 6-mm or 6.6-mm endotracheal tube can be cut and serve as a nasopharyngeal airway. With light lubrication and gentle insertion, there should be few problems with this airway (Figure 4-9). However, bleeding and trauma to the nasal mucosa are common. Mild

PEARLS
Preventing Deaths

- Become skilled at recognizing when:
  - Active airway management is necessary
  - The patient needs assistance with ventilation
  - An airway device is placed incorrectly
  - An airway device that was placed correctly has become displaced (The pulse oximeter and CO$_2$ monitor are critical for this.)
- Become competent in intubating the trachea. Be prepared to use a rescue airway (e.g., Combitube®, King LT-D™ airway) if you are unable to intubate.
- Prevent aspiration of gastric contents. Suction must be immediately available. Be prepared for equipment failure by having backup equipment available.
- Failure to manage the airway can be a fatal error.

hemorrhage from the nose after insertion of the airway is *not* an indication to remove it. In fact, it is probably better to keep an NPA in place so as not to disturb the clot or reactivate the bleeding. The NPA will be better tolerated than the oropharyngeal one and thus can usually be used in patients who still have a gag reflex.

Oropharyngeal Airways: Oropharyngeal airways (OPAs) are designed to keep the tongue off the posterior pharyngeal wall and thereby help maintain a patent airway (Figure 4-10). Patients who are easily able to tolerate an oropharyngeal airway should be considered candidates for endotracheal intubation, because their protective reflexes are so depressed that they cannot protect their lower airways from aspiration. Special OPAs are available. Some are designed as intubation guides, whereas others have proximal ends that protrude from the lips and are designed to be used with balloon masks that seal the mouth and nose.

Blind Insertion Airway Devices: Esophageal tracheal combitube (Combitube®), King LT-D™ airway, and the laryngeal mask airway (LMA) are all blind insertion airway devices (BIADs). These adjuncts are not as effective as endotracheal intubation in preventing aspiration or ensuring ventilation and thus are not recommended for advanced EMS providers except as rescue devices in cases in which you are unsuccessful in intubating the trachea (see Appendix A).

Endotracheal Intubation: Endotracheal intubation is the gold standard of airway care in patients who cannot protect their airways or in those needing assistance with breathing. Several problems will face you when you decide to intubate a trauma patient. Thus there are several methods used to perform endotracheal intubation. Intubation frequently must be done under the most difficult circumstances—on the side of the road, in a crashed vehicle, or under a train. In addition, the patient's spine may need to be motion restricted, with a cervical collar or other equipment in place. This may so restrict movement and visualization of the airway that you have to consider alternative methods of intubation.

Although the original method of intubation was clearly tactile or digital, this was later changed by the invention of the laryngoscope, which allowed visualization of the upper airway and placement of the tube under direct vision. The ability to see the actual passage of the tube through the glottic opening rendered tactile orotracheal intubation obsolete, and its practice largely died out until interest in it was revived in the last two decades.

There are several choices to facilitate intubation in the trauma patient, ranging from awake intubation using topical anesthetics to deep sedation and rapid sequence intubation (RSI). *Rapid sequence intubation* refers to the use of paralytic agents to quickly facilitate tube placement and to minimize the risk of aspiration. You must be cognizant of the fact that both deep sedation and RSI inhibit the normal muscle tone of the airway and thus may make it impossible to effectively mask-ventilate the patient. In this situation, it is necessary to immediately place an endotracheal tube to achieve successful ventilation. For this reason, you must be very familiar with the predictors of difficult laryngoscopy and intubation before deciding to intubate a patient who is already breathing on his own. *Remember, patients who have spontaneous yet inadequate respiratory effort are better off than the patient who has been given a paralytic and can neither be mask-ventilated nor intubated.*

Although it is not always possible to guess every time which patient will have a difficult airway, certain physical features allow us to predict which patients might potentially have difficult laryngoscopy and intubation. The mnemonic "MMAP" has been proposed to identify these features. MMAP stands for Mallampati, measurement 3-3-1, atlanto-occipital extension, and pathology:

M — *Mallampati.* The Mallampati score ranges from I to IV and is dependent on what structures can be viewed when the mouth is opened (Table 4-1). Generally, the higher the grade, the more difficult it will be to perform laryngoscopy.

M — *Measurement 3-3-1.* This measurement can also aid in predicting the difficult airway. Ideally, you should be able to fit three (*3*) fingers under the patient's chin between the hyoid bone and the mentum of the chin; the patient should be able to open his mouth so that three (*3*) fingers fit between the upper and lower incisors; and, lastly, the patient should be able to protrude the lower jaw such that the lower teeth are 1 cm (*1*) beyond the upper teeth.

A — *Atlanto-occipital junction.* In patients in whom cervical-spine injury is *not* suspected, the ability to extend the head at the atlanto-occipital junction to achieve the "sniffing position" will aid in visualizing the vocal cords.

P — *Pathology.* Finally, pathology refers to any clinical evidence of anatomic airway obstruction. Airway obstruction can result from medical or traumatic conditions, such as edema, infection, burns, penetrating or blunt injuries. This is particularly important as upper airway obstructive pathology is a relative contraindication to RSI.

As for all clinicians responsible for emergency airway management, the appropriate decision regarding whom and how to intubate will ultimately be related to several factors. These include the assessment of the patient and the particular clinical presentation, the skill set of the individual health-care professionals present, and the system in which they work. An additional factor unique to the prehospital setting is time. Ventilation with a bag-valve mask (BVM) and immediate transport of the patient may be a better option in certain instances than taking the additional time required to perform RSI.

Although *direct-vision orotracheal intubation* should be considered the primary method of placing a tube in the trachea, the procedure is not always easy, nor is it indicated in all patients. In the management of trauma patients particularly, options must be available to permit successful intubation in even the most challenging of situations and patients. There is evidence that the technique of *direct-vision orotracheal intubation* results in movement of the head and neck. The question therefore arises as to whether the use of this method presents an added risk in possible cervical-spine injuries. Controversy exists as to whether such movement is either substantial or of real clinical significance. In short, the method of intubation should be suited to each patient. Those with a low risk of cervical-spine injury can be intubated in the conventional way, using a laryngoscope. Intubation by the nasotracheal route, the tactile or transillumination methods, or a combination of the two

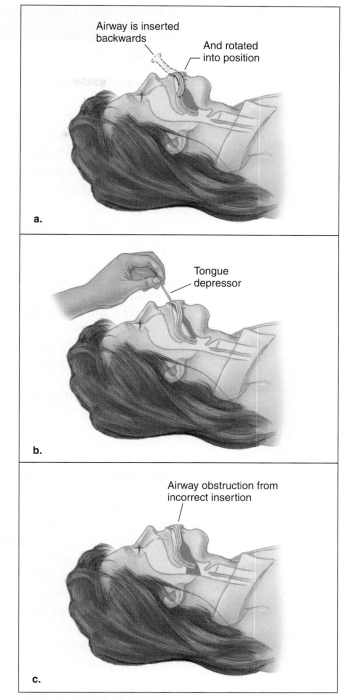

FIGURE 4-10 Insertion of an oropharyngeal airway.

TABLE 4-1 *Estimating Difficulty of Intubation*
Mallampati Score
View pharynx with mouth open and tongue not protruding.
Scoring:
I. Entire tonsil or tonsillar bed is visible.
II. Upper half of tonsil or tonsillar bed is visible.
III. Soft and hard palate are clearly visible.
IV. Only hard palate is visible.
The higher the score, the higher the degree of difficulty.

should be reserved for patients with specific indication for alternative techniques (see Chapter 5 and Appendix A).

Translaryngeal jet ventilation (TLJV) can provide a quick, reliable, and relatively safe temporary method of adequate oxygenation and ventilation when the airway cannot be maintained because of obstruction or partial obstruction above the cords, and access below the level of the cords is needed. A special cannula is inserted through the cricothyroid membrane, and the patient is ventilated using a special manual jet ventilator device (see Appendix A).

SUPPLEMENTAL OXYGEN

Patients who are injured need supplemental oxygen, especially if they are unconscious. It is well recognized that patients suffering from head injury are frequently hypoxic. Supplemental oxygen can be supplied by a simple face mask run at 10–12 liters per minute. This will provide the patient with about 40 to 50 percent oxygen. Nonrebreathing masks with a reservoir bag and oxygen flow rates into the bag of 12–15 liters per minute can provide 60 to 90 percent oxygen to the patient. These are recommended for all trauma patients requiring supplemental oxygen. Nasal oxygen cannulae are well tolerated by most patients, but provide only about 25 to 30 percent oxygen to the patient. They are recommended only for those patients who refuse to accept an oxygen mask.

Supplemental oxygen must be used to ensure adequate oxygenation when you perform positive pressure ventilation. Oxygenation must be supplemented during mouth-to-mask ventilation by running oxygen at 10–12 liters per minute through the oxygen nipple attached to most masks or by placing the oxygen tubing under the mask and running it at the same rate. Alternatively, you can increase the oxygen percentage delivered during mouth-to-mask breathing by placing a nasal cannula on yourself. This increases the delivered oxygen percentage from 17 percent to about 30 percent.

Bag-valve mask (BVM) devices or resuscitator bags with a large (2.5 liters) reservoir bag and an oxygen flow rate of 12–15 liters per minute will increase the delivered oxygen from 21 percent (air) to 90 or 100 percent. Adding a reservoir bag to a BVM will increase the delivered oxygen from 40 to 50 percent to 90 to 100 percent and thus should always be used.

Flow-restricted oxygen-powered ventilation devices (FROPVD) will provide 100 percent oxygen at a flow rate of 40 liters per minute at a maximum pressure of 50 cm ± 5 cm water.

VENTILATION

Normal Ventilation

The movement of air or gases in and out of the lungs is called *ventilation*. At rest, adults normally take in about 400 to 600 cc with each breath. This is called the *tidal volume*. Multiplying that value by the number of breaths per minute (the respiratory rate) gives the *minute volume*, the amount of air breathed in (and, of course, out) each minute. This is an important value and is normally 5–12 liters per minute. Normal ventilation by healthy lungs will produce an oxygen level of about 100 mmHg and a carbon dioxide level of 35 to 40 mmHg. A carbon dioxide level below 35 mmHg indicates hyperventilation, and values greater than 40 mmHg indicate hypoventilation.

The clinical terms *hypoventilation* and *hyperventilation* do not refer to oxygenation but to the level of carbon dioxide maintained. It is easier for carbon dioxide to diffuse across the alveolocapillary membrane of the lungs than it is for oxygen to do so. This makes it easier to excrete carbon dioxide than to oxygenate the blood. Thus, if the chest or lungs are injured, the body may be able to maintain normal levels of carbon dioxide in the blood and yet the cells can be hypoxic. A patient with a contused lung might have a respiratory rate of 36, a carbon dioxide level of 30 mmHg, and an oxygen level of only 80 mmHg. Although hyperventilating, this person is still hypoxic. He does not need to breathe faster; he needs to have supplemental oxygen. When in doubt, give your patient oxygen.

Devices to measure oxygen saturation (pulse oximeters) have been available for several years and expired CO_2 monitors (capnographs) are now available for prehospital use. *Pulse oximeters* measure oxygen saturation and should be used on almost all trauma patients, while CO_2 monitors are most useful for continuously monitoring endotracheal tube placement (though they have many other uses; see Chapters 8 and 10). These devices will be discussed in Chapter 5.

Positive Pressure (Artificial) Ventilation

Normal breathing takes place because the negative pressure inside the (potential) pleural space "draws" air in through the upper airway from the outside. In any patient who is unable to do this, or whose airway needs protecting, you may need to "pump" air or oxygen in through the glottic opening. This is called *intermittent positive pressure ventilation (IPPV)*. IPPV in trauma patients can take various forms, from mouth-to-mouth to bag-valve-endotracheal tube ventilation. *NOTE: "Pumping" air into the oropharynx is no guarantee that it will go through the glottic opening and into the lungs.*

The oropharynx leads to the esophagus. Pressure in the oropharynx of greater than 25 cm H_2O will open the esophagus and lead to air being pumped into the stomach (gastric insufflation). Bag-valve masks and FROPVDs can produce pressures greater than this, which is why the Sellick maneuver (posterior pressure on the cricoid cartilage) is so very important as a basic airway maneuver. When you need to ventilate a patient using IPPV, you should know approximately what the *delivered volume* is (how much volume you are delivering with each breath you give). You can estimate the minute volume by multiplying delivered volume by the ventilatory rate. A flow-restricted oxygen-powered ventilator device that delivers oxygen at the rate of 40 liters per minute will have a delivered volume of about 700 cc each second that the valve is activated. Unless the Sellick maneuver is used, delivering this volume at a pressure of 50 cm H_2O will almost guarantee gastric insufflation and all the complications resulting from it. BVM breathing is no better, because pressures generated by squeezing the bag may equal or exceed 60 cm H_2O.

Delivered volumes are usually less with bag resuscitators than with FROPVDs. There are two reasons for this. The average resuscitator bag holds only 1,800 cc of gas, which is the absolute limit to the volume that could be delivered if you were able to squeeze the bag completely. Using one hand, the best an average adult can squeeze is approximately 1,200 cc. Most people will squeeze only 800 to 1,000 cc with one hand. The other reason for greater delivered volumes with flow-restricted oxygen-powered ventilator devices is that a FROPVD has a trigger that allows the rescuer to hold a mask on the face with both hands, thus decreasing mask leak. Keep in mind that these volumes, delivered from the ventilating port of these devices, equal the volumes delivered to the patient only if an endotracheal tube is in place. In other words, they do not take into account mask leak. When performing IPPV with a mask, keep the following essentials in mind:

- Supplemental oxygen must be provided for the patient during IPPV.
- Suction must be *immediately* available.
- Ventilation must be done carefully to avoid gastric distension and to reduce the risk of regurgitation and possible aspiration. You can help prevent these complications by using the Sellick maneuver.
- Pulse oximetry and end-tidal CO_2 monitoring (capnography) are the most reliable methods of monitoring effectiveness of ventilation. The pulse oximeter measures the oxygen saturation of the blood and the capnograph measures the CO_2 level. Use the end-tidal CO_2 level to judge whether to increase or decrease the rate of ventilation. If you adjust your respiratory rate to keep the expired CO_2 level between 35–40, you can be sure you are neither hypo- or hyperventilating the patient.

In the case of bag-mask breathing, up to 40 percent mask leak can be expected. Balloon mask designs can reduce this, and a two-person technique, in which one rescuer holds the mask in place with both hands while a second squeezes the bag, may better ensure adequate delivered volumes. During the stress of an emergency situation, you will tend to ventilate patients at an increased rate. Normal rates should be 10 to 12 times per minute but, if the patient is intubated, the rate usually can be 8 to 10 times per minute. Your pulse oximeter and end-tidal CO_2 monitor are most important in getting the correct rate for each patient.

Compliance

When air, or air containing oxygen, is delivered by positive pressure into the lungs of a patient, the "give" or elasticity of the lungs and chest wall will influence how easily it will be for the patient to breathe. If you are performing mask ventilation, a normal elasticity of the lungs and chest wall will allow air to enter the glottic opening and little gastric distension should result. However, if the elasticity is poor, ventilation will be harder to achieve and gastric distension more likely. The ability of the lungs and chest wall to expand and therefore ventilate a patient is known as *compliance*. It is simpler to speak of "good compliance" or "bad compliance" rather than "high" or "low" compliance, since the latter terms can be somewhat confusing.

Compliance is an important concept, because it governs whether or not you can adequately ventilate a patient. Compliance can become bad (i.e., low) in some disease states of the lung or in patients who have an injury to the chest wall. In cardiac arrest, compliance will also become bad, due to poor circulation to the muscles. This makes ventilating the patient all the more difficult. With an endotracheal tube in place, the patient's compliance becomes an important clinical sign and may reveal airway problems. Keep in mind that with an endotracheal tube in place and with bag-valve ventilation, you have a kind of "pressure-detection" device much like a tire-pressure gauge. That is, you can "feel" with your fingers and hand a *change* in compliance, either worsening or improving. A worsening of compliance may be the first sign of a tension pneumothorax. Poor compliance also will be felt in right (or left) mainstem bronchus intubation—

pulling back on the tube will result in an immediate improvement in the ability to ventilate (i.e., better compliance).

Ventilation Techniques

Mouth to Mouth: Mouth-to-mouth ventilation is the most reliable and effective method, with the advantage of requiring no equipment and a minimum of experience and training. In addition, delivered volumes are consistently adequate because mouth seal is effectively and easily maintained. In addition, compliance can be "felt" more accurately, and high oropharyngeal pressures are therefore less likely. This method is almost never used because of the fear of disease transmission. However, it is appropriate for many patients, especially those with whom you are familiar (such as family members). Because of its effectiveness and universal availability, you should be familiar with the technique.

Mouth to Mask: Though not quite as effective as mouth-to-mouth ventilation, mouth-to-mask ventilation can overcome the slight danger of disease transmission by interposing a face mask between your mouth and that of the patient. Commercially designed pocket face masks, which fold into a small case that can be carried in your pocket, are particularly suited for the initial ventilation of many types of patients. Some have a side port for supplemental oxygen. Pocket ventilating masks have consistently been shown to deliver larger volumes than bag-mask devices and do so with a greater percentage of oxygen than mouth-to-mouth ventilation. Mouth-to-mask ventilation has significant advantages over bag-mask devices, and should be more widely used (see Chapter 5).

Flow-Restricted Oxygen-Powered Ventilating Device: In the past, the high-pressure, oxygen-powered ventilators (demand valves) were considered too dangerous to use in multiple-trauma patients. Experience with the newer flow-restricted oxygen-powered ventilator devices (FROPVDs) that meet American Heart Association guidelines (oxygen flow rate of 40 liters per minute at a maximum pressure of 50 ± 5 cm H_2O) suggests that these may now be the equal of bag-valve devices for ventilation (Figure 4-11). They have the advantage of delivering 100 percent oxygen and allowing use of two hands while using face-mask ventilation. FROPVDs are no worse than BVMs at producing gastric distention. However, because it is more difficult to feel lung compliance when ventilating with the FROPVD, there is still some controversy about its use. Follow your medical director's advice on the use of a FROPVD.

Bag-Valve Mask: The bag-valve mask, a descendant of the anesthetic bag, is a fixed-volume ventilator with an average delivered volume of about 800 cc. With a two-handed squeeze, over 1 liter can be delivered to the patient. It should be used with a reservoir bag or tubing. Plain BVMs without reservoir bag or tubing can only deliver 40 to 50 percent oxygen and thus should be replaced with reservoir bags.

The most important problem associated with the bag-valve mask device is the volume delivered. Mask leak is a serious problem, decreasing the volume delivered to the oropharynx by sometimes 40 percent or more. In addition, old masks of conventional design have significant dead space beneath them, thus increasing the challenge to provide an adequate volume to the patient. The newer balloon mask has a design that eliminates dead space beneath the mask and provides an improved seal over the nose and mouth. It has been

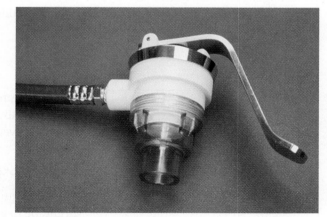

FIGURE 4-11 The flow-restricted oxygen-powered ventilation device. This valve delivers a set flow of 40 liters per minute at maximum pressure of 50 ± 5 cm H_2O. Do not use it unless it meets these standards and your medical director approves.

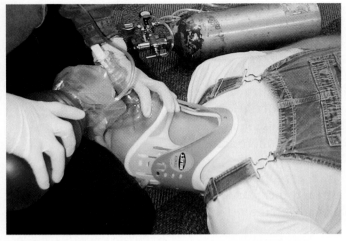

FIGURE 4-12 The inflated balloon mask has been shown to reduce mask leak and provide greater volumes during ventilation with bag-mask devices. *(Photo courtesy of Buddy Denson, EMT-P)*

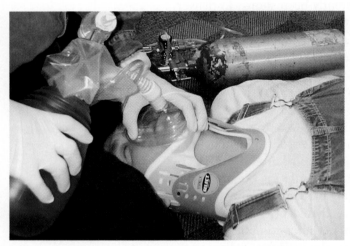

FIGURE 4-13 A ventilating port extension attached to a ventilating bag permits a better mask seal and therefore greater delivered volumes. When the bag is compressed against the thigh, as shown here, delivered volumes may be increased further. *(Photo courtesy of Buddy Denson, EMT-P)*

Increasing Difficulty ↓

- Reposition
- OPA/NPA
- Two-person bag
- Consider obstruction
- BIAD
- Laryngoscopy and intubation

FIGURE 4-14 Response to difficult bag-mask ventilation.

shown in mannequin studies to decrease mask leak and to improve ventilation. It is recommended particularly for trauma patients (Figure 4-12).

A better seal can sometimes be obtained, and larger volumes delivered, in either the balloon or conventional mask, with the use of extension tubing attached to the ventilating port of the bag-valve device. This permits the mask to be better seated on the face without a levering effect from the rigid ventilating port connector that tends to unseat the mask. With the extension in place, the bag can be more easily compressed, even against the knee or thigh, thus increasing the delivered volume and overcoming any mask leak (Figure 4-13).

Effective ventilation with a BVM requires a high degree of skill and is not without problems. Prehospital personnel must be prepared for situations where mask ventilation is difficult and be able to respond to these challenges. Predictors of difficult mask ventilation can be remembered using the "BOOTS" mnemonic.

B — *Beards*

O — *Obesity*

O — *Older patients*

T — *Toothlessness*

S — *Snores or stridor*

All these signs suggest that the patient will not be easy to ventilate. Facial hair and the lack of teeth make mask seal more difficult. Obesity increases both lung and chest compliance. In older patients and in those in whom cervical-spine control is essential, it is more difficult to get proper head and neck positioning. Finally, the presence of snoring or stridor should alert the rescuer to the presence of airway obstruction.

If unable to ventilate a patient using a BVM, the first step should be to reposition the airway and consider the use of an OPA or NPA. If you are still unsuccessful, the next step is to initiate two-person BVM ventilation with extra emphasis on the jaw-thrust maneuver to maximize airway opening. Continued problems with mask ventilation should prompt the consideration of airway obstruction as a potential cause. Ultimately, the placement of a BIAD or endotracheal tube may be required to definitively ventilate the patient in the worst-case scenario (Figure 4-14).

Airway Equipment

The most important rule to follow in regard to airway equipment is that it should be in good working order and immediately available. It will do the patient no good if you have to run back to the ambulance to get the suction apparatus. In other words, be prepared. This is not difficult. Five basic pieces of equipment are necessary for the initial response to all prehospital trauma calls.

- Personal protection equipment (see Chapter 1)
- Long backboard with attached head motion-restriction device
- Appropriately sized rigid cervical extrication collar
- Airway kit (see below)
- Trauma box (see Chapter 1)

The *airway kit* should be completely self-contained and should contain everything needed to secure an airway in any patient. Equipment now available is lightweight and portable. Oxygen cylinders are aluminum, and newer suction devices are less bulky and lighter. It is no longer acceptable to have suction units that are bulky and stored separately from a source of oxygen. Suction units should be contained in a kit with oxygen and other essential airway tools. A lightweight airway kit should consist of the following (Figure 4-15):

- Oxygen D cylinder, preferably aluminum
- Portable battery-powered and hand-powered suction units
- Oxygen cannulae and masks
- Endotracheal intubation kit
- Rescue airway device such as the esophageal tracheal combitube (Combitube®), King LT-D™ airway, or laryngeal mask airway (LMA)
- Bag-valve mask ventilating device (with reservoir bag)
- Pocket mask with supplemental oxygen intake
- Pulse oximeter
- CO_2 monitor
- Translaryngeal oxygen cannula and manual ventilator

The contents of the airway kit are critical. Check all equipment each shift and have a card attached to be initialed by the person checking it.

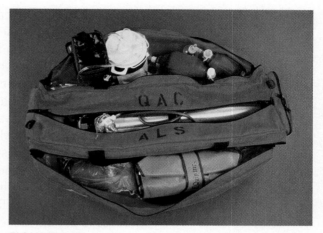

FIGURE 4-15 An airway kit containing the essentials for airway management. Note that portable suction is included in this design. The total weight (with aluminum "D" oxygen cylinder) is approximately 10 kg (22 lb), about the same as a steel "E" cylinder.

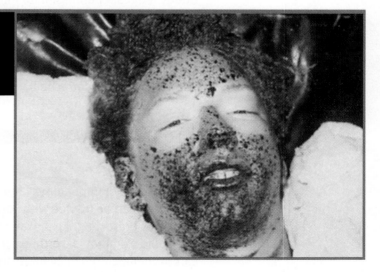

Case Study
continued

Dan, Joyce, and Buddy of the Emergency Transport System have been called to the scene of a house fire. Their Scene Size-up reveals that the fire department is present, the scene is safe, and there is only one victim. She had been asleep in a back bedroom and the firefighters pulled her out of a window. The general impression is poor because the patient is covered in soot, she is coughing, and she appears to be having some trouble breathing. Buddy is acting as team leader. The team dons personal protective equipment, gathers essential equipment, and approaches the patient.

Buddy begins his initial assessment by introducing the team, while Joyce prepares to apply a nonrebreather oxygen mask. When questioned about what happened, the young woman states she had some food simmering on the stove and decided to take a brief nap. When she awakened, the room was full of smoke, and when she opened the bedroom door the hallway was engulfed in flames. She slammed the door and was trying to climb out the window when the fire department arrived. She denies any history of asthma or lung disease and does not smoke. She complains of headache, persistent cough, and some dyspnea. Buddy notes she has a hoarse voice and her breathing is rapid and shallow. She has a strong rapid pulse at the wrist. Dan has the stretcher ready, and the patient climbs onto it. Because of the mechanism of injury, Buddy chooses to perform a focused exam for burns and airway injury. He has already determined that this is a priority patient because of the abnormal initial assessment. This is also a load-and-go situation because of the respiratory difficulty.

A brief exam of the head and face reveals erythema and blistering of the face and lips. Her hair is singed. There is also soot in the nose and mouth with singed hairs in her nose. There are no other burns but there is erythema (but no blistering) of the skin of the neck and exposed surfaces of her arms, with some singeing of the hair. The breath sounds are present and equal bilaterally but there is a slight expiratory wheeze.

The patient is immediately moved to the ambulance and transported. Dan drives; Buddy and Joyce provide patient care. While Buddy obtains the rest of the SAMPLE history and vital signs, Joyce starts a saline lock IV, applies a pulse oximeter, and performs a 12-lead EKG (reveals sinus tachycardia). The patient states that the oxygen helps her dyspnea, but Buddy notes that her voice is hoarser. She has no allergies. Her past medical history is negative for any serious illnesses and she takes no medications. Her last oral intake was noon. (It is now 6:00 PM.)

Vital signs are blood pressure 120/70, pulse 130, and respiratory rate 36 with expiratory wheezing. The pulse oximeter reading is 100 percent on 100 percent oxygen, but Buddy realizes that the pulse oximeter is not reliable in this situation. Buddy notifies medical direction that he has a patient who was asleep in a closed space with smoke and was briefly exposed to flames. She is now dyspneic and coughing with bilateral expiratory wheezing and a hoarse voice. She also has a headache. Joyce has already given a nebulized bronchodilator treatment with only slight improvement. Buddy requests permission to intubate because of the danger of losing the airway. This is accomplished using nasotracheal intubation because the patient still has a gag reflex.

After arrival at the emergency department, the patient is found to have a carboxyhemoglobin level of 25 percent and also upper airway burns. She required several days of endotracheal intubation until her airway swelling decreased.

Case Study Wrap-up

This is a case of upper airway burns and smoke inhalation. The carbon monoxide poisoning can be treated with 100 percent oxygen; hyperbaric oxygen can be used if available. Protecting the airway and maintaining oxygenation are the keys to recovery. The pulse oximeter is worthless in this situation, as it does not recognize carboxyhemoglobin or cyanide poisoning and will give falsely high readings. Unless you have the capability to perform rapid sequence intubation, you will usually have to perform nasotracheal intubation in this situation.

SUMMARY

Trauma patients provide the greatest challenge in airway management. To be successful you must have a clear understanding of the anatomy of the airway and be proficient in techniques to open and maintain your patient's airway. You must have the correct equipment organized in a kit that is immediately available when you begin assessment of the trauma patient. To provide adequate ventilation for your patient, you must understand the concepts of tidal volume, minute volume, and lung compliance. Finally, you must become familiar with the various options for control of the airway and develop and maintain expertise in performing them.

BIBLIOGRAPHY

1. American College of Emergency Physicians Policy Statement. Verification of endotracheal tube placement. http://www.acep.org/webportal/PracticeResources/PolicyStatements/pracmgt/VerificationofEndotrachealTubePlacement.htm
2. Biebuyck, J. F. 1991. Management of the difficult adult airway. *Anesthesiology* 75: 1087–1110.
3. International Liaison Committee on Resuscitation. 2005. International Consensus on Cardiopulmonary Resuscitation and Emergency Cardiovascular Care Science with Treatment Recommendations. *Circulation* 112: III-1-III-136.
4. Kovacs, G., A. Law. *Airway management in emergency medicine.* 1st ed. McGraw-Hill. In Press.
5. Langeron, O., E. Masso, C. Huraux, M. Guggiari, A. Bianchi, B. Coriat, et al. 2000. Prediction of difficult mask ventilation. *Anesthesiology* 92(5): 1229–36.
6. Mosesso, V. N., K. Kukitsch, et al. 1994. Comparison of delivered volumes and airway pressures when ventilating through an endotracheal tube with bag-valve versus demand-valve. *Prehospital and Disaster Medicine* 9(1): 24–28.
7. O'Connor, R. E., R. A. Swor. 1999. Verification of endotracheal tube placement following intubation. National Association of EMS Physicians Standards and Clinical Practice Committee. *Prehospital Emergency Care.* 3:248–50. [III]
8. Ravussin, P., J. Freeman. 1985. A new transtracheal catheter for ventilation and resuscitation. *Canadian Anaesthesiology Society Journal* 32: 60–64.
9. Robinson, N., M. Clancy. 2001. In patients with head injury undergoing rapid sequence intubation, does pretreatment with intravenous lignocaine/lidocaine lead to an improved neurological outcome? A review of the literature. *Emergency Medicine Journal* 18(6): 453–57.
10. Salem, M. R., A. Y. Wong, M. Mani, et al. 1974. Efficacy of cricoid pressure in preventing gastric inflation during bag-mask ventilation in pediatric patients. *Anesthesiology* 40: 96–98.
11. Sivestri, S., G. Ralls, B. Krauss, et al. 2005. The effectiveness of out-of-hospital use of continuous end-tidal carbon dioxide monitoring on the rate of unrecognized misplaced intubation within a regional emergency medical services system. *Annals of Emergency Medicine* 45(5): 497–503.
12. Stewart, R. D., R. M. Kaplan, B. Pennock, et al. 1985. Influence of mask design on bag-mask ventilation. *Annals of Emergency Medicine* 14: 403–6.
13. Stockinger, Z. T., N. E. McSwain. 2004. Prehospital endotracheal intubation for trauma does not improve survival over bag-valve-mask ventilation. *Journal of Trauma* 56(3): 531–36.
14. Ufbert J., J. Bushra, D. Karras, et al. 2005. Aspiration of gastric contents: Association with prehospital intubation. *The American Journal of Emergency Medicine* 23: 379–82.
15. Wang, H., T. Sweeney, R. O'Conner, et al. 2001. Failed prehospital intubations: An analysis of emergency department courses and outcomes. *Prehospital Emergency Care* 5(2): 131–41.
16. White, S. J., R. M. Kaplan, R. D. Stewart. 1987. Manual detection of decreased lung compliance as a sign of tension pneumothorax (abstr). *Annals of Emergency Medicine* 16: 518.

Airway Management Skills

Donna Hastings, EMT-P
Bob Page, EMT-P

OBJECTIVES

Upon completion of this chapter, you should be able to:

1. Suction the airway.
2. Insert a nasopharyngeal and oropharyngeal airway.
3. Use the pocket mask.
4. Use the bag-valve mask.
5. Use the pulse oximeter.
6. Properly prepare for endotracheal intubation.
7. Perform laryngoscopic orotracheal intubation.
8. Perform nasotracheal intubation.
9. Confirm placement of the endotracheal tube.
10. Use capnography to confirm placement of the endotracheal tube.
11. Properly anchor the endotracheal tube.

BASIC AIRWAY MANAGEMENT

PROCEDURES

❋ Suctioning the Airway

1. Attach the suction connecting tubing to the portable suction machine.
2. Turn the device on and test it.
3. Insert the suction tip through the nose (soft or whistle tip) or mouth (soft or rigid) without activating the suction.
4. Activate the suction and withdraw the suction tube.
5. Repeat the procedure as necessary.

NOTE: Although the intent is to suction foreign matter, air and oxygen are also being suctioned out of the patient. Never suction for greater than 15 seconds. After suctioning, reoxygenate the patient as soon as possible.

❋ Inserting the Nasopharyngeal Airway (NPA)

The nasopharyngeal airway (NPA) is made to go into the right nostril. Do not use it if the patient has facial fractures or racoon eyes. To insert the NPA into the patient's right nostril:

1. Choose the appropriate size. It should be as large as possible but still fit easily through the patient's external nares. The size of the patient's little finger can be used as a rough guide.
2. Lubricate the tube with a water-based lubricant.
3. Insert the tube straight back through the right nostril with the beveled edge of the airway toward the septum.
4. Gently pass it into the posterior pharynx with a slight rotating motion until the flange rests against the nares.

To insert the NPA into the left nostril:

1. Turn the airway upside down so that the bevel is toward the septum.
2. Insert straight back through the nostril until you reach the posterior pharynx.
3. Turn the airway over 180 degrees and insert it down the pharynx.

NOTE: If the tongue is occluding the airway, a jaw thrust or chin lift must be done to allow the nasopharyngeal airway to go under the tongue.

❋ Inserting the Oropharyngeal Airway (OPA)

1. Choose the appropriate-size OPA. The distance from the corner of the mouth to the lower part of the external ear is a good estimate.
2. Open the airway.
   a. Scissor maneuver
   b. Jaw lift
   c. Tongue blade
3. Insert the airway gently without pushing the tongue back into the pharynx.
   a. Insert the airway under direct vision using a tongue blade. This is the preferred method and is safe for adults or children.
   b. Insert the airway upside down or sideways and rotate into place. This method should not be used for children.
4. If the oropharyngeal airway causes gagging, remove it and replace it with an NPA.

✴ Using a Pocket Mask with Supplemental Oxygen

1. Stabilize the patient's head in a neutral position.
2. Connect the oxygen tubing to the oxygen cylinder and the mask.
3. Open the oxygen cylinder and set the flow rate at 12 liters per minute.
4. Open the airway.
5. Insert an OPA or NPA.
6. Place the mask on the face and establish a good seal.
7. Ventilate mouth-to-mask with enough volume (about 800–1,000 cc oxygen) to cause adequate chest rise. Ventilate at a rate of 8 to 10 breaths per minute. The inspiratory phase should last 1.5 to 2 seconds. Let the patient exhale for 1.5 to 4 seconds.

✴ Using the Bag-Valve Mask

1. Stabilize the patient's head in a neutral position.
2. Connect the oxygen, connecting tubing to the bag-valve system and oxygen cylinder.
3. Attach the oxygen reservoir to the bag-valve mask.
4. Open the oxygen cylinder and set the flow rate at 12 liters per minute.
5. Select the proper size mask and attach it to the bag-valve device.
6. Open the airway.
7. Insert an OPA (or an NPA, if the patient has a gag reflex).
8. Place the mask on the face and have your partner establish and maintain a good seal.
9. Using both hands, ventilate with about 800 to 1,000 cc oxygen at a rate of 8 to 10 breaths per minute.
10. If you are forced to ventilate without a partner, use one hand to maintain a face seal and the other hand to squeeze the bag. This decreases the volume of ventilation because less volume is produced by only one hand squeezing the bag.

The Pulse Oximeter

A pulse oximeter is a noninvasive photoelectric device that measures the arterial oxygen saturation and pulse rate in the peripheral circulation. It consists of a portable monitor and a sensing probe that clips onto the patient's finger, toe, or earlobe (Figure 5-1). The device displays the pulse rate and the arterial oxygen saturation in a percentage value (% SaO_2). This useful device should be used on all patients with any type of respiratory compromise. The pulse oximeter is useful to assess the patient's respiratory status, the effectiveness of oxygen therapy, and the effectiveness of BVM or FROPVD ventilation.

Remember that the device measures percent of SaO_2, not the arterial partial pressure of oxygen (PaO_2). The hemoglobin molecule is so efficient at carrying oxygen that it is 90 percent saturated (90 percent SaO_2) when the partial pressure of oxygen is only 60 mmHg (100 is normal). If you are used to thinking about PaO_2 (where 90–100 mmHg is normal), then you may be fooled into thinking that a SaO_2 reading (pulse oximeter) of 90 percent is normal when it is actually critically low. As a general rule, any pulse oximeter reading below 92 percent is cause for concern and requires some sort of intervention (such as opening the airway, suction, oxygen, assisted ventilation, intubation, decompression of tension pneumothorax). A pulse oximeter reading below 90 percent is critical and requires immediate intervention to maintain adequate tissue oxygenation. Try to maintain a pulse oximeter reading of 95 percent or higher. However, do not withhold oxygen from a patient with a pulse oximeter reading above 95 percent who also shows signs and symptoms of hypoxia or difficulty breathing.

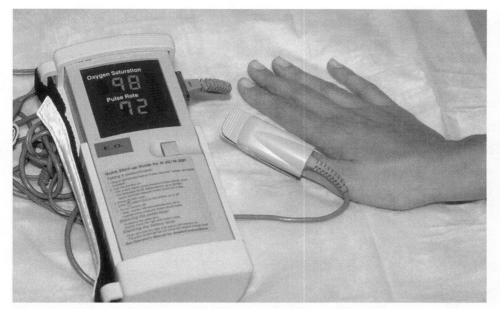

FIGURE 5-1 Portable pulse oximeter. *(Photo courtesy of David Effron, MD)*

The following are conditions that make the pulse oximeter reading unreliable.

- *Poor peripheral perfusion* (shock, vasoconstriction, hypotension). Do not attach the sensing probe onto an injured extremity. Try not to use the sensing probe on the same arm that you are using to monitor the blood pressure. Be aware that the pulse oximeter reading will go down while the blood pressure cuff is inflated.
- *Severe anemia.*
- *Carbon monoxide poisoning.* This will give falsely high readings because the sensing probe cannot distinguish between oxyhemoglobin and carboxyhemoglobin.
- *Hypothermia.*
- *Excessive patient movement.*
- *High ambient light* (bright sunlight, high-intensity light on area of the sensing probe).
- *Nail polish or a dirty fingernail* if you are using a finger probe. Use acetone to clean the nail before attaching the probe.

To use the pulse oximeter, turn on the device, clean the area that you are to monitor (earlobe, fingernail, or toenail), and attach the sensing clip to the area.

Remember that while very useful, the pulse oximeter is just another tool to help you assess the patient. Like all tools, it has limitations and should not replace careful physical assessment.

ADVANCED AIRWAY MANAGEMENT

Preparations

Whatever the method of intubation used, both patients and rescuers should be prepared for the procedure. The following equipment is considered basic to all intubation procedures (Figure 5-2).

- *Gloves.* Latex or nitrile examining (not necessarily sterile) gloves should be worn for all intubation procedures.

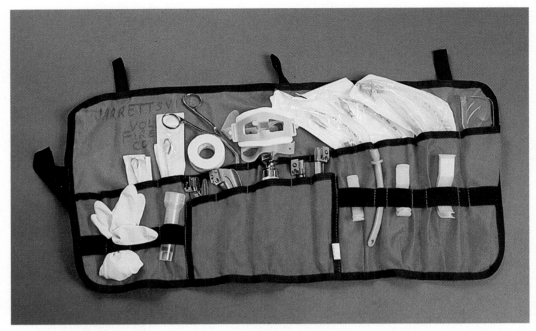

FIGURE 5-2 An intubation wrap contains the essentials for carrying out endotracheal intubation. The kit folds on itself and is compact and portable. When opened, it provides a clean working surface.

- *Eye protection.* Providers must wear goggles or face shield.
- *Oxygenation.* All patients should be ventilated or should breathe high-flow oxygen (12 liters per minute) for several minutes prior to the attempt.
- *Equipment.* Check all equipment, and keep at hand in an organized kit. For laryngoscopic intubation, the endotracheal tube should be held in a "field hockey stick" or open "J" shape by a malleable stylet that is first lubricated and inserted until the distal end is just proximal to the side hole of the endotracheal tube. Check the cuff of the endotracheal tube by inflating it with 10 cc of air. Completely remove the air and leave the syringe filled with air attached to the pilot tube. Lubricate the cuff and distal end of the tube.
- *Suction.* Suction must be immediately at hand.
- *Assistant.* An assistant should be available to help in the procedure and may apply the Sellick maneuver during ventilation and the subsequent intubation attempt. The assistant may also help hold the head and neck in a neutral position. Some intubators like the assistant to count aloud to 30 during the intubation procedure. You may prefer to simply hold your breath (when you need to breathe, the patient really needs a breath) while performing intubation.
- *Lidocaine.* Topical lidocaine sprayed into the posterior pharynx before intubation attempts can decrease the adverse cardiovascular and intracranial pressure effects of the intubation procedure.

Laryngoscopic Orotracheal Intubation

For laryngoscopic orotracheal intubation, the upper airway and the glottic opening are visualized and the tube is slipped gently through the cords. The advantages of this method include the ability to see obstructions and to visualize the accurate placement of the tube. It has the disadvantage of requiring a relatively relaxed patient without anatomic distortion and with minimal bleeding or secretions.

Equipment:

- A straight (Miller) or curved (Macintosh) blade and laryngoscope handle, all in good working order (checked daily)
- A transparent endotracheal tube, 28 to 33 cm in length and 7, 7.5, or 8 mm in internal diameter for the adult patient
- A stylet to help mold the tube into a field hockey stick shape
- A water-soluble lubricant—no need for it to contain a local anesthetic
- A 10 or 12 cc syringe
- Magill forceps
- Tape and tincture of benzoin or endotracheal tube holder
- Suction equipment in good working order
- Pulse oximeter and CO_2 detector or monitor
- If available, a bougie for difficult intubations

PROCEDURE

✴ Laryngoscopic Orotracheal Intubation

Intubation in the trauma patient differs from usual endotracheal intubation in that the patient's neck must be stabilized during the procedure. Following ventilation and initial preparations, the following steps should be carried out (Figure 5-3; Scan 5.1).

1. An assistant holds the head, performs the Sellick maneuver, and counts slowly aloud to 30 (if you request).

2. Pull down on the chin and slide the blade into the right side of the patient's mouth. Push the tongue to the left and "inch" the blade down along the tongue in an attempt to see the epiglottis. A key maneuver must be performed here: The blade must pull forward on the tongue to lift up the epiglottis and bring it into view.

3. Use the laryngoscope blade to lift the tongue and epiglottis up and forward in a straight line. "Levering" the blade is a common error with novices and can result in broken teeth and other trauma. The laryngoscope is essentially a "hook" to lift the tongue and epiglottis up and out of the way so that the glottic opening can be identified.

4. Advance the tube along the right side of the oropharynx once the epiglottis is seen. When the glottic opening (or even just the arytenoid cartilages) is identified, slip the tube through to a depth of about 5 cm beyond the cords.

5. While the tube is still held firmly, remove the stylet, inflate the cuff, attach a bag-valve device, and check the tube for placement using the immediate confirmation protocol given in the paragraphs that follow.

6. Begin ventilation using adequate oxygen concentration and tidal volume.

   For difficult intubations where you cannot see the cords or where the angle is such that it is difficult to get the tube through the cords, a bougie can be very helpful. Insert the bougie through the cords and then slip the tube over the bougie and slide it down through the cords (Scan 5.2). Then remove the bougie and perform steps 5 and 6 above.

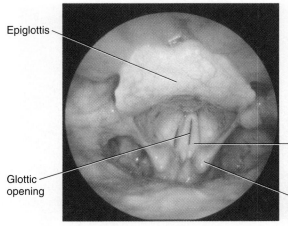

FIGURE 5-3 Landmarks during intubation.

SCAN 5.1

OROTRACHEAL INTUBATION

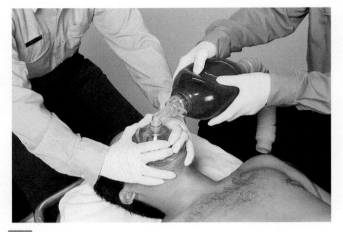

1 Ventilate the patient with 100 percent oxygen.

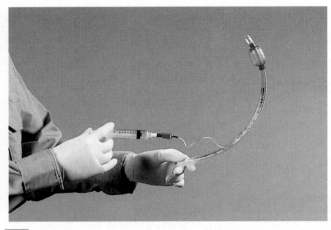

2 Assemble, prepare, and test all equipment.

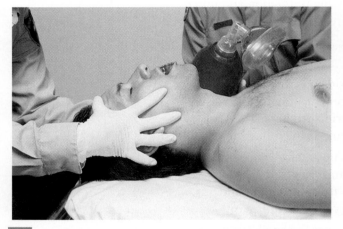

3 Position the patient's head. The trauma patient would have his neck stabilized from below.

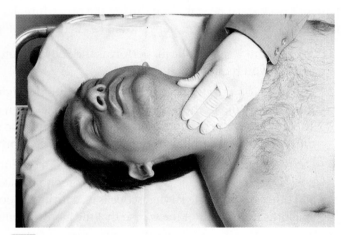

4 A second rescuer should perform the Sellick maneuver during intubation to prevent vomiting and improve visualization of the cords.

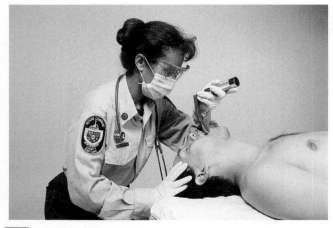

5 Prepare to insert laryngoscope blade.

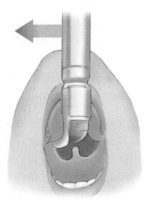

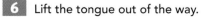

6 Lift the tongue out of the way.

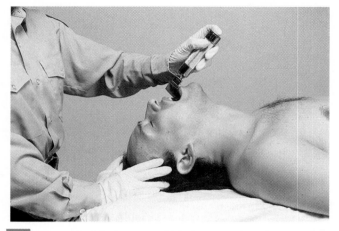

7 Insert the blade (curved blade into vallecula; straight blade under epiglottis) and lift to bring the glottic opening into view.

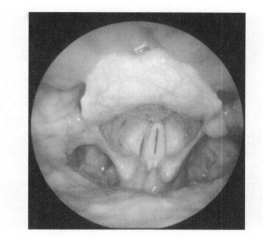

8 Visualize the cords and glottic opening.

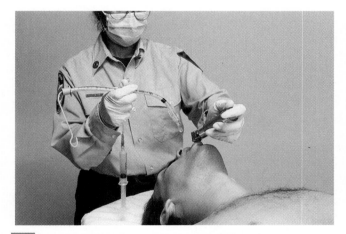

9 Insert endotracheal tube with stylet.

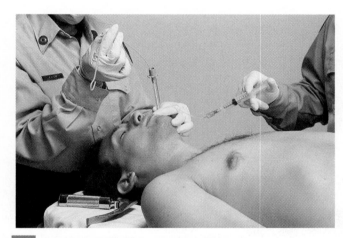

10 With tube held firmly, remove the stylet and inflate the cuff with 5–10 cc of air.

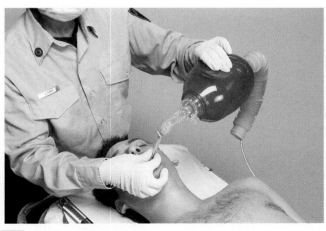

11 Attach a bag-valve unit or other ventilation device to tube.

(continued next page)

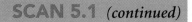

SCAN 5.1 *(continued)*

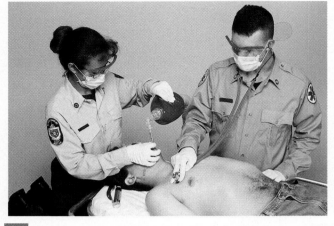

12 Perform immediate confirmation of tube placement.

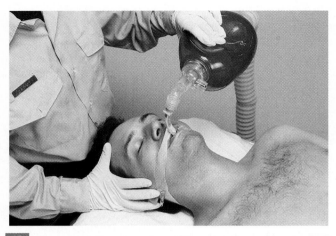

13 If correct placement is confirmed, secure the tube in place.

SCAN 5.2

OROTRACHEAL INTUBATION USING BOUGIE

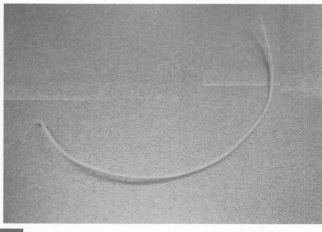

1 Bougie. *(Photo courtesy of Roy Alson, MD)*

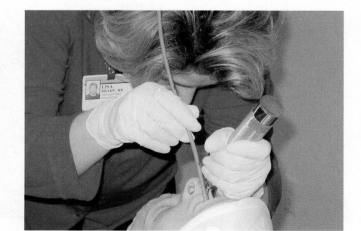

2 Inserting the bougie into the trachea. *(Photo courtesy of Roy Alson, MD)*

Nasotracheal Intubation

The nasotracheal route of endotracheal intubation in a prehospital setting may be justified when you cannot open the adult patient's mouth because of clenched jaws and when you cannot ventilate the patient by other means. The greatest disadvantage of this method is its relative difficulty, depending as it does upon the appreciation of the intensity of the breath sounds of spontaneously breathing patients. It is a blind procedure and as such requires extra skill and care to successfully perform proper intratracheal placement.

Guidance of the tube through the glottic opening is a question of you perceiving the intensity of the sound of the patient breathing out. You can, with some difficulty, guide the tube toward the point of maximum intensity and slip it through the cords. You can better hear and feel the breath sounds with your ear placed against the proximal opening of the tube. Commercial adaptors are now available to do this without contaminating yourself or your equipment (Figure 5-4).

The success of this method will also depend upon an anterior curve to the tube that will prevent its passing into the esophagus. Prepare two tubes prior to carrying out the intubation attempt. Insert the distal end of the 7-mm tube into its proximal opening, thus molding it into a formed circle. Preparing two tubes allows the immediate use of the second, more rigid tube should the first plastic tube become warm with body temperature, thus losing its anterior curve. Displacing the tongue and jaw forward may also help in achieving placement, since this maneuver lifts the epiglottis anteriorly out of the way of the advancing tube.

PROCEDURE
✳ Nasotracheal Intubation

1. Perform routine preparation procedures.
2. Lubricate the cuff and distal end of a 7-mm or 7.5-mm endotracheal tube. With the bevel against the floor or septum of the nasal cavity, slip the tube distally through the largest naris. Insert along the floor of the nasal cavity (at a 90-degree angle to the face).

SCAN 5.2 *(continued)*

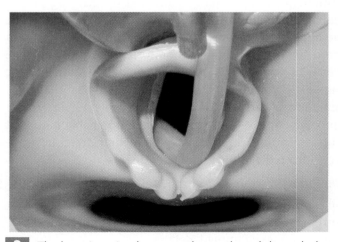

3 The bougie going between the cords and through the glottic opening. *(Photo courtesy of Roy Alson, MD)*

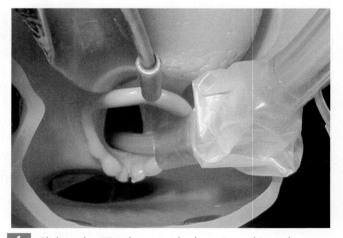

4 Sliding the ET tube over the bougie and into the trachea. *(Photo courtesy of Roy Alson, MD)*

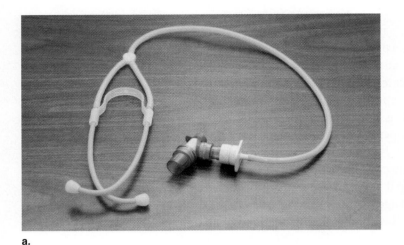

a.

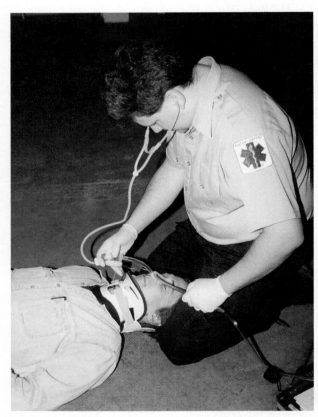

b.

FIGURE 5-4 (a) Example of a commercial nasotracheal tube auscultation device (Burden nasoscope) used to (b) better hear breath sounds while inserting the naso-tracheal tube. *(Photos courtesy of Brant Burden, EMT-P)*

3. When the tube tip reaches the posterior pharyngeal wall, take great care on "rounding the bend" and then direct the tube toward the glottic opening.

4. By watching the neck at the laryngeal prominence, you can judge the approximate placement of the tube; tenting of the skin on either side of the prominence indicates that the tube is caught up in the pyriform fossa, a problem solved by slight withdrawal and rotation of the tube to the midline. Bulging and anterior displacement of the laryngeal prominence usually indicate that the tube has entered the glottic opening and has been correctly placed. At this point the patient, especially if not deeply comatose, will cough, strain, or both. This may be alarming to the novice intubator, who might interpret this as laryngospasm or misplacement of the tube. The temptation may be to pull the tube and ventilate, since the patient may not breathe immediately. Holding your hand or ear over the opening of the tube to detect airflow may reassure you that the tube is correctly placed, and you may inflate the cuff and begin ventilation.

5. Confirm tube placement using the immediate confirmation protocol below.

Immediate Confirmation of Tube Placement

One of the greatest challenges of intubation is ensuring the correct intratracheal placement of endotracheal tubes. An un-recognized esophageal intubation is a lethal complication of this life-saving procedure. Every effort must be made to avoid this catastrophe, and a strict protocol must be followed to re-duce the risk.

Although the most reliable method of ensuring proper placement is actually visualizing the tube passing through the glottic opening, even this is not 100 percent sure. The gold standard for confirming and monitoring endotracheal tube placement is waveform capnography (see discussion starting on page 90). If you do not have capnography available, the fol-lowing protocol can be used but is not reliable. When you use this protocol, you should recognize the unreliable nature of auscultation as the sole method of confirming intratracheal placement. Correct intratra-cheal placement should be suspected from the following initial signs.

■ *An anterior displacement of the laryngeal prominence* as the tube is passed distally

■ *Coughing, bucking, or straining* on the part of the patient. Note: Phonation—any noise made with the vocal cords—is absolute evidence that the tube is in the esophagus, and the tube should be removed immediately.

■ *Breath condensation on the tube with each ventilation*—not 100 percent reliable, but very suggestive of intratracheal placement

- *Normal compliance with bag ventilation.* (The bag does not suddenly "collapse," but rather there is some resilience to it and resistance to lung inflation.)
- *No cuff leak after inflation.* (Persistent leak indicates esophageal intubation until proven otherwise.)
- *Adequate chest rise with each ventilation.*

The following procedure should then be carried out immediately to prove correct placement.

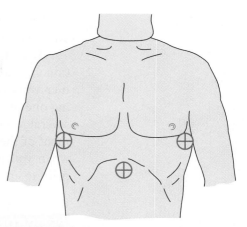

FIGURE 5-5 Sites to auscultate when performing immediate confirmation of ET tube placement.

PROCEDURE
❈ Immediate Confirmation of Tube Placement

1. Auscultate three sites as shown in Figure 5-5.
   a. Epigastrium—the most important; should be silent, with no sounds heard
   b. Right and left midaxillary lines
2. Inspect for full movement of the chest with ventilation.
3. Check position using suction bulb or syringe or one of the CO_2 detecting devices.
4. Watch for any change in the patient's color or in the pulse oximeter reading. Also observe the EKG monitor for changes.

Commercial suction bulbs or syringes are available for confirming tube placement (Figure 5-6). They are almost as reliable as capnography for confirming initial tube placement. (Capnography is superior for constant monitoring of tube position.) To use a bulb detector, squeeze the bulb and insert the end into the 15-mm adapter on the endotracheal tube. Release the bulb. If the tube is in the trachea, the bulb will expand immediately. If the tube is in the esophagus, the bulb will remain collapsed. If you are using the detector syringe, you will be able to withdraw the syringe plunger easily if the tube is in the trachea, but you will not be able to withdraw the plunger if the tube is in the esophagus.

Commercial CO_2 detectors are also available to attach in-line between the endotracheal tube and the BVM or FROPVD. Three different kinds are available.

- Qualitative (colorimetric) CO_2 detectors
- Quantitative CO_2 monitors
- Quantitative waveform CO_2 monitors

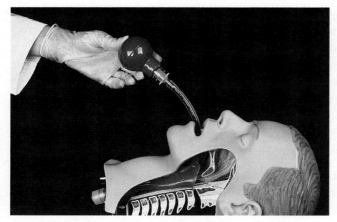

FIGURE 5-6a Esophageal intubation detector device, bulb style.

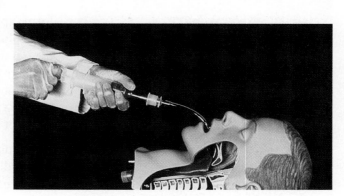

FIGURE 5-6b Esophageal intubation detector device, syringe style.

See the detailed discussion of these monitors in the following section, "Using Capnometry and Capnography to Confirm and Monitor ET Tube Position."

Apply the protocol for confirmation of tube placement immediately following intubation. If you are using a quantitative CO_2 monitor or quantitative waveform CO_2 monitor, then you may continue monitoring ET tube position with these devices. If you are not using one of these devices, then repeat the ET tube position reconfirmation protocol after several minutes of ventilation. Thereafter, repeat the reconfirmation protocol after movement of the patient from the ground to the stretcher, after loading onto the ambulance, when you perform the ITLS Secondary Survey and Ongoing Exams, and immediately prior to arrival at the hospital.

PROCEDURE

✳ Reconfirming ET Tube Position

1. Auscultate six sites as shown in Figure 5-7.
   a. Epigastrium—it should be silent with no sounds heard
   b. Right and left apex
   c. Right and left midaxillary lines
   d. Sternal notch—"tracheal" sounds should be readily heard here

2. Inspect the chest for full movement of the chest with ventilation.

3. Gently palpate the tube cuff in the sternal notch while compressing the pilot balloon between the index finger and thumb. A pressure wave should be felt in the sternal notch.

4. Use adjuncts such as a suction bulb or CO_2 detectors to help confirm placement.

Any time placement is still in doubt in spite of the above protocol, visualize directly or remove the tube. Never assume that the tube is in the right place—always be sure and record that the protocol has been carefully followed.

Using Capnometry and Capnography to Confirm and Monitor ET Tube Position: Capnometry represents a major clinical upgrade in the assessment, diagnostics, and ventilatory status in the monitoring of patients. It is important for you to understand the differences between simple detection of end-tidal CO_2 (ETCO$_2$) called colorimetric or qualitative capnometry, quantitative capnometry (a value without a waveform), and the most useful and diagnostic form known as quantitative waveform capnography.

Colorimetric CO_2 detectors (qualitative capnometry) are simple devices designed to detect ETCO$_2$ (Figure 5-8). They do not accurately measure the amount of CO_2. Typically, these devices use a special piece of "litmus paper" that changes color from purple to yellow as it detects CO_2. If a device of this type is used as a confirming device, you must be aware of the following:

■ It may not be accurate in poor perfusion states, such as shock or cardiac arrest, due to very small amounts of CO_2 returning to the lungs. In these cases, another confirming device is necessary. In cases of cardiac arrest, best results will be obtained if good compressions are being done at the time the device is used.

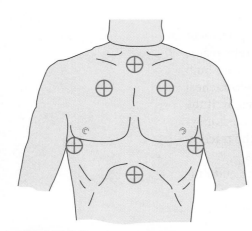

FIGURE 5-7 Sites to auscultate when performing reconfirmation of ET tube placement.

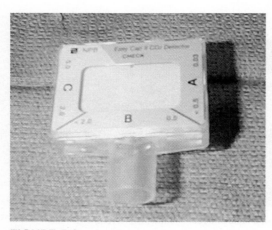

FIGURE 5-8 Colorimetric CO_2 detector.

- You must bag six breaths through it before using it to confirm the CO_2 as being from the trachea. It is a fact that CO_2 can be detected from the esophagus, and it would take about six breaths to purge it.
- If the device gets wet, it will not be useful.
- Once intubated, the device can be used for spot checks only, as it will stay yellow after a few minutes of continuous use, not changing colors with each breath.
- Since the device only detects $ETCO_2$, it cannot be used as a monitor of ventilation.

Quantitative capnometry actually measures the amount of CO_2 in expired air ($ETCO_2$). More than just detection, the device can be used to monitor the adequacy of ventilations and help the provider to accurately "titrate" the $ETCO_2$ levels in patients where CO_2 levels are critical, such as those with closed head injuries. They are often combined with a pulse oximeter (Figure 5-9). Quantitative capnometry means $ETCO_2$ measurement without a waveform. If these devices are used to confirm tube placement, you must be aware of the following limitations.

- In poor perfusion states or arrest, the numbers will be very low, and may take up to 30 seconds to display a number. If this is the case, it may not be useful to initially confirm; rather, it could be used to monitor the tube after that.

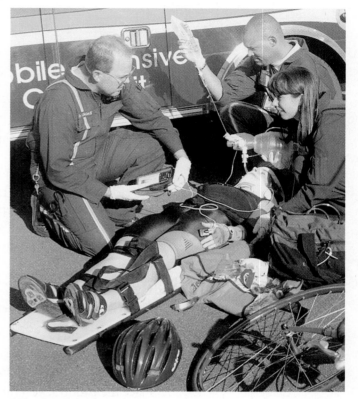

FIGURE 5-9 Combined quantitative CO_2 monitor and pulse oximeter. *(Photo courtesy of Nonin Medical, Inc.)*

- As in colorimetric devices, these devices can also detect esophageal CO_2, so six breaths are necessary to actually confirm tracheal CO_2.
- In cases of cardiac arrest, best results are obtained if good compressions are being performed while the device is being used.

Quantitative waveform capnography is the ultimate confirmation device and is a standard of care in surgical suites and many EMS systems. These devices not only detect and measure the $ETCO_2$, but they also provide you with a diagnostic waveform that can confirm (by the shape of the waveform) endotracheal placement even in low perfusion states. These waveforms will appear within 2 seconds of the actual breath. Furthermore, these devices can be built into existing cardiac monitors, which will allow you to continuously monitor the waveform and value (Figure 5-10). They also will allow you to print out a real-time waveform that is time and date stamped for absolute documentation of correct tube placement. Capnography has many other uses in nonintubated patients, including perfusion monitor, airway monitor, and ventilation monitor.

In using capnography to confirm endotracheal tube placement, you must be aware of the following limitations.

- Like all CO_2 detection devices, low perfusion states will result in low CO_2 readings and subsequently small waveforms (Figure 5-11). In arrest situations, good compressions should be done as the waveforms are being evaluated. This will increase the size of the waveform.

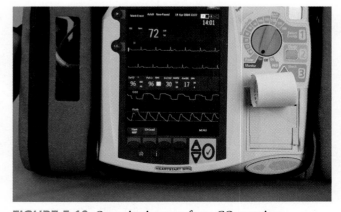

FIGURE 5-10 Quantitative waveform CO_2 monitor incorporated into cardiac monitor.

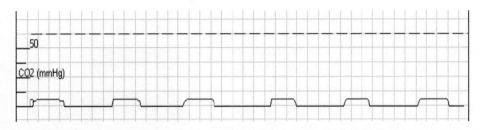

FIGURE 5-11 Small capnography waveform means poor perfusion or severe acidosis.

- To use the devices in conjunction with your cardiac monitors, you must enable the waveform display on the monitor screen before intubation. A delay of 10 to 30 seconds for warm-up (depending on the monitor) will ensue if you wait to activate it after placing the tube. For best results, have the capnography waveform default when the monitor is turned on.

PROCEDURE

Confirming and Monitoring ET Tube Placement with Capnography

1. Prepare all equipment for intubation. Turn on monitor and attach capnography filter line or wires to the monitor. (This will vary depending on the brand of capnograph.)
2. Place the endotracheal tube and inflate the cuff. In cases of arrest, compressions should not be interrupted to perform this procedure.
3. Attach the capnography airway adapter on the endotracheal tube and then attach the BVM to the airway adapter.
4. Ventilate the patient and observe the waveform. The presence of a "square" pattern confirms tracheal placement (Figure 5-12). Print out the waveform, if possible (for documentation). If the waveform is nonexistent, or appears in gross and irregular waveform patterns, the tube is possibly in the esophagus or hypopharynx.

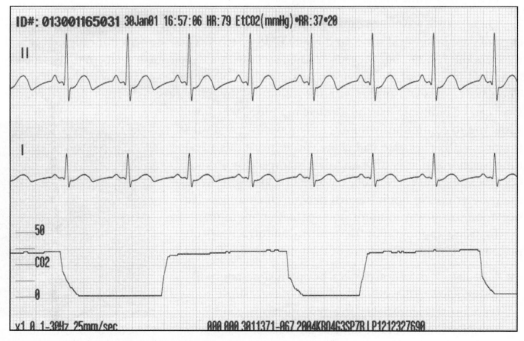

FIGURE 5-12 "Square" waveform is normal.

5. Listen for breath sounds midaxillary on each side to rule out right mainstem intubation.

6. Secure the tube and continually monitor the waveforms during transport.

7. On arrival at the receiving facility, print out another waveform (if available) to prove correct placement at the time of patient transfer.

8. On your run report, document the visualization of the vocal cords, attach the waveform printout(s) or document the presence, and document equal breath sounds.

Troubleshooting while monitoring:

- *Loss of waveform completely:* apnea, or tube is dislodged or obstructed
- *Waveforms and values getting smaller:* hyperventilation (check the depth and rate of ventilation) or hypoperfusion (shock, or loss of pulses)

Anchoring the Tube

Anchoring a tube can be a frustrating exercise. Not only does it require some fine movements of the hands when we appear to be all thumbs, but it is difficult to perform when ventilation, movement, or extrication is being carried out. Keep one thing in mind: There is no substitute for the human anchor. That is, Rescuer 2 should be held responsible for ensuring that the tube is held fast and that it does not migrate in or out of the airway. To lose a tube can be a catastrophe, especially if the patient is rather inaccessible or the intubation was a difficult one to begin with.

Fixing the endotracheal tube in place is important for several reasons. First, movement of the tube in the trachea will produce more mucosal damage and may increase the risk of postintubation complications. In addition, movement of the tube will stimulate the patient to cough, strain, or both, leading to cardiovascular and intracranial pressure changes that could be detrimental. Most important, there is a greater risk in the prehospital setting of dislodging a tube and losing control of the airway if it is not anchored solidly in place.

The endotracheal tube can be secured in place by either tape or a commercially available holder. While taping a tube in place is convenient and relatively easily done, it is not always effective. There is often a problem with the tape sticking to skin wet with rain, blood, airway secretions, or vomitus. If you are using tape, several principles should be followed:

- Insert an oropharyngeal airway to prevent the patient from biting down on the tube.
- Dry the patient's face and apply tincture of benzoin to better ensure proper adhesion of the tape.
- Carry the tape right around the patient's neck when anchoring the tube. Do not move the neck. Do not tie it so tight that it occludes the external jugular veins.
- Anchor the tube at the corner of the mouth, not in the midline.

Because of the difficulty of fixing the tube in place with tape, it may be better to use a commercial endotracheal tube holder that uses a strap to fix the tube in a plastic holder, which also acts as a bite block (Figure 5-13). Because flexion or extension of the patient's head can move the tube in or out of the airway by 2 or 3 cm, it is good practice to restrict head and neck movement of any patient who has an endotracheal tube in place (even more important in children). If the patient is spinal motion-restricted because of the risk of cervical-spine injury, flexion and extension should be less of a concern.

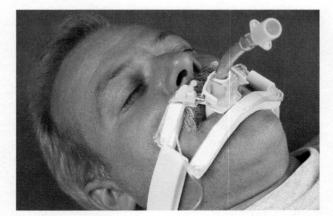

FIGURE 5-13 A commercial endotracheal tube holder.

Thoracic Trauma

Andrew B. Peitzman, MD, FACS
Paul Paris, MD, FACEP

OBJECTIVES

Upon completion of this chapter, you should be able to:

1. Identify the major symptoms of thoracic trauma.
2. Describe the signs of thoracic trauma.
3. State the immediate life-threatening thoracic injuries.
4. Explain the pathophysiology and management of an open pneumothorax.
5. Describe the clinical signs of a tension pneumothorax in conjunction with appropriate management.
6. List three indications to perform emergency chest decompression.
7. Explain the hypovolemic and respiratory compromise pathophysiology and management in massive hemothorax.
8. Define flail chest in relation to associated physical findings and management.
9. Identify the triad of physical findings in the diagnosis of cardiac tamponade.
10. Explain the cardiac involvement and management associated with blunt injury to the chest.
11. Summarize other thoracic injuries and their appropriate management.

(© Eddie Sperling Photography)

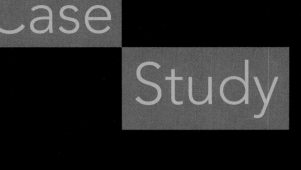

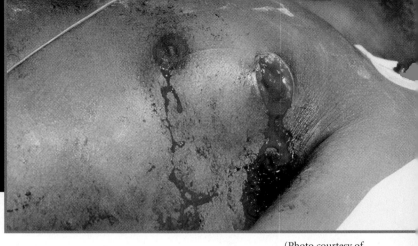

(Photo courtesy of
Roy Alson, MD)

Dan, Joyce, and Buddy of the Emergency Transport System (ETS) have been called to a bar where a patron has been stabbed. The Scene Size-up reveals that the police are on scene, have cleared the bar, and are questioning bystanders outside. There is a single male victim who is sitting in a chair and holding his chest. Since the scene is safe and the mechanism of injury (stab wound) is readily apparent, the team dons personal protective equipment. As they approach the patient, each carries essential trauma care equipment. *How would you approach this patient? What type of assessment would you perform? What would you do first? Is this a load-and-go situation?* Keep these questions in mind as you read the chapter. Then, at the end of the chapter, find out how the rescuers completed this call.

INTRODUCTION

Major thoracic injury may result from MVCs, falls, gunshot wounds, crush injuries, stab wounds, or other mechanisms. Of all trauma patients, half of those with multiple injuries have an associated thoracic injury. Of all trauma deaths, 25 percent are due entirely to thoracic injuries. Of all patients with potentially fatal thoracic injury, two-thirds are alive when they reach the emergency department, but only 15 percent of them require surgery. This suggests that patients with potentially fatal thoracic injuries can usually be saved by good prehospital and emergency department care. The goal of this chapter is to enable you to recognize the signs and symptoms of such injuries and to provide the appropriate emergency treatment.

ANATOMY OF THE CHEST

The thorax is a bony cavity that is formed by 12 pairs of ribs, which join posteriorly with the thoracic spine and anteriorly with the sternum. The intercostal neurovascular bundle runs along the inferior surface of each rib (Figure 6-1).

The inner side of the thoracic cavity and the lung itself are lined with a thin layer of tissue, the pleura. The space between the two pleural layers is normally only a potential space. However, a pneumothorax is formed when this space is occupied by air. A hemothorax is formed when it is filled with blood. This potential space can hold 3 liters of fluid on each side in an adult.

As shown in Figure 6-2, one lung occupies each thoracic cavity. Between the two chest cavities is the mediastinum, which contains the heart, aorta, superior and inferior vena cava, trachea, major bronchi, and esophagus. The spinal cord is protected by the vertebral column. The diaphragm separates the thoracic organs from the abdominal cavity. The upper abdominal organs, including the spleen, liver, kidneys, pancreas, and stomach, are

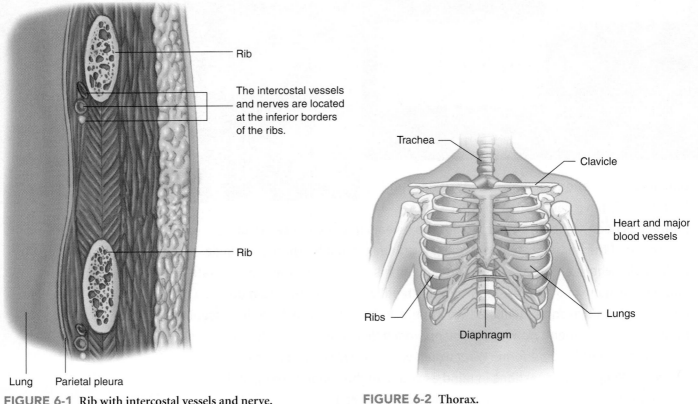

Rib

The intercostal vessels and nerves are located at the inferior borders of the ribs.

Rib

Lung   Parietal pleura

FIGURE 6-1 Rib with intercostal vessels and nerve.

Trachea

Clavicle

Heart and major blood vessels

Lungs

Ribs

Diaphragm

FIGURE 6-2 Thorax.

protected by the lower rib cage (Figure 6-3). Any patient with a penetrating thoracic wound at the level of the nipples (fourth intercostal space) or lower should be assumed to have an abdominal injury as well as a thoracic injury. Similarly, blunt deceleration injuries, such as steering wheel injuries, often affect both thoracic and abdominal structures.

Penetrating wounds that traverse the mediastinum have a particularly high potential for life-threatening injury because of the vital cardiovascular and tracheobronchial structures within this area.

PATHOPHYSIOLOGY

When evaluating a patient with probable thoracic trauma, always follow the ITLS Primary Survey (Chapter 2) to avoid missing life-threatening injuries. During the ITLS Primary Survey, search for the most dangerous injuries first to give your patient the best chance for survival. As with any trauma patient, the mechanism of injury is very important in caring for the thoracic trauma patient. Thoracic injuries may be the result of blunt or penetrating trauma. With blunt trauma, the force is distributed over a large area, and visceral injuries occur from deceleration, shearing forces, compression, or bursting. Penetrating injuries, usually gunshot wounds or stab wounds, distribute the forces of injury over a smaller area. However, the trajectory of a bullet is often unpredictable, and all thoracic structures are at risk.

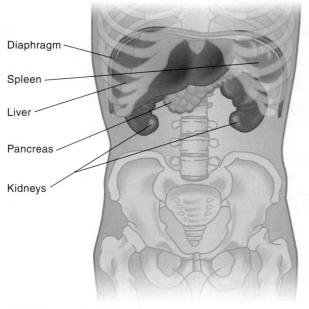

Diaphragm

Spleen

Liver

Pancreas

Kidneys

FIGURE 6-3 Intrathoracic abdomen.

The common end point in thoracic injury is tissue hypoxia. Tissue hypoxia may result from the following:

- Inadequate oxygen delivery to the tissues secondary to airway obstruction
- Hypovolemia from blood loss
- Ventilation/perfusion mismatch from lung parenchymal injury
- Changes in pleural pressures from tension pneumothorax
- Pump failure from severe myocardial injury

EMERGENCY CARE OF CHEST INJURIES

The major symptoms of chest injury are shortness of breath and chest pain. The signs indicative of chest injury found on inspection include hemoptysis, cyanosis, distended neck veins, tracheal deviation, asymmetrical chest movement, including paradoxical motion, chest wall contusion, open wounds, subcutaneous emphysema, and shock. In addition, palpation may reveal tenderness, instability, and crepitation (TIC). Listen to the lung fields for the presence and equality of breath sounds. Using the ITLS Primary Survey, including the Rapid Trauma Survey, will guide you in an organized fashion to discovery of these injuries (Figure 6-4).

Life-threatening thoracic injuries should be identified immediately during the ITLS Primary Survey. Major thoracic injuries to identify are listed below and may be remembered as the "deadly dozen."

- The following injuries must be detected and treated during the ITLS Primary Survey:
    1. Airway obstruction
    2. Open pneumothorax
    3. Flail chest
    4. Tension pneumothorax
    5. Massive hemothorax
    6. Cardiac tamponade
- Life-threatening injuries that are more likely to be detected during the ITLS Secondary Survey or during hospital evaluation are the following:
    7. Myocardial contusion
    8. Traumatic aortic rupture
    9. Tracheal or bronchial tree injury
    10. Diaphragmatic tears
    11. Esophageal injury
    12. Pulmonary contusion

Airway Obstruction

Airway management remains a major challenge in the care of any multiple-trauma patient. Hypoxia secondary to airway obstruction (foreign body, tongue, aspiration of vomitus, or blood) is a common cause of preventable trauma death. Management of the airway has been discussed in Chapter 4, so nothing further will be added here other than to stress its importance.

Open Pneumothorax

An open pneumothorax is caused by a penetrating thoracic injury and may present as a sucking chest wound. The signs and symptoms are usually proportional to the size of the chest wall defect (Figure 6-5).

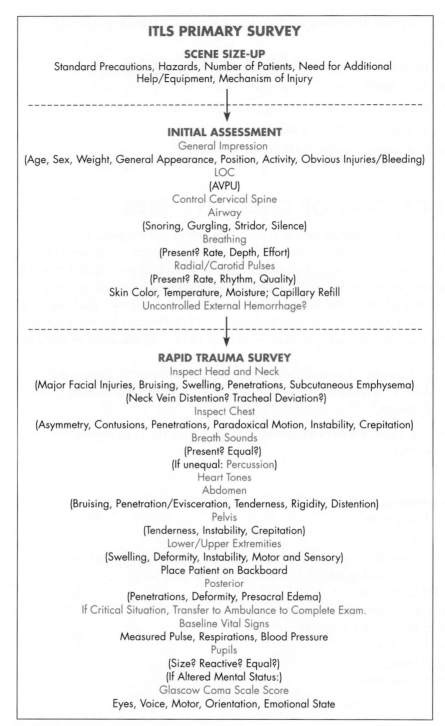

ITLS PRIMARY SURVEY

SCENE SIZE-UP
Standard Precautions, Hazards, Number of Patients, Need for Additional
Help/Equipment, Mechanism of Injury

INITIAL ASSESSMENT
General Impression
(Age, Sex, Weight, General Appearance, Position, Activity, Obvious Injuries/Bleeding)
LOC
(AVPU)
Control Cervical Spine
Airway
(Snoring, Gurgling, Stridor, Silence)
Breathing
(Present? Rate, Depth, Effort)
Radial/Carotid Pulses
(Present? Rate, Rhythm, Quality)
Skin Color, Temperature, Moisture; Capillary Refill
Uncontrolled External Hemorrhage?

RAPID TRAUMA SURVEY
Inspect Head and Neck
(Major Facial Injuries, Bruising, Swelling, Penetrations, Subcutaneous Emphysema)
(Neck Vein Distention? Tracheal Deviation?)
Inspect Chest
(Asymmetry, Contusions, Penetrations, Paradoxical Motion, Instability, Crepitation)
Breath Sounds
(Present? Equal?)
(If unequal: Percussion)
Heart Tones
Abdomen
(Bruising, Penetration/Evisceration, Tenderness, Rigidity, Distention)
Pelvis
(Tenderness, Instability, Crepitation)
Lower/Upper Extremities
(Swelling, Deformity, Instability, Motor and Sensory)
Place Patient on Backboard
Posterior
(Penetrations, Deformity, Presacral Edema)
If Critical Situation, Transfer to Ambulance to Complete Exam.
Baseline Vital Signs
Measured Pulse, Respirations, Blood Pressure
Pupils
(Size? Reactive? Equal?)
(If Altered Mental Status:)
Glasgow Coma Scale Score
Eyes, Voice, Motor, Orientation, Emotional State

FIGURE 6-4 ITLS Primary Survey.

Normal ventilation involves a negative pressure being generated inside the chest by diaphragmatic contraction. As air is drawn through the upper airway, the lungs expand. With a large open wound of the chest (larger than the trachea or about the size of the patient's little finger), the path of least resistance for airflow is through the chest wall defect. Air going in and out of this opening makes a sucking sound (from which the term "sucking chest wound" comes), and bubbles on expiration. This air will enter only the pleural dead space. It will not enter the lung and therefore will not contribute to oxygenation of the blood. Ventilation is impaired and hypoxia results.

An open pneumothorax may be identified during the ITLS Primary Survey (Figure 6-6).

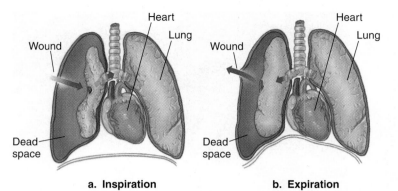

a. Inspiration   **b. Expiration**

FIGURE 6-5 Open pneumothorax. If the wound is larger than the opening to the trachea, air will preferentially go into dead space rather than the lung.

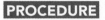
Management of Open Pneumothorax

1. Ensure an open airway.

2. Promptly close the chest wall defect by any available means. You may initially accomplish this with your hand and then with a defibrillation pad, Vaseline gauze, rubber glove, or plastic dressing. However, using an occlusive dressing carries the risk of a tension pneumothorax. To circumvent this problem, tape the occlusive dressing on three sides to produce a flutter valve, which will allow air to escape from the chest but not enter it (Figure 6-7). A commercial chest seal with a one-way valve is now available (Asherman Chest Seal®) and is currently the best device with which to close an open chest wound (Figure 6-8). A chest tube will be needed ultimately, followed by operative closure of the chest wall defect.

3. Administer high-flow oxygen.

4. Insert a large-bore IV.

5. Monitor the heart and note heart tones for comparison later.

6. Monitor oxygen saturation with a pulse oximeter.

7. Transport rapidly to the appropriate hospital.

8. Notify medical direction early.

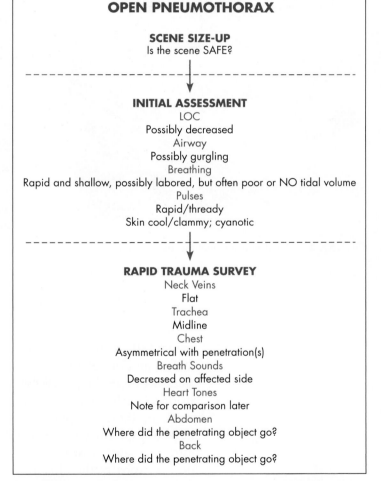

FIGURE 6-6 An open pneumothorax may be identified during the ITLS Primary Survey.

Flail Chest

Flail chest occurs when three or more adjacent ribs are fractured in at least two places (Figure 6-9). The result is a segment of the chest wall that is not in continuity with the thorax. A lateral flail chest or anterior flail chest (sternal separation) may result. With posterior rib fractures, the heavy musculature usually prevents the occurrence of a flail

a. On inspiration, dressing seals wound, preventing air entry

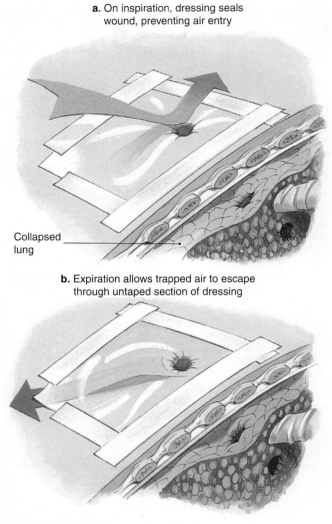

Collapsed lung

b. Expiration allows trapped air to escape through untaped section of dressing

FIGURE 6-7 Treatment of sucking chest wound.

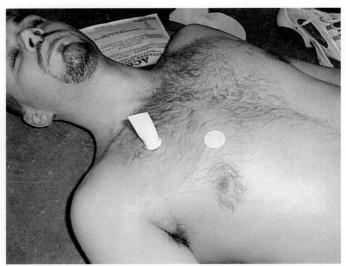

a.

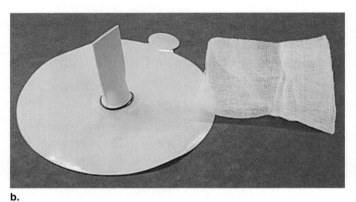

b.

FIGURE 6-8 Sealing a sucking chest wound with Asherman Chest Seal®.

segment. If the patient is breathing spontaneously, the flail segment moves with para-doxical motion relative to the rest of the chest wall (Figures 6–10 and 6–11). The force necessary to produce this injury also bruises the underlying lung tissue (pulmonary con-tusion), which will contribute to the hypoxia. This patient is at risk for the development of a hemothorax or pneumothorax. With a large flail segment, the patient may be in marked respiratory distress, and probably will have very little tidal volume, so will re-quire ventilatory assistance and, at some point, intubation. Pain from the chest wall in-jury exacerbates the already impaired respiration from paradoxical motion and the underlying lung contusion. Palpation of the chest wall may reveal crepitation in addi-tion to the abnormal respiratory motion (Figure 6-12).

Flail chest may be identified during the ITLS Primary Survey (Figure 6-13).

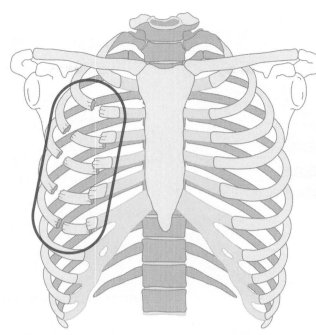

FIGURE 6-9 Flail chest occurs when three or more adjacent ribs fracture in two or more places.

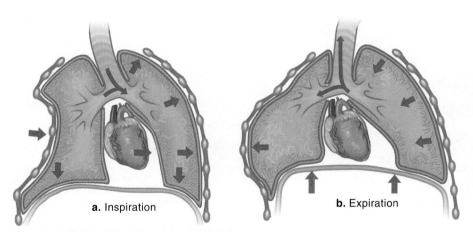

a. Inspiration   **b.** Expiration

FIGURE 6-10 Pathophysiology of flail chest.

PROCEDURE
✳ Management of Flail Chest

1. Ensure an open airway.
2. Assist ventilation.
3. Administer high-flow oxygen.
4. Initially, stabilize the flail segment with manual pressure. Then stabilize it with bulk dressings taped to the chest wall (Figure 6-14). However, this is usually not necessary

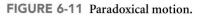

Inspiration
Ribs rise

Flail
section
sucks
in

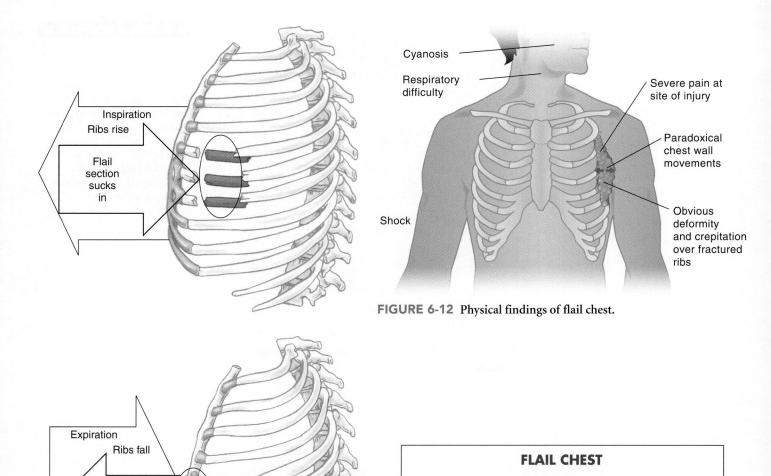

Cyanosis

Respiratory
difficulty

Severe pain at
site of injury

Paradoxical
chest wall
movements

Shock

Obvious
deformity
and crepitation
over fractured
ribs

FIGURE 6-12 Physical findings of flail chest.

Expiration
Ribs fall

Flail
section
bulges
out

FIGURE 6-11 Paradoxical motion.

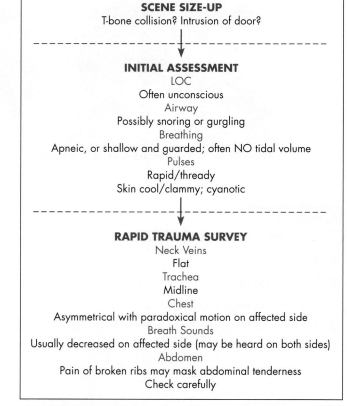

FLAIL CHEST

SCENE SIZE-UP
T-bone collision? Intrusion of door?

INITIAL ASSESSMENT
LOC
Often unconscious
Airway
Possibly snoring or gurgling
Breathing
Apneic, or shallow and guarded; often NO tidal volume
Pulses
Rapid/thready
Skin cool/clammy; cyanotic

RAPID TRAUMA SURVEY
Neck Veins
Flat
Trachea
Midline
Chest
Asymmetrical with paradoxical motion on affected side
Breath Sounds
Usually decreased on affected side (may be heard on both sides)
Abdomen
Pain of broken ribs may mask abdominal tenderness
Check carefully

FIGURE 6-13 Flail chest may be identified during the ITLS Primary Survey.

until the patient is placed on a backboard. Remember that trying to maintain manual pressure on a flail segment while performing a log roll can compromise a stable spine.

5. Load and go.

6. If shock is present, use care to prevent fluid overload, which could worsen hypoxemia.

7. Consider intubation early in order to provide positive end-expiratory pressure (PEEP). Continuous positive airway pressure (CPAP) could be used here if available.

8. Monitor oxygenation with pulse oximeter and expiratory CO_2 with capnography (if available).

9. Transport rapidly to the appropriate hospital.

10. Notify medical direction early.

Remember that intubation and positive pressure ventilation is the best way to stabilize a flail chest, but this may be very difficult in the field if the patient still has a gag reflex. Also keep in mind that a pneumothorax is commonly associated with a flail chest; be alert for development of tension pneumothorax.

Tension Pneumothorax

A tension pneumothorax is an injury that occurs when a one-way valve is created from either blunt or penetrating trauma. Air can enter but not leave the pleural space (Figure 6-15). This causes an increase in the intrathoracic pressure, which will collapse the affected lung and

Tape pad in place, extending tape to both sides of chest

Intubation and positive pressure ventilation is the best stabilization

FIGURE 6-14 Stabilizing flail chest.

PEARLS
Tension Pneumothorax

The diagnosis of tension pneumothorax requires several findings. Patients with simple rib fractures but no pneumothorax will have decreased breath sounds on the affected side due to splinting to relieve the pain. Never decompress a chest unless the criteria for decompression are present. Identify dyspnea, tachypnea, diminished breath sounds, hyperresonance to percussion on affected side, hypotension, distended neck veins, and decreased lung compliance if intubated. Tracheal deviation is a late sign and is more often seen on x-ray than clinically.

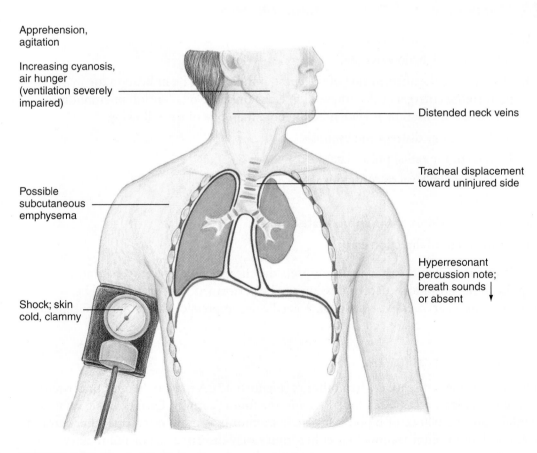

Apprehension, agitation

Increasing cyanosis, air hunger (ventilation severely impaired)

Possible subcutaneous emphysema

Shock; skin cold, clammy

Distended neck veins

Tracheal displacement toward uninjured side

Hyperresonant percussion note; breath sounds ↓ or absent

FIGURE 6-15 Physical findings of tension pneumothorax.

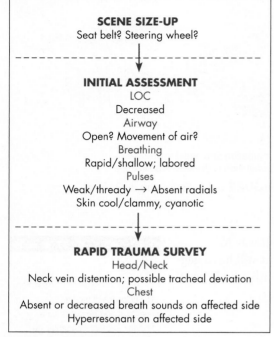

FIGURE 6-16 The tension pneumothorax may be identified during the ITLS Primary Survey.

will then exert pressure on the mediastinum. This pressure will eventually collapse the superior and inferior vena cava, resulting in a loss of venous return to the heart. A shift of the trachea and mediastinum away from the side of the tension pneumothorax will also compromise ventilation of the other lung, although this is a late phenomenon and usually cannot be detected except by x-ray.

Clinical signs of a tension pneumothorax include dyspnea, anxiety, tachypnea, distended neck veins, and possibly tracheal deviation away from the affected side. Auscultation will reveal diminished breath sounds on the affected side and will be accompanied by hyperresonance when percussed. Shock with hypotension will follow. In a review of 108 field patients diagnosed with tension pneumothorax and requiring needle decompression, none were recorded as having a deviated trachea.

The development of decreased lung compliance (difficulty in squeezing the bag-valve device) in the intubated patient should always alert you to the possibility of a tension pneumothorax. Intubated patients with a history of chronic obstructive pulmonary disease (COPD) or asthma are at increased risk for development of tension pneumothorax from positive pressure ventilation.

The tension pneumothorax may be identified during the ITLS Primary Survey (Figure 6-16).

PROCEDURE

✳ Management of Tension Pneumothorax

1. Establish an open airway.
2. Administer high-flow oxygen.
3. Decompress the affected side of the chest, if indicated. The indication for performing emergency decompression is the presence of a tension pneumothorax with decompensation as evidenced by more than one of the following:
   a. Respiratory distress and cyanosis
   b. Loss of the radial pulse (late shock)
   c. Decreasing level of consciousness
4. Load and go.
5. Rapidly transport to the appropriate hospital.
6. Notify medical direction early.

If you are not authorized to decompress the chest, the patient must be transported rapidly to the hospital so decompression can be performed. A chest tube will be necessary upon arrival to the hospital. A needle decompression is a temporary, but life-saving, measure.

Massive Hemothorax

Blood in the pleural space is a hemothorax (Figure 6-17). A massive hemothorax occurs as a result of at least a 1,500 cc blood loss into the thoracic cavity. Each thoracic cavity may contain up to 3,000 cc of blood. Massive hemothorax is more often due to penetrating trauma than to blunt trauma, but either injury may disrupt a major pulmonary or systemic vessel. As blood accumulates within the pleural space, the lung on the affected side

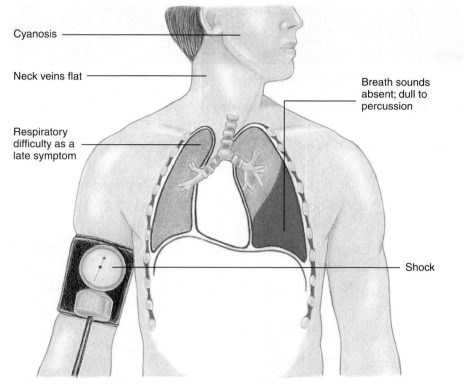

Cyanosis

Neck veins flat

Breath sounds absent; dull to percussion

Respiratory difficulty as a late symptom

Shock

FIGURE 6-17 Physical findings of massive hemothorax.

is compressed. If enough blood accumulates (rare), the mediastinum will be shifted away from the hemothorax. The inferior and superior vena cava and the contralateral lung are compressed. Thus, the ongoing blood loss is complicated by hypoxemia.

Signs and symptoms of massive hemothorax are produced by both hypovolemia and respiratory compromise. The patient may be hypotensive from blood loss and compression of the heart or great veins. Anxiety and confusion are produced by hypovolemia and hypoxemia. Clinical signs of hypovolemic shock may be apparent. The neck veins are usually flat secondary to profound hypovolemia, but may very rarely be distended due to mediastinal compression. Other signs of hemothorax include decreased breath sounds and dullness to percussion on the affected side. See Table 6-1 for comparison of tension pneumothorax and massive hemothorax.

PROCEDURE
✳ Management of Massive Hemothorax

1. Secure an open airway.
2. Apply high-flow oxygen.
3. Load and go.
4. Notify medical direction early.
5. Treat for shock. Replace volume carefully after IV insertion en route. Try to keep the blood pressure just high enough to maintain a peripheral pulse (90–100 mmHg systolic). While the major problem in massive hemothorax is usually hemorrhagic shock, elevating the blood pressure will increase the bleeding into the chest.
6. Observe closely for the possible development of a tension hemopneumothorax, which would require acute chest decompression.

TABLE 6-1 *Primary Survey of Tension Pneumothorax Contrasted to Massive Hemothorax*

	Tension Pneumothorax	Massive Hemothorax
Scene Size-up	Seat belt? Steering wheel?	Scene safe? Penetrating vs. blunt trauma?
Level of consciousness (LOC)	Decreased	Decreased
Breathing	Rapid/shallow; labored	Rapid/shallow; labored
Pulses	Weak/thready; absent radials	Weak/thready; absent radials
Skin	Cool/clammy/diaphoretic; cyanotic	Cool/clammy/diaphoretic; pale/ashen
Neck	Neck vein distension; rare tracheal deviation	Neck veins flat; trachea midline
Breath sounds	Decreased or absent breath sounds on affected side	Decreased or absent breath sounds on affected side
	Hyperresonant to percussion on affected side	Dull to percussion on affected side

Cardiac Tamponade

Cardiac tamponade is usually due to penetrating injury. The pericardial sac is an inelastic membrane that surrounds the heart. If blood collects rapidly between the heart and pericardium from a cardiac injury, the ventricles of the heart will be compressed. A small amount of pericardial blood may compromise cardiac filling. As the compression of the ventricles increases, the heart is less able to refill and cardiac output falls.

Diagnosis of cardiac tamponade classically relies upon the triad of hypotension, distended neck veins, and muffled heart sounds (Beck's triad). Muffled heart sounds may be very difficult to appreciate in the prehospital setting, but if you briefly listen to the heart when performing the primary survey you may notice a change later. The patient may have a paradoxical pulse. If the patient loses his peripheral pulse during inspiration, this is suggestive of a paradoxical pulse and the presence of cardiac tamponade. The major differential diagnosis in the field is tension pneumothorax. With cardiac tamponade, the patient will be in shock with a midline trachea and equal breath sounds (Figure 6-18), unless there is an associated pneumothorax or hemothorax.

The cardiac tamponade may be identified during the ITLS Primary Survey (Figure 6-19).

PROCEDURE
❖ Management of Cardiac Tamponade

1. Ensure an open airway.
2. Administer high-flow oxygen.
3. Load and go!

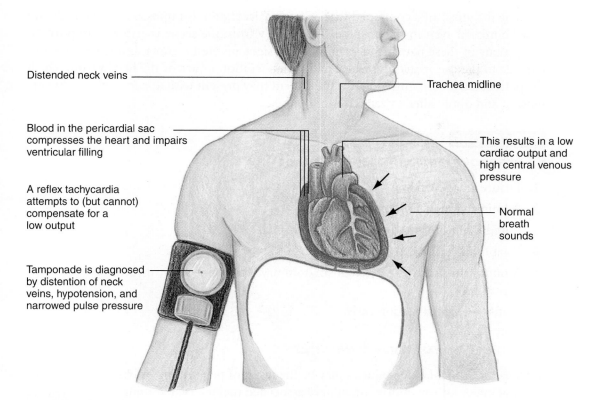

Distended neck veins

Trachea midline

Blood in the pericardial sac compresses the heart and impairs ventricular filling

This results in a low cardiac output and high central venous pressure

A reflex tachycardia attempts to (but cannot) compensate for a low output

Normal breath sounds

Tamponade is diagnosed by distention of neck veins, hypotension, and narrowed pulse pressure

FIGURE 6-18 Pathophysiology and physical findings of cardiac tamponade.

4. Transport rapidly to the appropriate hospital.

5. Notify medical direction early.

6. Monitor the heart early, especially with chest pain or an irregular pulse.

7. Treat for shock. An IV infusion of electrolyte solution (en route) may increase the filling of the heart and increase cardiac output. However, since there may be associated intrathoracic bleeding, give only enough fluid to maintain a pulse (90–100 mmHg systolic).

8. Treat dysrhythmias as they present.

9. Watch for other complications, including hemothorax and pneumothorax.

Traumatic Aortic Rupture

A traumatic aortic rupture is the most common cause of immediate death in motor-vehicle collisions or falls from heights. Ninety percent of these patients die immediately. For the survivors, salvage is feasible with prompt diagnosis and surgery. Traumatic thoracic aortic tears usually are due to deceleration injury with the heart and aortic arch moving suddenly anteriorly (third collision), transecting the aorta where it is fixed at the ligamentum arteriosum. In the 10 percent of patients who do not exsanguinate promptly, the aortic tear will be contained temporarily by surrounding tissues and the adventitia. However, this will usually rupture within hours unless surgically repaired.

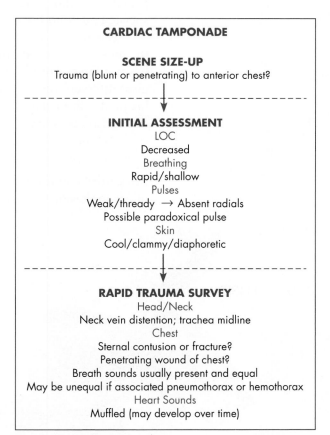

CARDIAC TAMPONADE

SCENE SIZE-UP
Trauma (blunt or penetrating) to anterior chest?

- -

INITIAL ASSESSMENT
LOC
Decreased
Breathing
Rapid/shallow
Pulses
Weak/thready → Absent radials
Possible paradoxical pulse
Skin
Cool/clammy/diaphoretic

- -

RAPID TRAUMA SURVEY
Head/Neck
Neck vein distention; trachea midline
Chest
Sternal contusion or fracture?
Penetrating wound of chest?
Breath sounds usually present and equal
May be unequal if associated pneumothorax or hemothorax
Heart Sounds
Muffled (may develop over time)

FIGURE 6-19 The cardiac tamponade may be identified during the ITLS Primary Survey.

The diagnosis of a contained thoracic aortic laceration is impossible in the field and may be missed even in the hospital. The history from the scene is critically important, since many of these patients have no obvious signs of chest trauma. Information about damage to the car or steering wheel with a deceleration injury or the height from which the patient fell is vital. Infrequently, the patient may present with upper extremity hypertension and diminished lower extremity pulses.

PROCEDURE
❊ Management of Potential Aortic Tears

1. Ensure an open airway.
2. Administer high-flow oxygen.
3. Rapidly transport to the appropriate hospital.
4. Establish IV access.
5. Monitor the heart. The mechanism of injury is the same as for myocardial contusion.
6. Notify medical direction early.

Tracheal or Bronchial Tree Injury

Tracheal or bronchial tree injuries may be the result of penetrating or blunt trauma. Penetrating upper airway injuries often have associated major vascular injuries and extensive tissue destruction. Blunt trauma may present with subtle findings. Blunt injury usually ruptures the trachea or mainstem bronchus near the carina. Presenting signs of blunt or penetrating injury include subcutaneous emphysema of the chest, face, or neck or an associated pneumothorax or hemothorax.

Securing the airway in the patient with a laryngeal or tracheal injury may challenge the most experienced care provider. Ideally, a cuffed endotracheal tube should be passed beyond the site of the rupture. However, this may not be possible, and emergency surgical intervention may be needed to obtain an airway. Thus, prompt transport to the hospital is important. Observing the patient for signs of a pneumothorax or hemothorax is also necessary.

Myocardial Contusion

Myocardial contusion is a potentially lethal lesion resulting from blunt chest injury. Blunt injury to the anterior chest is transmitted via the sternum to the heart, which lies immediately posterior to it (Figure 6-20). Cardiac injuries from this mechanism may include valvular rupture, pericardial tamponade, or cardiac rupture, but contusion of the right atrium and right ventricle occurs most commonly (Figure 6-21). This bruising of the heart is basically the same injury as an acute myocardial infarction and likewise presents with chest pain, dysrhythmias, or cardiogenic shock (rare). In the field, cardiogenic shock cannot be distinguished from cardiac tamponade. The chest pain may be difficult to differentiate from the associated musculoskeletal discomfort that the patient also suffers as a result of the injury. All patients with blunt anterior chest trauma should be presumed to have a myocardial contusion. The management is the same as for cardiac tamponade above.

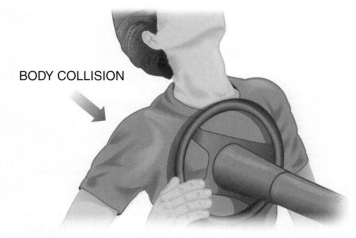

BODY COLLISION

FIGURE 6-20 Pathophysiology of myocardial contusion.

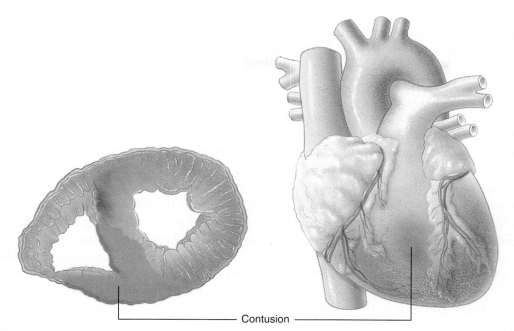

Contusion

FIGURE 6-21 Myocardial contusion most frequently affects the right atrium and ventricle as they collide with the sternum.

Diaphragmatic Tears

Tears in the diaphragm may result from a severe blow to the abdomen. A sudden increase in intra-abdominal pressure, such as a seat-belt injury or kick to the abdomen, may tear the diaphragm and allow herniation of the abdominal organs into the thoracic cavity. This occurs more commonly on the left than the right, since the liver protects the right hemidiaphragm. Blunt trauma produces large radial tears in the diaphragm. Penetrating trauma may also produce holes in the diaphragm, but these tend to be small.

Traumatic diaphragmatic hernia is difficult to diagnose even in the hospital. The herniation of abdominal contents into the thoracic cavity may cause marked respiratory distress. On examination, the breath sounds may be diminished and, infrequently, bowel sounds may be heard when the chest is auscultated. The abdomen may appear scaphoid if a large quantity of abdominal contents is in the chest.

PROCEDURE

✠ Management of Diaphragmatic Rupture

1. Ensure an open airway.
2. Assist ventilation as necessary
3. Administer high-flow oxygen.
4. Transport the patient to the appropriate hospital.
5. Treat shock. Insert an IV en route. Associated injuries are common and hypovolemia may occur.
6. Notify medical direction early.

Pulmonary Contusion

A very common chest injury resulting from blunt trauma, a pulmonary contusion takes hours to develop and rarely develops during prehospital care, unless very long transport or delayed discovery of the victim occurs. Contusion of the lung may produce marked hypoxemia. Management consists of intubation and/or assisted ventilation if indicated, oxygen administration, transport, and IV insertion.

Other Chest Injuries

Impaled Objects: Penetrating objects, such as a knife, may cause impalement injuries of the chest. As in other areas of the body, the object should not be removed in the field. Stabilize the object, ensure an airway, insert an IV, and transport the patient.

Traumatic Asphyxia: Traumatic asphyxia is an important set of physical findings. However, the term *traumatic asphyxia* is a misnomer, because the condition is not caused by asphyxia. The syndrome results from a severe compression injury to the chest, such as from a steering wheel, conveyor belt, or heavy object. The sudden compression of the heart and mediastinum transmits this force to the capillaries of the neck and head. The patients appear similar to those of strangulation, with cyanosis and swelling of the head and neck. The tongue and lips are swollen, and conjunctival hemorrhage is evident. The skin below the level of the crush injury to the chest will be pink unless there are other problems.

Traumatic asphyxia indicates that the patient has suffered a severe blunt thoracic injury, and major thoracic injuries are likely to be present. Management includes airway maintenance, IV access, treating other injuries, and rapid transport.

PEARLS
Simple Pneumothorax
Reassess patients with chest injuries frequently to prevent progression of a simple pneumothorax or open pneumothorax to a tension pneumothorax. The pulse oximeter is very helpful.

Simple Pneumothorax: Simple pneumothorax may result from blunt or penetrating trauma. Fractured ribs are the usual cause in blunt trauma. Pneumothorax is caused by accumulation of air within the potential space between the visceral and parietal pleura. The lung may be totally or partially collapsed as the air continues to accrue in the thoracic cavity. In a healthy patient this should not acutely compromise ventilation, if a tension pneumothorax does not evolve. Patients with less respiratory reserve may not tolerate even a simple pneumothorax.

Diagnosis of a pneumothorax is based on pleuritic chest pain, dyspnea, decreased breath sounds on the affected side, and hypertympany to percussion. Close observation is required in anticipation of the patient developing a tension pneumothorax.

Sternal Fractures: Sternal fractures also indicate that the patient has suffered marked blunt trauma to the anterior chest. These patients should be presumed to have a myocardial contusion. Diagnosis of sternal fracture may be made by palpation.

Simple Rib Fracture: Simple rib fracture is the most frequent injury to the chest. If the patient does not have an associated pneumothorax or hemothorax, the major problem is pain. This pain will prohibit the patient from breathing adequately. On palpation, the area of rib fracture will be tender and may be unstable. Give oxygen and monitor for pneumothorax or hemothorax while encouraging the patient to breathe deeply.

Case Study *continued*

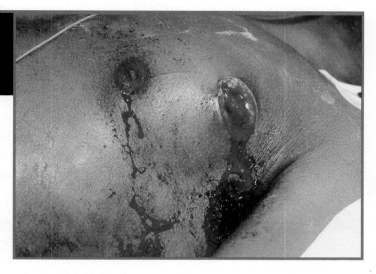

(Photo courtesy of Roy Alson, MD)

Dan, Joyce, and Buddy of the Emergency Transport System have been called to a local bar where a patron has been stabbed. The Scene Size-up reveals that the police are on-scene and have cleared the bar and are questioning bystanders outside. There is a single male victim who is sitting in a chair and holding his chest. Since the scene is safe and the mechanism of injury (stab wound) is readily apparent, the team dons personal protective equipment and each carries their essential trauma care equipment as they approach the patient. The patient, a male in his twenties, states that he was stabbed twice in the left chest but has no other injuries. He states that during an argument his drinking buddy stabbed him twice in the left anterior chest before bystanders could take the knife away from him. The patient denies falling or any other injuries.

Joyce is acting as team leader and as she begins the initial assessment, her general impression is good. The patient is sitting in a chair and is awake and answering appropriately. He does not appear to be in any distress. Respiration appears to be fast and shallow and when his hand is removed from his left chest, there are two stab wounds. One of the wounds is small but the other is about 5 cm long and obviously sucks when he inhales. The radial pulse is rapid but strong. Joyce immediately asks Dan to apply a nonrebreather oxygen mask and then clean the chest and apply an Asherman Chest Seal®. Because of the nature of the injury she decides to do a focused exam. Exam of the airway is normal, with good movement of air and a normal speaking voice. The neck veins are flat and the trachea is in the midline. The breath sounds are not present on the left (except for the sucking sound) but are normal on the right. Respiration is rapid and shallow. The two wounds (no longer bleeding) are as mentioned above. Percussion of the chest reveals dullness to percussion on the left. Heart sounds are normal but rapid. The abdomen is soft and nontender. There are no other wounds. Vital signs are pulse 140, respiration 36/minute, blood pressure 90/60. As soon as Dan seals the sucking chest wound, the patient is placed on a stretcher (no backboard or packaging) and moved to the ambulance.

He is treated with 100 percent oxygen by nonrebreather mask. Two large-bore IVs are started during transport but, because the blood pressure is not below 90 mmHg systolic, Joyce keeps the flow rates just fast enough to keep the veins open. She is concerned about causing worsening of any intrathoracic bleeding.

The history reveals:

S — Pain in left chest, shortness of breath, and weakness

A — None

M — None

P — No history of serious illness.

L — Just ate some Slim Jims and pickled eggs; admits to drinking "three beers"

E — States he was drinking with his friend, who became upset when they got into an argument over football. In a snit, his friend stabbed him with a large pocketknife. His friend is now outside talking to the police and is crying and protesting that he never meant to hurt the patient.

Buddy applies a cardiac monitor and a pulse oximeter (98 percent on 100 percent oxygen). Joyce notifies medical direction that they will be arriving in 5 minutes with a young male with a sucking chest wound, a hemothorax, and early shock. She is told to watch the vital signs but not to give a bolus of saline unless the blood pressure drops below 80 mmHg systolic. Joyce performs the Detailed Exam and finds everything normal except what was noted on the Focused Exam. The ITLS Ongoing Exam was not performed, since they arrived at the emergency department before she had time to do one. While in the emergency department, the patient had a chest tube inserted and 1,000 cc of blood evacuated. There was no further bleeding, so the patient did not have to go to surgery. He was in the hospital for 5 days and had an uneventful recovery.

Case Study Wrap-up

This is one of the few examples of a Focused Exam being adequate for a trauma patient. Note that even a Focused Exam requires that both the chest and the abdomen be examined because the diaphragm rises so high in the chest that a midchest stab wound may go through the diaphragm and cause abdominal injuries. A sucking chest wound can be closed using an occlusive dressing taped on only three sides so that air can escape (preventing development of a tension pneumothorax) but air cannot enter the chest. The commercially available Asherman Chest Seal® has a built-in flutter valve and is currently the best way to seal a sucking chest wound, or the decompression needle for a tension pneumothorax.

Studies have found that for penetrating wounds of the chest, the pneumatic antishock garment or IV fluids may significantly worsen survival (Chapter 8). Thus, the PASG is contraindicated and IV fluids should only be used to maintain sufficient perfusion to keep the patient alive to reach the trauma center.

SUMMARY

Chest injuries are common and often life threatening in the multiple-trauma patient. If you follow the ITLS Primary Survey, you will identify the injuries. These are often load-and-go patients. Primary goals in treating the patient with chest trauma are the following:

1. Ensure an open airway while protecting the cervical spine.
2. Administer high-flow oxygen and ventilate if necessary.
3. Stabilize flail segments.
4. Seal sucking chest wounds.
5. Decompress the chest if needed.
6. Load and go.
7. Notify medical direction early.
8. Obtain IV access.

The thoracic injuries discussed are life threatening, but treatable by prompt intervention and transport to the appropriate hospital. It is mandatory that the injuries presented are recognized in the field and treated appropriately to salvage these patients.

BIBLIOGRAPHY

1. American College of Surgeons Committee on Trauma. 2004. *Advanced trauma life support.* Chicago: American College of Surgeons, 103–15.
2. Eckstein, M., D. Suyehara. 1998. Needle thoracostomy in the prehospital setting. *Prehospital Emergency Care* 2(2): 132–35.
3. Leppaniemi, A., R. Haapiainen. 2003. Occult diaphragmatic injuries caused by stab wounds. *Journal of Trauma* 55: 646–50.
4. McGwin G., J. Metzger, S. Moran, et al. 2003. Occupant- and collision-related risk factors for blunt thoracic aorta injury. *Journal of Trauma* 54: 655–63.
5. Spodick, D. 2003. Acute cardiac tamponade. *New England Journal of Medicine* 349: 684–90.
6. Vles, W., F. Veen, J. Roukema, et al. 2003. Consequences of delayed diagnoses in trauma patients, a prospective study. *Journal of the American College of Surgeons* 197: 596–602.

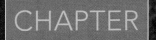
Thoracic Trauma Skills

Donna Hastings, EMT-P

Upon completion of this chapter, you should be able to:

1. Describe the indications for emergency decompression of a tension pneumothorax.
2. Explain the complications of needle decompression of a tension pneumothorax.
3. Perform needle decompression of a tension pneumothorax.

(© Eddie Sperling Photography)

CHEST DECOMPRESSION

Indications

As with all advanced procedures, this technique must be accepted local protocol and you must obtain medical direction before performing it. The conservative management of tension pneumothorax is oxygen, ventilatory assistance, and rapid transport. The indication for performing emergency decompression is the presence of a tension pneumothorax with decompensation as evidenced by more than one of the following:

▪ Respiratory distress and cyanosis

▪ Loss of the radial pulse (late shock)

▪ Decreasing level of consciousness

Complications

▪ Laceration of the intercostal vessels may cause hemorrhage. The intercostal artery and vein run around the inferior margin of each rib. Poor needle placement can lacerate one of these vessels.

▪ Creation of a pneumothorax may occur if not already present. If your assessment was incorrect, you may give the patient a pneumothorax when you insert the needle into the chest.

▪ Laceration of the lung is possible. Poor technique or inappropriate insertion (no pneumothorax present) can cause laceration of the lung, with subsequent bleeding and an air leak.

▪ Risk of infection is a consideration. Adequate skin preparation with an antiseptic will usually prevent this.

PROCEDURE

✷ Performing a Chest Decompression

1. Assess the patient to make sure that his condition is due to a tension pneumothorax.
   a. Decreased level of consciousness (LOC)
   b. Open airway
   c. Rapid shallow respiration; respiratory distress
   d. Weak/thready pulses; possible absent radial pulse
   e. Skin is cool, clammy, diaphoretic; pale or cyanotic
   f. Neck vein distention (may not be present if there is associated severe hemorrhage)
   g. Possible tracheal deviation away from the side of the injury (almost never present)
   h. Absent or decreased breath sounds on the affected side
   i. Tympany (hyperresonance) to percussion on the affected side

2. Give the patient high-flow oxygen and ventilatory assistance.

3. Determine that indications for emergency decompression are present. Then obtain medical direction to perform the procedure.

4. Identify the second or third intercostal space on the anterior chest at the midclavicular line on the same side as the pneumothorax. This may be done by

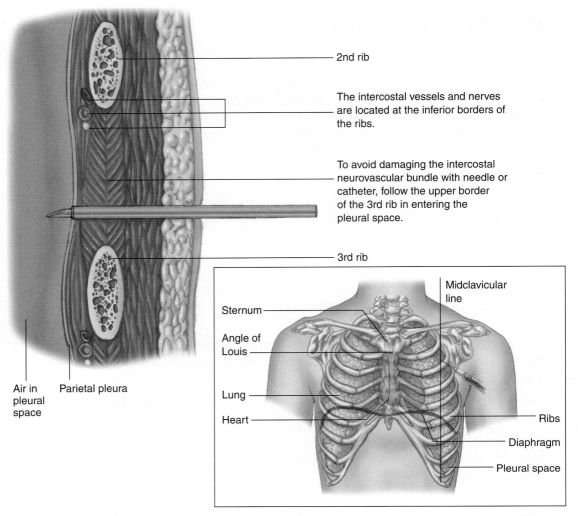

FIGURE 7-1 Needle decompression of a tension pneumothorax.

feeling for "angle of Louis," the bump located on the sternum about a quarter of the way from the suprasternal notch (Figure 7-1). The anterior site is preferred because the supine patient has a better chance of having accumulated air in the pleural space removed when decompressing at the midclavicular area as opposed to the midaxillary area. Monitoring of the site is also easier if performed in the anterior site because the catheter is not as likely to be unintentionally dislodged when the patient is moved. However, if there is significant anterior chest trauma, the alternate site may be used: the midaxillary line, fourth or fifth intercostal space directly above the fifth or sixth rib (the nipple is over the fifth rib).

5. Quickly prepare the area with an antiseptic.

6. Remove the plastic cap from a 2-inch (5-cm) large-bore catheter. This allows air to exit the needle as it passes into the pleural space. Use a catheter that is long enough to enter the pleural space. One study found that the chest wall thickness in the anterior chest varies from 1.3 cm to 5.2 cm, with a mean of 3.2 cm. The minimum catheter length should be 5 cm. Insert the needle into the skin over the superior border of the third rib, midclavicular line, and direct it into the intercostal space at a 90-degree angle to the third rib (Figures 7-1 and 7-2). Direction of the bevel is irrelevant to successful results. As the needle enters the pleural space, there will be a "pop." If a tension pneumothorax is present, there will be a hiss of air as the

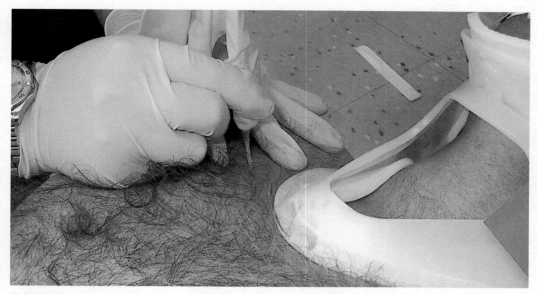

FIGURE 7-2 **Needle decompression by the anterior approach.** *(Photo courtesy of Jere Baldwin, MD)*

pneumothorax is decompressed. If using an over-the-needle catheter, advance the catheter into the skin. Remove the needle and leave the catheter in place. The catheter hub must be stabilized to the chest with tape.

7. Place a one-way valve on or over the decompressing needle. The Asherman Chest Seal® will go over the needle and provide a one-way valve. Other one-way valves can be made but should be tested before using (a needle through the finger of a rubber glove will not work as a one-way valve). Young healthy patients will tolerate having no valve at all on the decompressing needle.

8. Leave the plastic catheter in place until it is replaced by a chest tube at the hospital.

9. Intubate the patient if indicated. Monitor closely for recurrence of the tension pneumothorax.

BIBLIOGRAPHY

1. American College of Surgeons Committee on Trauma. 2004. *Advanced trauma life support.* Chicago: American College of Surgeons, 127.
2. Eckstein, M., D. Suyehara. 1998. Needle thoracostomy in the prehospital setting. *Prehospital Emergency Care* 2(2): 132–35.

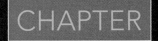

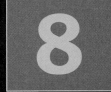

CHAPTER 8

Shock Evaluation and Management

Raymond L. Fowler, MD, FACEP
Paul E. Pepe, MD, MPH, FACEP, FCCM
John T. Stevens, EMT-P

OBJECTIVES

Upon completion of this chapter, you should be able to:

1. List the four components of the vascular system necessary for normal tissue perfusion.

2. Describe the symptoms and signs of shock in the order that they develop, from the very least to the very worst.

3. Describe the three common clinical shock syndromes.

4. Explain the pathophysiology of hemorrhagic shock, and compare it to the pathophysiology of neurogenic shock.

5. Describe the management of the following:
   a. Hemorrhage that can be controlled
   b. Hemorrhage that cannot be controlled
   c. Nonhemorrhagic shock syndromes

6. Discuss the use of hemostatic agents for uncontrolled extremity hemorrhage.

7. Discuss the current indications for the use of IV fluids in the treatment of hemorrhagic shock.

(© Eddie Sperling Photography)

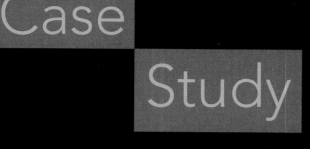

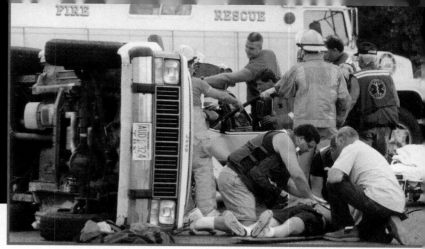

Dan, Joyce, and Buddy of the Emergency Transport System have been called to the scene of a high-speed side-impact auto collision. *What injuries might they anticipate in a collision of this type? Would the victim likely develop shock? What type of interventions might they likely have to make?* Keep these questions in mind as you read the chapter. Then, at the end of the chapter, find out how the rescuers completed this call.

INTRODUCTION

The management of shock has been the subject of intensive research for decades and, as a result, changes have been made in the recommendations for prehospital treatment of the patient with hemorrhagic shock. The experience of the United States and the United Kingdom in the Iraq war has led to new thinking in the management of exsanguinating hemorrhage. This chapter will review the present knowledge about the pathophysiology and treatment of shock in the traumatized patient and in patients with various other shock states.

BASIC PATHOPHYSIOLOGY

The normal perfusion of body tissues requires four intact components.

- An intact vascular system to deliver oxygenated blood throughout the body: the blood vessels
- Adequate air exchange in the lungs to allow oxygen to enter the blood: oxygenation
- An adequate volume of fluid in the vascular system: blood cells and plasma
- A functioning pump: the heart

It is important to remember that blood pressure requires a "steady state" activity of all of the above factors. The heart must be pumping, the blood volume must be adequate, the blood vessels must be intact, and the lungs must be oxygenating the blood. An important formula regarding the maintenance of blood pressure should be fresh in the mind of every emergency medical provider:

$$\text{Blood Pressure} = \text{Cardiac Output} \times \text{Peripheral Vascular Resistance}$$

In addition, the formula for cardiac output is written as follows:

$$\text{Heart Rate} \times \text{Stroke Volume} = \text{Cardiac Output}$$

Thus, if cardiac output falls (either due to falling heart rate or lowered stroke volume) or if peripheral vascular resistance falls (such as in the dilated arteries that occur in neurogenic shock), then blood pressure will fall.

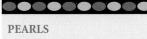

The preservation of these components can be related to the basic rules of shock management, which are: maintain the airway, maintain oxygenation and ventilation, control bleeding where possible, and maintain circulation through an adequate heart rate and intravascular volume.

The term *shock* describes a condition that occurs when the perfusion of the body's tissues with oxygen, electrolytes, glucose, and fluid becomes inadequate. Several processes cause this drop in perfusion. The loss of red blood cells in hemorrhaging patients results in less oxygen transport to the body tissues. Decreased circulating blood volume leads to lowered glucose, fluid volume, and electrolytes to the cells. These circulatory disturbances result in the cells of the body becoming "shocked," and grave changes in body tissue begin to occur. Eventually, cell death follows.

Deprived of oxygen, cells begin to use "backup" processes that utilize energy sources less efficiently, producing toxic by-products such as lactic acid. Although these backup (anaerobic) processes may postpone cellular death for a time, the lack of oxygen is compounded by these toxic by-products because they can poison certain cellular functions, such as the production of energy by mitochondria. Eventually, accumulating lactic acid in the blood and organs creates a systemic acidosis that further disrupts cellular activity. Respiratory muscle function also weakens, and respiratory failure develops, which worsens hypoxia.

In response to inadequate oxygen delivery, the body responds with increased activity of the sympathetic nervous system (called "increased sympathetic tone"), resulting in the increased release of circulating catecholamines (epinephrine and norepinephrine). These hormones increase both the rate and strength of the heart's contractions and constrict peripheral arterial blood vessels. The midbrain responds to the progressive hypoxia and acidosis with an increase in the respiratory rate.

As you can see, shock is a condition that begins with an injury, spreads throughout the body as a multisystem insult to major organs, and results in specific symptoms that you can detect at the bedside as the patient becomes progressively sicker. Thus, shock is a cellular process with clinical manifestations. The patient with shock may be pale, diaphoretic, and tachycardic. At the cellular level, the patient's cells are starving for oxygen and nutrients. Shock, therefore, is a condition in which poor tissue perfusion can severely and possibly permanently damage the organs of the body, causing disability or death. The clinical signs and symptoms of the patient in shock imply that critical processes are threatening every vulnerable cell in the patient's body, particularly those in vital organs.

ASSESSMENT AND SHOCK

When first considering the concept of shock, you must understand that shock produces signs and symptoms that you can observe during patient assessment. The initial diagnosis of the shock state can often be made from the physical assessment findings. Although blood pressure should be monitored frequently to help determine whether organ perfusion is adequate, remember that assessment tools other than measuring the blood pressure must also be used to recognize shock in the trauma patient.

Humans vary as to the blood pressure required to maintain adequate perfusion. The question "How low can you go?" while maintaining adequate perfusion has not yet been answered. We know that the healthy young patient can often maintain adequate perfusion in the face of hypotension whereas older patients, hypertensive patients, and those with head injury often cannot tolerate hypotension for even short periods. It is vital that you work with your medical director to stay up to date on recommendations for shock management as new research is completed.

Although this text is about trauma, shock is a clinical condition associated with more medical problems than just trauma. Following is a discussion of shock syndromes, many of which are caused by traumatic conditions. The take-home point, though, is that the shock state is one of low tissue perfusion (from many causes) in which the body usually demonstrates similar signs of its response to this perfusion-deprived condition. The body may not always demonstrate similar signs. See, for example, the discussion of high-space shock that follows. Therefore, the stabbed and bleeding patient in hemorrhagic shock often shows many of the same signs as the burned or dehydrated patient with low blood volume that is NOT due to hemorrhage.

Compensated and Decompensated Shock

Generally, the onset of the symptoms and signs of hypovolemic shock (including hemorrhagic shock) occur in the following order.

Compensated Shock

- *Weakness and lightheadedness*—caused by decreased blood volume
- *Thirst*—caused by hypovolemia (especially with relatively low fluid amounts in the blood vessels)
- *Pallor* (pale, white color of the skin)—caused by catecholamine-induced vasoconstriction and/or loss of circulating red blood cells
- *Tachycardia*—caused by the effect of catecholamines on the heart as the brain increases the activity of the sympathetic nervous system
- *Diaphoresis* (sweating)—caused by the effects of catecholamines on sweat glands
- *Tachypnea* (elevated respiratory rate)—caused by the brain elevating the respiratory rate under the influence of stress, catecholamines, acidosis, and hypoxia
- *Decreased urinary output*—caused by hypovolemia, hypoxia, and circulating catecholamines (important to remember in interfacility transfers)
- *Weakened peripheral pulses*—the "thready" pulse (thready means "threadlike," meaning the arteries actually shrink in width as intravascular volume is lost); caused by vasoconstriction, tachycardia, and loss of blood volume

NOTE: The symptoms and signs listed above are in the order of progressive "compensation," as the body attempts to deal with the cause of shock. Beginning with the next item, hypotension, the body is no longer able to maintain perfusion, and the shock condition is now "decompensated."

Decompensated Shock

- *Hypotension*—caused by hypovolemia, either absolute or relative (see later paragraphs for a discussion of relative hypovolemia), and/or by the diminished cardiac output seen in "obstructive" or "mechanical" shock
- *Altered mental status* (confusion, restlessness, combativeness, unconsciousness)—caused by decreased cerebral perfusion, acidosis, hypoxia, and catecholamine stimulation
- *Cardiac arrest*—caused by critical organ failure secondary to blood or fluid loss, hypoxia, and occasionally arrhythmia caused by catecholamine stimulation and/or low perfusion

To summarize, many of the symptoms of shock of any etiology, including the classic hemorrhagic shock picture, are caused by the release of catecholamines. When the brain senses that perfusion to the tissues is insufficient, it sends messages down the spinal cord to the sympathetic nervous system and the adrenal glands, causing a release of catecholamines (epinephrine and norepinephrine) into the circulation. The circulating catecholamines cause the tachycardia, anxiousness, diaphoresis, and vasoconstriction. The vasoconstriction in the arterioles shunts blood away from the skin and intestines to the heart, lungs, and brain. Close monitoring early in the shock syndrome may allow you to detect an initial rise in the blood pressure due to this shunting, though this does not always happen. There will almost always be an initial narrowing of the pulse pressure because vasoconstriction raises the diastolic pressure more than the systolic. The shunting of blood from the skin and the loss of circulating red blood cells cause the pallor of shock.

Decreased perfusion causes weakness and thirst initially, and then later, an altered level of consciousness (confusion, restlessness, or combativeness) and worsening pallor. As shock continues, the prolonged tissue hypoxia leads to worsening acidosis. This acidosis can ultimately cause a loss of response to catecholamines, worsening the drop in blood pressure. This is often the point at which the patient in "compensated" shock suddenly "crashes." Eventually, the hypoxia and acidosis cause cardiac dysfunction, including cardiac arrest, and ultimately death.

Although the individual response to post-traumatic hemorrhage may vary, many patients will have the following classic patterns of "early" and "late" shock.

- *Early shock* (loss of approximately 15 to 25 percent of the blood volume), enough to stimulate slight to moderate tachycardia, pallor, narrowed pulse pressure, thirst, weakness, and possibly delayed capillary refill. In "early shock," the body is "compensating" for the physical insult that is causing the problem (hemorrhage, dehydration, tension pneumothorax, and so on).

- *Late shock* (loss of approximately 30 to 45 percent of the blood volume), enough to cause hypotension as well as the other symptoms of hypovolemic shock listed earlier. When "late shock" has occurred, this means that the body's ability to compensate for the physical insult has failed. As mentioned above, hypotension is the first sign of "late shock." The hypotensive patient, then, is near death, requiring aggressive assessment and management by the provider to prevent death of the patient.

Note that during the Initial Assessment, early shock presents as a fast pulse with pallor and diaphoresis, while late shock may present as weak pulse or loss of the peripheral pulse. One useful tip is to remember that the radial pulse appears at a systolic pressure of about 80, the femoral pulse appears at a systolic pressure of about 70, and the carotid pulse appears at a systolic pressure of about 60. Thus, if you had a trauma victim with a carotid pulse but no radial pulse, you could estimate that the patient's systolic pressure was between 60 and 80. A scientific study (see reference 5 at the end of the chapter) suggests that these numbers are slightly high. Nevertheless, weakened pulses taken with other signs of shock (such as those listed below) should quickly lead you to suspect decompensated shock. The aggressiveness with which you treat the shock will depend on a number of factors and will be guided by the patient's systolic blood pressure.

Prolonged capillary refill time was previously thought to be very useful for detecting early shock. Capillary refill time is tested by pressing on the palm of the hand or, in a child, squeezing the whole foot. The test is suspicious for shock if the blanched area remains pale for longer than 2 seconds. Scientific evaluation of this test has shown it to have a high correlation with late shock but to be of little value for detecting early shock. The test was associated with both frequent false-positive and false-negative results. Low blood volume, cold temperatures, and catecholamine-induced vasoconstriction can all cause decreased perfusion of the capillary bed in the skin and thus cause abnormal results. Measurement of capillary refill is useful for small children in whom it is difficult to get an accurate blood pressure, but it is of little use for detecting early shock in adults.

Evaluation of Tachycardia

One of the first signs of illness, and arguably one of the most common, is that of tachycardia. You will frequently be confronted with the patient with an elevated pulse rate, and you must make some sort of distinction as to the cause.

PEARLS
Tachycardia

A persistently elevated pulse rate while at rest is ALWAYS an indication of something medically wrong with the patient, including the possibility of occult hemorrhage.

First, remember that you must always attempt to explain why a patient has tachycardia. An elevated pulse rate (generally considered to be above 100 in an adult and higher at younger ages) is never normal. Humans can transiently raise their pulses in the setting of anxiety, but such elevation quickly returns to normal or fluctuates in rate depending on the waxing and waning of the anxiety state.

Second, remember that an elevated pulse rate is one of the first signs of shock. Any adult trauma patient with a sustained pulse rate above 100 must be suspected of having occult hemorrhage until proven otherwise. However, during the ITLS Primary Survey, a pulse rate greater than 120 should be a red flag for possible shock.

Finally, some patients who are in shock may not develop a tachycardia. It has been reported that a "relative bradycardia" may develop in patients with traumatic hypotension. So, the absence of tachycardia in an injured patient does not rule out that the patient is in shock.

Capnography

The heart delivers oxygen and nutrients to the cells of the body by way of blood vessels. The cells "burn" the nutrients in the presence of oxygen to produce energy, water, and carbon dioxide (CO_2). The water and CO_2 move into the bloodstream, the CO_2 being carried to the lungs by the red blood cells for excretion during exhalation. CO_2 then is the exhaled by-product of metabolism. Put another way, the level of exhaled CO_2 indicates how brightly the fire of metabolism is burning in the cells. When measured moment to moment at the airway, the level of CO_2 being excreted may be graphed as a waveform.

Devices are now commonly available either separately or on EKG monitors that measure waveform capnography. The typical exhaled CO_2 is approximately 40 mmHg. Falling measured CO_2 indicates either that the patient is hyperventilating (from anxiety or acidosis) or that the amount of oxygen being supplied to the cells is falling. You might say it this way: A falling exhaled CO_2 level suggests that the fire of metabolism in the patient may be burning low.

Patients in shock have decreased oxygen being supplied to their cells. Thus, if you are monitoring a patient who appears to be in shock or at risk of going into shock, monitor the level of exhaled CO_2. A level of exhaled CO_2 that falls much under 40—especially if it falls into the 20s or below—may be an indication of circulatory collapse and thus can be an additional warning sign of worsening shock (see Chapter 5, Figures 5-11 and 5-12).

PEARLS
Capnography
Falling waveform capnography may be one of the first indicators that a patient is going into a shock state.

The Shock Syndromes

Although the most common shock state seen in trauma patients is associated with hemorrhage and the accompanying hypovolemia, there are actually three major classifications of shock. These "types of shock" relate directly to the blood pressure equation discussed earlier in this chapter (Blood Pressure = Cardiac Output × Peripheral Vascular Resistance). These three shock states can be categorized according to their causes as follows:

■ *Low-volume shock* (absolute hypovolemia) is caused by hemorrhage or other major body fluid loss (diarrhea, vomiting, and "third spacing" due to burns, peritonitis, and other causes).

■ *High-space shock* (relative hypovolemia) is caused by spinal injury, vasovagal syncope, sepsis, and certain drug overdoses.

■ *Mechanical shock* (cardiogenic shock, also known as obstructive shock) is caused by pericardial tamponade, tension pneumothorax, massive pulmonary embolism, or conditions weakening the heart muscle, such as myocardial contusion or infarction.

There are notable differences in the appearance of patients with these conditions, and it is critical that you be aware of the signs and symptoms that accompany each one.

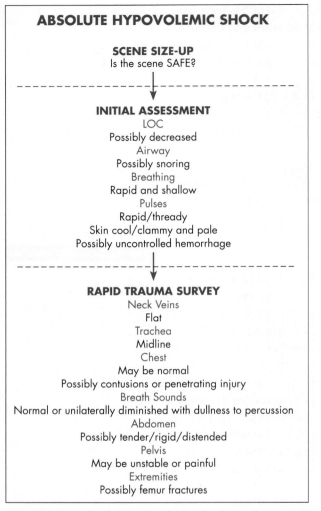

FIGURE 8-1 Absolute hypovolemic shock may be identified during the ITLS Primary Survey.

Low-Volume Shock (Absolute Hypovolemia): Loss of blood from injury is called *post-traumatic hemorrhage*. In addition to head injury, hemorrhagic shock is the number-one cause of preventable death from injury. The amount of volume that the blood vessels can hold is many liters more than that which actually flows through the vasculature. The sympathetic nervous system keeps the vessels constricted, reducing their volume and maintaining blood pressure high enough to perfuse vital organs. If blood volume is lost, "sensors" in the major vessels signal the adrenal gland and the nerves of the sympathetic nervous system to secrete catecholamines, which cause vasoconstriction and thus further shrink the vascular space and maintain perfusion pressure to the brain and heart. If the blood loss is minor, the sympathetic system can shrink the space enough to maintain blood pressure. If the loss is severe, the vascular space cannot be shrunk down enough to maintain blood pressure, and hypotension occurs.

Normally, the blood vessels are elastic and are distended by the volume that is in them. This produces a radial artery pulse that is full and wide. Blood loss allows the artery to shrink in width, becoming more threadlike in size; hence the term "thready" pulse in shock, as discussed previously.

Hypovolemic shock victims usually have tachycardia, are pale, and have flat neck veins. So, if you come upon a trauma victim who is pale, tachycardic, with weak radial pulses, and flat neck veins, this patient is probably bleeding from some injury.

Absolute hypovolemic shock may be identified in your patient during the ITLS Primary Survey (Figure 8-1).

High-Space Shock (Relative Hypovolemia): As mentioned earlier, the volume that the blood vessels can hold is many liters more than the blood volume in the blood vessels. Again, it is the steady-state action of the sympathetic nervous system that keeps the arterioles of the vascular bed constricted in the normal state in order to maintain perfusion to the heart and brain. Anything that interrupts the outflow from the sympathetic nervous system and causes the loss of this normal vasoconstriction allows the vascular space to dilate, becoming much "too large" for the amount of blood in the vascular system. If blood vessels dilate, the 5 liters or so of blood flowing through the normal adult's vascular space may not be sufficient to maintain blood pressure and vital tissue perfusion. The condition causing the vascular space to be too large for a normal amount of blood has been called high-space shock or relative hypovolemia (also known as "vasodilatory shock"). Although several causes of high-space shock exist (such as sepsis syndrome and drug overdose), neurogenic shock, commonly called *spinal shock*, is addressed here because it may be caused by trauma.

The nerves of the sympathetic nervous system come off of the spinal cord in the thoracic (chest) and lumbar area. This is why the sympathetic nervous system is often called the "thoracolumbar autonomic nervous system." Neurogenic shock occurs most typically after an injury to the spinal cord. An injury to the spinal cord in the neck can prevent the brain from being able to send out the sympathetic nervous system signals. Thus, a cervical spinal-cord injury can prevent the brain from raising the pulse rate, from raising the strength of the heart's contraction, or from constricting the peripheral arterioles (the vessels that maintain blood pressure). Although circulating catecholamines already present in the bloodstream may preserve the blood pressure for a short time, the disruption of the sympathetic nervous system outflow from the spinal cord results in loss of the normal vascular tone and in the inability of the body to compensate for any accompanying hemorrhage.

The clinical presentation of neurogenic shock differs from hemorrhagic shock in that there is no catecholamine release, thus no pallor, tachycardia, or sweating. The patient will have a decreased blood pressure, but the heart rate will be normal or slow, and the skin is usually warm, dry, and pink. The patient may also have accompanying paralysis and/or sensory deficit corresponding to the spinal-cord injury. You may also see a lack of chest wall movement and only simple diaphragmatic movement when the patient is asked to take a deep breath, seen as protruding of the abdomen during inspiration. The important point is that neurogenic shock does not have the typical picture of hemorrhagic shock, even when associated with severe bleeding. The neurologic assessment is therefore very important, and you should not rely on typical shock symptoms and signs to suspect internal bleeding or accompanying hemorrhage-associated shock. Neurogenic shock patients may "look better" than their actual condition really is.

Certain drug overdoses and chemical exposures can also result in shock from vasodilatation and relative hypovolemia. Very often injuries result after such intoxication, and their effect on typical clinical signs and symptoms (like neurogenic shock) should be considered. Examples of drug overdoses and chemical exposures that may produce the relative hypovolemia syndrome include nitroglycerin, calcium channel blockers, antihypertensive medications, and cyanide.

Whereas neurogenic shock (due to spinal-cord injury) is bradycardic, pink, and has flat neck veins, the other forms of high-space shock (drug overdoses, cyanide, sepsis) typically are tachycardic, pale or flushed, and have flat neck veins.

Relative hypovolemia due to neurogenic (spinal) shock may be identified in your patient during the ITLS Primary Survey (Figure 8-2).

Mechanical (Cardiogenic or Obstructive) Shock: The heart is a pump. Like any pump, it has a "power" stroke and a "filling" stroke, just like a piston moving up and down in the cylinder of a motor. In the normal adult's resting state, the heart pumps out about 5 liters of blood per minute. This means, of course, that the heart also must take in about 5 liters of blood per minute. Therefore, any traumatic or medical condition that slows or prevents the venous return of blood can cause shock by lowering cardiac output and thus oxygen delivery to the tissues. Likewise, anything that obstructs the flow of blood to or through the heart can cause shock.

The following are traumatic conditions that can cause mechanical shock.

- *Tension pneumothorax* is so named because of the high air tension (pressure) that may sometimes develop in the pleural space (between the lung and chest wall) due to a lung injury. This very high positive pressure collapses the low-pressure superior and inferior vena cava, preventing the return of venous blood to the heart. Shifting of mediastinal structures may also lower venous return by impinging on the superior and inferior vena cava, also causing a deviation of the trachea away from the affected

PEARLS
Mechanical or High-Space Shock
Look for signs of mechanical or high-space shock, especially if there is no bleeding.

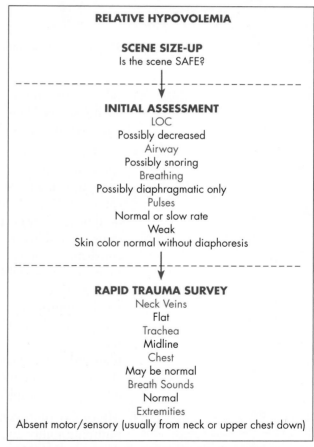

RELATIVE HYPOVOLEMIA

SCENE SIZE-UP
Is the scene SAFE?

INITIAL ASSESSMENT
LOC
Possibly decreased
Airway
Possibly snoring
Breathing
Possibly diaphragmatic only
Pulses
Normal or slow rate
Weak
Skin color normal without diaphoresis

RAPID TRAUMA SURVEY
Neck Veins
Flat
Trachea
Midline
Chest
May be normal
Breath Sounds
Normal
Extremities
Absent motor/sensory (usually from neck or upper chest down)

FIGURE 8-2 Relative hypovolemia due to neurogenic (spinal) shock may be identified during the ITLS Primary Survey.

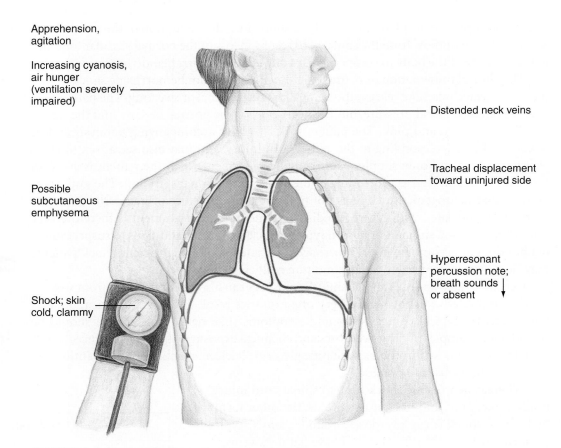

Apprehension, agitation

Increasing cyanosis, air hunger (ventilation severely impaired)

Possible subcutaneous emphysema

Shock; skin cold, clammy

Distended neck veins

Tracheal displacement toward uninjured side

Hyperresonant percussion note; breath sounds ↓ or absent

FIGURE 8-3 Physical findings of tension pneumothorax.

side. Decreased venous return results in lower cardiac output and the development of shock. (See Figure 8-3 and Chapters 6 and 7 for a complete description of the signs, symptoms, and treatment of tension pneumothorax.)

■ *Cardiac tamponade* (or "pericardial tamponade") occurs when blood fills the "potential" space between the heart and the pericardium, squeezing the heart and preventing the heart from filling (Figure 8-4). This decreased filling of the heart causes cardiac output to fall, resulting in the development of shock. Pericardial tamponade may occur in more than 75 percent of cases of penetrating cardiac injury. The signs and symptoms of tamponade have been labeled as "Beck's triad," consisting of shock, muffled heart tones, and distended neck veins. On-scene interventions should be avoided if the diagnosis is suspected, because any time wasted on-scene could result in death of the patient. Definitive surgical care in the nearest appropriate facility for pericardial decompression may be the only life-saving measure available. Using intravenous fluids to increase filling pressure of the heart may possibly be of some value, but IV fluids could also worsen the condition if there is an additional internal exsanguinating injury. Use of IV fluids in this situation should be during transport and only on the order of medical direction. (See Chapter 6 for a more complete discussion.)

■ *Myocardial contusion* can result in diminished cardiac output because the heart loses pumping ability due to direct injury to the heart muscle (Figure 8-5) and/or cardiac dysrhythmias (Figure 8-6). Myocardial contusion often cannot be differentiated from cardiac tamponade in the field. Therefore, rapid transport, supportive care, and cardiac monitoring are the mainstays of therapy.

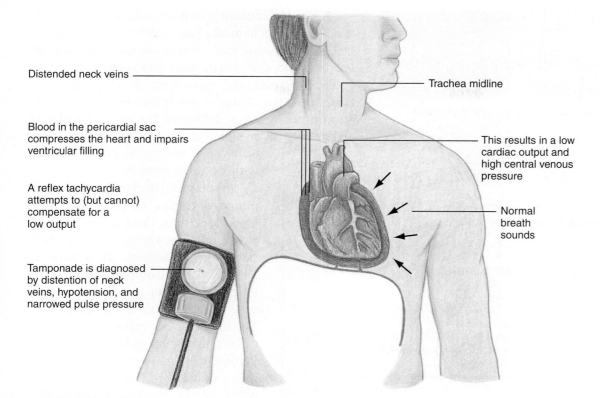

Distended neck veins

Trachea midline

Blood in the pericardial sac compresses the heart and impairs ventricular filling

This results in a low cardiac output and high central venous pressure

A reflex tachycardia attempts to (but cannot) compensate for a low output

Normal breath sounds

Tamponade is diagnosed by distention of neck veins, hypotension, and narrowed pulse pressure

FIGURE 8-4 Pathophysiology and physical findings of cardiac tamponade.

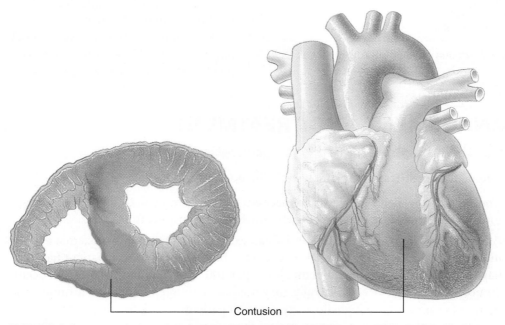

Contusion

FIGURE 8-5 Myocardial contusion most frequently affects the right atrium and ventricle as they collide with the sternum.

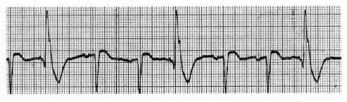

FIGURE 8-6 Myocardial contusion may cause ventricular ectopy.

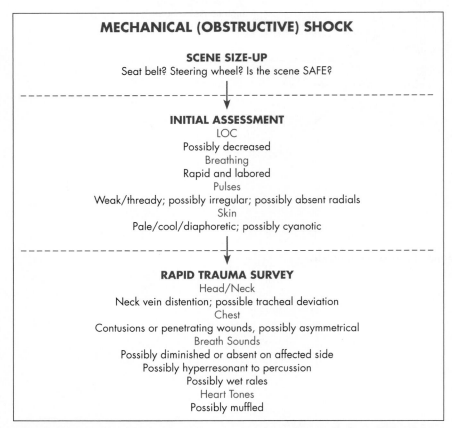

MECHANICAL (OBSTRUCTIVE) SHOCK

SCENE SIZE-UP
Seat belt? Steering wheel? Is the scene SAFE?

- -

INITIAL ASSESSMENT
LOC
Possibly decreased
Breathing
Rapid and labored
Pulses
Weak/thready; possibly irregular; possibly absent radials
Skin
Pale/cool/diaphoretic; possibly cyanotic

- -

RAPID TRAUMA SURVEY
Head/Neck
Neck vein distention; possible tracheal deviation
Chest
Contusions or penetrating wounds, possibly asymmetrical
Breath Sounds
Possibly diminished or absent on affected side
Possibly hyperresonant to percussion
Possibly wet rales
Heart Tones
Possibly muffled

FIGURE 8-7 Mechanical (obstructive) shock may be identified during the ITLS Primary Survey.

A word of caution is important here. Patients with shock from mechanical causes can be very near death. Delay on the scene may prevent salvage of the patient. For example, one urban study has suggested that, in applicable cases, the time from development of a tamponade to circulatory arrest may be as little as 5 to 10 minutes. Survival following traumatic circulatory arrest, even in the best of trauma systems, is rarely achieved if surgery is not performed within 5 to 10 minutes.

Mechanical shock is caused by a diminished cardiac output rather than blood loss; thus, these patients usually have a different appearance at the bedside than hemorrhagic shock patients. Since the cardiac output is diminished, the blood backs up into the venous system, resulting in distended neck veins. The lungs are not being perfused well, causing the patient to become cyanotic. Because the patient is in shock with an intact spinal cord, catecholamines are released and the patient develops pallor, tachycardia, and diaphoresis. Thus, mechanical shock patients are pale and cyanotic with distended neck veins and tachycardia. A post-trauma patient with these signs is near death, requiring rapid transport to a trauma center. In the setting of a tension pneumothorax, needle decompression of the affected side of the thorax can be life saving.

Mechanical (obstructive) shock may be identified in your patient during the ITLS Primary Survey (Figure 8-7).

MANAGEMENT AND TREATMENT
General Management of Post-Traumatic Shock States

Management of post-traumatic shock states includes the following:

1. *Control bleeding.* Red blood cells are necessary to carry oxygen. Control of bleeding must be obtained either by direct pressure or rapid transport to surgery.

2. *Administer high-flow oxygen.* Cyanosis is an extremely late sign of hypoxemia and may not occur at all if there has been extensive blood loss. Indeed, a patient has to have 5 grams of deoxygenated hemoglobin per 100 cc of blood for cyanosis to occur. Someone bleeding to death, literally, may not have enough hemoglobin around to manifest cyanosis. Give high-flow oxygen to all patients at risk for shock. Try to maintain a pulse oximeter reading greater than 95 percent.

3. *Load and go.* Trauma patients in shock from any cause are considered to be in the load-and-go category. Transport as soon as you finish the ITLS Primary Survey

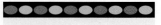

PEARLS
Hemorrhage

Control hemorrhage. If it cannot be done in the field, the patient needs to be in the operating room as soon as possible.

(Initial Assessment and Rapid Trauma Survey). Almost all critical interventions should be done in the ambulance (see Chapter 2).

Treatment of Post-Traumatic Hemorrhage

Specific prehospital management of the patient in shock remains both controversial and the subject of ongoing research. There is no question of the need for control of hemorrhage, supplemental oxygen, and early transport, but the indications for most other therapies are still being debated. For example, the National Institutes of Health is sponsoring a major international clinical trial at this time to determine the optimal treatment for hemorrhagic shock due to trauma (and traumatic brain injury) in the prehospital environment.

Since the early days of modern shock treatment (about the middle of the 20th century), intravenous crystalloid solutions (and sometimes colloid) have been tested and/or utilized to reverse the effects of hypovolemia. In addition, it has been previously proposed that intra-abdominal and pelvic bleeding may possibly be diminished by use of the pneumatic antishock garment (PASG; or military antishock trousers, MAST). Research showed that the PASG seemed to cause a worsening death rate when the garment was applied to patients with uncontrolled bleeding. Indeed, current research into the management of hemorrhagic shock due to trauma suggests a modified approach.

Patients in hypovolemic shock due to hemorrhage may be generally thought of as falling into one of the following two categories: those with bleeding that you can control (such as many extremity injuries) and those with bleeding that you cannot control (such as internal injuries).

Hemorrhage That Can Be Controlled: A patient with controllable bleeding is fairly easy to manage. Most bleeding can be stopped with direct pressure. In some situations (usually blast or tactical injuries) there may be exsanguinating hemorrhage that you cannot control with direct pressure. In these most extreme circumstances you should not hesitate to apply a tourniquet. A tourniquet is rarely needed but when it is needed, it should be applied quickly.

If the patient has clinical evidence of shock that persists after direct control of the bleeding, you should take the steps described below.

PROCEDURE

Managing Shock When Bleeding Has Been Controlled

1. Put the patient's body in a horizontal or slightly head-down position.
2. Administer high-flow oxygen, preferably using a nonrebreather mask with a reservoir.
3. Transport immediately and in a safe, rapid manner.
4. Obtain IV access with large-bore catheters (16 gauge or greater). Consider intraosseous vascular access if the patient is critical and you are unable to establish an intravenous line.
5. Using normal saline, give a bolus of 20 mL/kg IV rapidly and then repeat the ITLS Ongoing Exam. If shock symptoms persist, continue to administer fluid in boluses and reassess. In some cases of very severe hemorrhage, because of the substantial loss of red blood cells and markedly impaired oxygen delivery to the tissues, shock symptoms and signs may persist despite hemorrhage control and IV volume infusion. These patients need the rapid transfusion of blood and/or blood products.

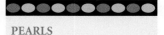

PEARLS

IV Access

Do not waste scene time to establish IV access. Consider the use of intraosseous vascular access if the patient is critical and you cannot obtain IV access.

6. Place the patient on an EKG monitor early during evaluation and treatment.

7. Apply pulse oximetry and, if available, waveform capnography.

8. Perform Ongoing Exams, and observe closely, especially for any return of bleeding.

Hemorrhage That Cannot Be Controlled

External Hemorrhage. A patient with external hemorrhage that is not controlled by direct pressure must be rapidly transported to an appropriate facility where necessary procedures to gain surgical hemostasis can be performed. Although most physicians advocate fluid resuscitation to treat hemorrhagic shock, you must also remember that elevating blood pressure can increase uncontrolled hemorrhage. To manage this patient, you should take the following steps.

PROCEDURE

✺ Managing Shock Due to Exsanguinating External Hemorrhage That You Cannot Control

1. Apply direct pressure on the bleeding site (e.g., femoral artery, facial hemorrhage). Substantial pressure may be required. Releasing of direct pressure may result in the continuation of bleeding.

2. Put the patient's body in a horizontal or slightly head-down position.

3. Apply tourniquets to a bleeding extremity only as a critical attempt to stop severe bleeding that cannot be otherwise controlled (discussed earlier).

4. If you cannot stop severe bleeding with pressure and cannot use a tourniquet (groin, axilla, neck, face, scalp), you should use one of the hemostatic agents such as QuikClot 1st Response or Celox (see Chapter 14). Pack the hemostatic agent in the wound and hold firm pressure.

5. Administer high-flow oxygen through a nonrebreather mask with a reservoir.

6. Transport immediately and in a rapid, safe manner.

7. Gain IV access when en route. Consider intraosseous vascular access if patient is critical and you are unable to establish an intravenous line.

   a. Give only enough normal saline to maintain a blood pressure high enough for adequate peripheral perfusion. Maintaining peripheral perfusion may be defined as producing a peripheral pulse (such as a radial pulse), maintaining consciousness (assuming a traumatic brain injury is not also present), and maintaining an "adequate blood pressure." The definition of an adequate blood pressure ("How low can you go?") remains controversial and will continue to be subject to change based upon ongoing research. Certainly most young patients can maintain adequate perfusion with a blood pressure of 80 to 90 mmHg systolic, but some experts now advocate even lower pressures. Keep in mind that a higher systolic pressure may be required in the setting of head injury with increased intracerebral pressure (see Chapter 10) and in patients with a history of hypertension. Rely on local medical direction for guidelines in this area.

   b. Early blood transfusion is the most important fluid replacement in severe cases.

   c. Finally, substantial research into the use of hypertonic saline for uncontrolled hemorrhage suggests promising evidence that small volumes of concentrated saline may support the vascular status of the bleeding patient by pulling interstitial fluid into the vascular space. It is unclear at this time whether hypertonic saline is safe for use via intraosseous access. Also, early work at this time indicates a potential role in the future for artificial blood products that carry oxygen to the tissues.

8. Monitor the heart, and apply pulse oximetry and waveform capnography (if available).

9. Perform ITLS Ongoing Exams, and observe closely.

NOTE: If assistance is not available, control of hemorrhage, even if minimal, should remain the priority. Other procedures become secondary if they interrupt attempts to maintain hemorrhage control. In the case of wounds with exsanguinating hemorrhage, the military has changed the initial assessment from ABC (airway, breathing, and circulation) to CAB, making control of the hemorrhage the first priority.

Internal Hemorrhage. The patient with uncontrolled internal hemorrhage is the classic critical trauma victim who will almost certainly die unless you promptly transport to an appropriate facility where rapid operative hemostasis can be obtained. The results of the most current medical research on the management of patients with exsanguinating internal hemorrhage is that there exists no substitute for gaining surgical control of bleeding. Recent work on the administration of IV fluids and the use of the PASG (pneumatic antishock garment) in shock patients with presumed internal hemorrhage suggests the following:

■ Use of the PASG in the setting of uncontrolled internal exsanguination due to penetrating injury may increase mortality, especially in the setting of intrathoracic hemorrhage. The PASG raises blood pressure, and raising blood pressure in the setting of bleeding vessels within the thorax, abdomen, and pelvis probably increases internal bleeding, raising the chance of death due to exsanguination.

■ Likewise, the use of large amounts of IV fluids in the setting of uncontrolled internal hemorrhage may also increase internal bleeding and mortality. IV fluids increase the blood pressure (like the PASG), but fluids may also dilute clotting factors. Furthermore, IV fluids carry almost no oxygen and are not a replacement for red blood cells. Early blood transfusion is very important in severe cases of hemorrhagic shock.

■ Any delay in providing rapid transport of such patients should not occur unless absolutely unavoidable, as in the case of a patient requiring prolonged extrication. Always document such circumstances carefully in the Patient Care Report.

■ Moribund trauma patients (ones in very deep shock with blood pressures under 50 mmHg systolic, i.e., nonpalpable pulses) usually die, but fluid administration may be indicated to maintain some degree of circulation. Treatment of this extreme amount of hemorrhage may override the concerns for increased hemorrhage secondary to the use of these interventions. However, this approach is still controversial. Local medical direction should guide such therapy pending further research.

The recommendations, therefore, for a patient with probable exsanguinating internal hemorrhage secondary to penetrating injuries are described below.

PROCEDURE

❇ Managing Shock Due to Internal Hemorrhage

1. Transport immediately and in a rapid, safe manner.

2. Put the patient's body in a horizontal or slightly head-down position.

3. Administer high-flow oxygen.

4. Gain IV access with large-bore catheters. Consider intraosseous vascular access if unable to establish an intravenous line.

5. Administer sufficient normal saline to maintain peripheral perfusion. Local medical direction should guide what is acceptable practice in this setting. Many experts now recommend that fluid resuscitation be kept to a minimum until hemorrhage control is obtained (operative intervention). Hemostatic agents cannot be used for internal hemorrhage. Again, substantial research into the use of hypertonic saline for uncontrolled hemorrhage suggests promising evidence that small volumes of concentrated saline may support the vascular status of the bleeding patient by pulling interstitial fluid into the vascular space. Research into the use of artificial blood products continues.

6. Monitor the heart, and apply pulse oximetry and waveform capnography (where available).

7. Perform ITLS Ongoing Exams, and observe closely.

Current published research has not yet adequately addressed the treatment of the patient with presumed internal hemorrhage in the setting of blunt injuries (MVCs, falls, and so on). This creates a dilemma because many patients with blunt injuries can lose a significant amount of blood and fluid from the intravascular space into the sites of large-bone fractures (hematoma and edema). This loss can be enough to cause shock, and yet the blood loss from these fractures is usually self-limited, with the exception of pelvic fractures. Pelvic fractures can result in exsanguination and death. In theory, this situation should be treated with oxygen and intravascular volume expansion (IV fluids).

However, if the blunt injury patient has a tear of a large internal blood vessel or a laceration or avulsion of an internal organ, raising the blood pressure prior to surgical intervention may also result in accelerated bleeding or a secondary hemorrhage. Therefore, if an internal hemorrhage is not suspected (patient is alert and oriented and has no apparent chest, abdominal, or pelvic injuries), fluids may be used judiciously for fractures and externally controlled hemorrhage. In the case of a severe mechanism of injury and/or inability to assess the patient, use fluids judiciously. Administer enough fluids to maintain peripheral perfusion. Remember that early blood transfusion, when available, is the most appropriate fluid replacement of severe blood loss. Frequent patient assessments and local EMS medical direction should guide therapy.

Special Situations in Hypovolemic Shock

Head Injury: The patient with severe head injury (Glasgow Coma Scale score of 8 or less) and shock is a special situation (see Chapter 10). These patients do not tolerate hypotension. Therefore, if necessary, adults with suspected hemorrhagic shock in addition to head injury should be fluid resuscitated to a blood pressure of 120 mmHg systolic to maintain a cerebral perfusion pressure of at least 60 mmHg.

Nonhemorrhagic Hypovolemic Shock: The patient who has low-volume shock syndrome not due to hemorrhage can generally be managed in the same manner as a patient with shock due to bleeding that can be controlled. An example of this type of patient would be one with shock due to fluid loss from burns or severe diarrhea. Low-volume shock is the usual cause of death in these patients. Since the loss of volume in this case is not from an injured vascular system, it is reasonable to treat such patients with aggressive volume replacement to restore vital signs toward normal. Just beware: Hemorrhagic shock due to a bleeding internal organ (such as a bleeding ulcer or a ruptured ectopic pregnancy) may be rapidly lethal, and the bleeding may not be at all apparent from the physical examination. So, if you see signs of shock present, follow the basic rules of shock management until you have explained the cause. For example, an unconscious, pale young woman of childbearing age is bleeding to death from a ruptured ectopic pregnancy until proved otherwise.

Treatment of Nonhemorrhagic Shock Syndromes

Treatments for the other shock syndromes, namely, mechanical (cardiogenic) and high-space (relative hypovolemia) are somewhat different. All patients require high-flow oxygen, rapid transport, shock positioning, and IV line placement (usually en route).

Mechanical Shock: The patient with mechanical shock must first be accurately assessed to determine the cause of the problem. The patient with tension pneumothorax needs prompt decompression of the elevated pleural pressure. (See Chapter 7 for indications and procedure for decompression.)

The patient with suspected pericardial tamponade must be rapidly transported to an appropriate facility, because the time from onset of tamponade to the time of cardiac arrest can be a matter of minutes. While anecdotal support exists in the literature for use of an intravenous volume challenge in such patients as a temporizing measure, no clear evidence exists that such treatment will improve survival. Use of IV fluids in this situation should be during transport and only on the order of medical direction. Obtaining IV access certainly should not delay direct transport or airway/oxygen interventions. Consider intraosseous vascular access if unable to establish an intravenous line. Bear in mind that trauma is not the only cause of tamponade. Metastatic cancer and other diseases resulting in pericardial effusion may also cause tamponade.

Myocardial contusion rarely causes shock. Recent reports indicate that most contusions cause little or no clinical findings. However, severe contusion may cause acute heart failure, manifested by distended neck veins, tachycardia, cyanosis, and possibly arrhythmias. These are the same signs seen with pericardial tamponade. These patients require rapid transport for proper care. Give high-flow oxygen and perform cardiac monitoring on the patient with suspected myocardial contusion. IV fluids may cause worsening of the patient's condition.

High-Space Shock: High-space shock, in theory, resembles controlled hemorrhage, in that there is relative hypovolemia with an "intact" vascular system (no "leaks"). Therefore, initial management includes IV fluid boluses. Consider intraosseous vascular access if the patient is critical and you are unable to establish an intravenous line.

In the absence of a head injury, the patient's level of consciousness is a useful monitor of the success or failure of resuscitation. Be alert for possible occult internal injuries, and keep in mind that raising the blood pressure may increase internal bleeding in that situation. An argument can be made for the use of vasopressors in patients with vasodilatory shock, such as in calcium channel blocker overdose or sepsis.

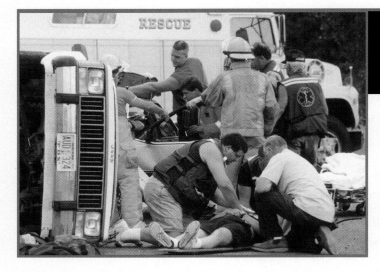

(Photograph © Craig Jackson/
In the Dark Photography)

Dan, Joyce, and Buddy of the Emergency Transport System have been called to the scene of a single vehicle, high-speed, side-impact auto collision. They are informed that a rescue truck is on-scene and attempting to extricate the driver. While driving to the scene, they decide that Buddy will act as team leader on this call.

On arrival Buddy gets the trauma box and cervical collars and begins the Scene Size-up. Dan gets the oxygen and airway equipment and Joyce gets the backboard. Buddy notes that the police are on-scene and they signal that the scene is safe. The team dons personal protective equipment, and each carries his or her part of the essential equipment as they approach.

The driver of the car had lost control on a wet road and hydroplaned. The car rolled over several times and then side-impacted a tree, finally coming to rest on its left side. The driver has been extricated but is dead on-scene. The restrained front-seat passenger is alert and oriented but complains of chest and abdominal pain. After extrication, Buddy's Rapid Trauma Assessment reveals facial lacerations but an open airway, tender lower ribs (no crepitation) on the right with a tender abdomen. He also has deformity and instability of the right thigh. Breath sounds are present and equal and the pelvis is stable and nontender. The patient has a strong regular pulse and a normal respiratory rate with good air movement. Because of the tender abdomen, they quickly package the patient and immediately load and go. In the ambulance the vital signs are pulse 110, respiration 22, BP 120/90. The patient states he has no allergies, takes no medications, and has always been healthy. Last food was about 4 hours ago.

After applying a traction splint to the right leg, Dan starts two large-bore IVs of normal saline at a KVO (keep vein open) rate. Buddy calls his on-line medical direction (OLMD) and reports that he is transporting a patient who has been in a high-speed MVC in which the driver was killed. He suspects that the patient has rib fractures, intra-abdominal injuries, and a fractured femur. OLMD instructs them to limit IV fluids unless the patient becomes hypotensive and then only give enough to maintain systolic BP of 90 mmHg. They are to transport the patient to the local level-one trauma center. OLMD also instructs the team to monitor waveform capnography, and the current reading on exhalation is 40 mmHg.

The ITLS Ongoing Exam performed 5 minutes later reveals that the patient's condition has changed. The pulse has increased to 140, the blood pressure has dropped to 70/40 with an absent radial pulse, and the waveform capnography is now 25 on exhalation. The abdomen has become distended and rigid. The lungs are still clear. Buddy gives 250-cc boluses of normal saline until the systolic blood pressure is 90 mmHg and a radial pulse returns. The trauma team is mobilized and waiting when they arrive. The patient is found to have a fractured right femur and a lacerated liver, but no other major injuries. His liver laceration is repaired and he receives six units of blood, but recovers uneventfully.

The mechanism of injury in this scenario is both rollover and lateral impact, with the driver receiving the brunt of the forces from the lateral impact. The driver died from major chest injuries. The passenger received serious injuries but was saved because he was restrained. Though his vital signs were good when EMS arrived, they recognized the tender abdomen was suggestive of internal injuries and were prepared for the development of hemorrhagic shock. IV fluids were given to maintain perfusion to vital organs but they did not try to raise the blood pressure to normal levels because of the danger of increasing intra-abdominal bleeding. The fractured femur was also a factor here, as there is usually a loss of one or two units of blood into the soft tissue of the thigh after a femur fracture. Falling waveform capnography provided additional verification of the patient's worsening shock state.

SUMMARY

A patient with shock must be diagnosed early. The early signs and symptoms of shock may be subtle, and when the later signs such as hypotension develop, the patient may be near death. The importance of careful assessment and reassessment cannot be overemphasized. You must understand the risk of any of the shock states to your patient. Further, you need to study and memorize the shock syndromes, especially in regard to the rapid provision of the proper treatment for such conditions as internal hemorrhage, pericardial tamponade, and tension pneumothorax. Finally, you should be aware of the controversy on the use of IV fluid resuscitation for cases of uncontrolled hemorrhage. Rely on your local medical direction to help keep you current on the standard of care in these areas.

BIBLIOGRAPHY

1. Bickell, W. H., M. J. Wall, P. E. Pepe, et al. 1994. Immediate versus delayed fluid resuscitation for hypotensive patients with penetrating torso injury. *New England Journal of Medicine* 331 (October): 1105–9.
2. Champion, H. 2003. Combat fluid resuscitation. *Supplement to the Journal of Trauma* 54.
3. Chiara, O., P. Pelosi, L. Brazzi, et al. 2003. Resuscitation from hemorrhagic shock: Experimental model comparing normal saline, dextran, and hypertonic saline solutions. *Critical Care Medicine* 31: 1915–22.
4. Demetriades, D., L. S. Chan, P. Bhasin, et al. 1998. Relative bradycardia in patients with traumatic hypotension. *Journal of Trauma* 45(3): 534–39.
5. Kowalenko, T., S. Stern, S. Dronen, X. Wang. 1992. Improved outcome with hypotensive resuscitation of uncontrolled hemorrhagic shock in a swine mode. *Journal of Trauma* 33: 349–53.
6. Mapstone, J., I. Roberts, P. Evans. 2003. Fluid resuscitation strategies: A systematic review of animal trials. *Journal of Trauma* 55: 571–91.
7. Mattox, K. L., W. H. Bickell, P. Pepe, et al. 1989. Prospective MAST study in 911 patients. *Journal of Trauma* 29: 1104–12.
8. Moore, E. 2003. Blood substitutes: The future is now. *Journal of the American College of Surgeons* 196: 1–16.
9. Schriger, D. L., L. J. Baraff. 1991. Capillary refill—Is it a useful predictor of hypovolemic states? *Annals of Emergency Medicine* 20: 601–5.

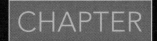

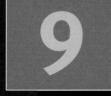

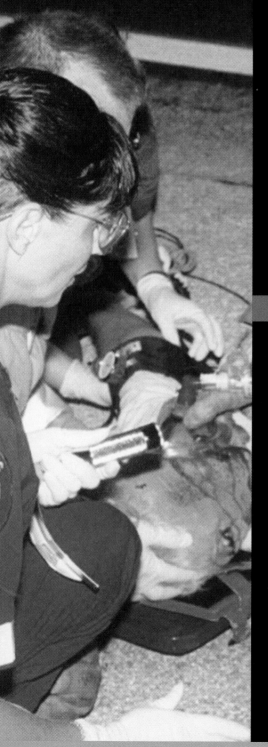

Fluid Resuscitation Skills

Donna Hastings, EMT-P

OBJECTIVES

Upon completion of this chapter, you should be able to:

1. Perform the technique of cannulation of the external jugular vein.
2. Recite indications for the use of intraosseous infusion.
3. Perform intraosseous infusion.
4. Use length-based resuscitation tape to estimate the weight of a child.

All students of this course are expected to be familiar with the technique of inserting an IV cannula in the veins of the lower arm or antecubital space; thus these sites will not be discussed here.

CANNULATION OF THE EXTERNAL JUGULAR VEIN

The external jugular vein runs in a line from the angle of the jaw to the junction of the medial and middle third of the clavicle (Figure 9-1). This vein is usually easily visible through the skin; pressing on it just above the clavicle will make it more prominent. It runs into the subclavian vein.

Indication for cannulation of the external jugular vein is the pediatric or adult patient who needs IV access and in whom no suitable peripheral vein is found.

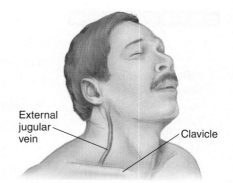

FIGURE 9-1 Anatomy of the external jugular vein.

PROCEDURE
❄ Performing External Jugular Cannulation

1. The patient must be in the supine position, preferably head down, to distend the vein and to prevent air embolism.

2. If no suspicion of cervical-spine injury exists, turn the patient's head to the opposite side. If there is a danger of cervical-spine injury, one rescuer must stabilize the head (it must not be turned) while the IV is being started. The cervical collar should be opened or the front removed during the procedure.

3. Quickly prepare the skin with an antiseptic and then align the cannula with the vein. The needle will be pointing at the clavicle at the junction of the middle and medial thirds.

4. With one finger, press on the vein just above the clavicle. This should make the vein more prominent.

5. Insert the needle into the vein at about the midportion and cannulate in the usual way.

6. If not already done, draw a 30 cc sample of blood and store it in the appropriate tubes.

7. Tape down the line securely. If there is danger of cervical-spine injury, a cervical collar can be applied over the IV site.

INTRAOSSEOUS INFUSION

The technique of bone marrow infusion of fluid and drugs is not new. It was first described in 1922 and was used commonly in the 1930s and 1940s as an alternative to IV infusion of crystalloids, drugs, and blood. The technique was "rediscovered" in the 1980s, and studies have confirmed it to be a fast, safe, and effective route to infuse medications, fluids, and blood. Intraosseous (IO) infusion can be used for giving medications in both adults and children, but because the flow rate is not as rapid as peripheral venous infusions, it cannot be used for rapid volume replacement in adults. Newer techniques for IO insertion may prove to offer adequate flow rates for adult volume resuscitation. Intraosseous infusion has the advantage of being quick and simple to perform while providing a stable (anchored in bone) access that is not easily dislodged during transport.

Indications

Indications for the use of intraosseous infusion include the pediatric or adult patient who is in cardiac arrest and in whom you cannot quickly obtain peripheral venous access, and the hypovolemic pediatric patient who has a prolonged transport (you do not need an IV if the transport is short) and in whom you are unable to quickly obtain peripheral venous access.

Potential Complications

Studies have shown that the following complications are rare. However, good aseptic technique is important, just as it is with IV therapy. Potential complications of IO infusion include:

- Subperiosteal infusion due to improper placement
- Osteomyelitis
- Sepsis
- Fat embolism
- Marrow damage
- Tibial fracture if needle is too large

PROCEDURE

✴ Performing Intraosseous Infusion in a Child

(See Appendix A for the technique of adult IO.)

1. Determine the need for this procedure; obtain permission from medical direction if required.
2. Have all needed equipment ready prior to bone penetration.
   a. 16–18 gauge intraosseous needles
   b. 10 cc syringe
   c. Antiseptic solution to prep the skin
   d. IV tubing and IV fluids
   e. Tape and dressing material to secure the IO needle
   f. BP cuff or commercial pressure device to infuse fluid under pressure
3. Identify the site, which is proximal tibia, one fingerbreadth below the tibial tuberosity either midline or slightly medial to the midline (Figure 9-2).
4. Prep the skin with an appropriate antiseptic (very important).
5. Obtain the proper needle. The needle must have a stylet so that it does not become plugged with bone. While 13-, 18-, and 20-gauge spinal needles will work, they are difficult and uncomfortable to grip during the insertion process. Long spinal needles tend to bend easily, so if you use spinal needles, try to obtain the short ones. The preferred needle is a 14- to 18-gauge intraosseous needle, but bone marrow needles can also be used.
6. Using aseptic technique, insert the needle into the bone marrow cavity. Insert the needle perpendicular to the skin, directed away from the epiphyseal plate (Figure 9-2), and advance to the periosteum. Penetrate the bone with a slow boring or twisting motion until you feel a sudden "give" (decrease in resistance) as the needle enters the marrow cavity. This can be confirmed by removing the stylet and aspirating blood and bone marrow (Figures 9-3 and 9-4).
7. Attach standard IV tubing and infuse fluid and/or medications (Figure 9-5). You may have to infuse fluid

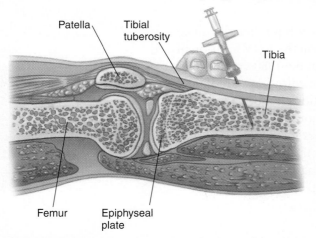
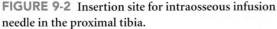

FIGURE 9-2 Insertion site for intraosseous infusion needle in the proximal tibia.

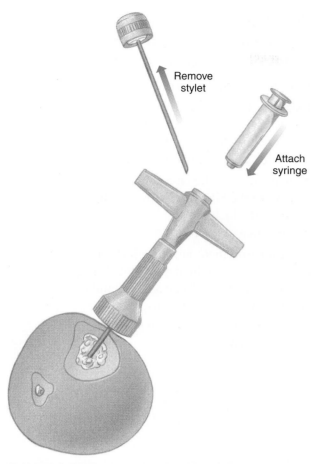

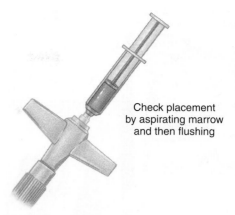

FIGURE 9-4 To check needle placement, aspirate approximately 1 cc of bone marrow.

FIGURE 9-3 Remove stylet from the needle and attach syringe.

under pressure (BP cuff blown up around IV bag) to obtain an adequate infusion rate.

8. Tape the tubing to the skin and secure the bone marrow needles as if to secure an impaled object (gauze pads taped around the insertion site).

LENGTH-BASED RESUSCITATION TAPES

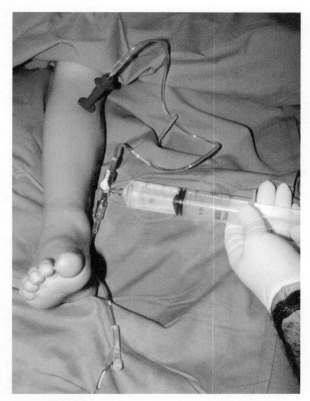

FIGURE 9-5 Intraosseous needle in child's tibia being used for fluid infusion. *(Photo courtesy of Bob Page, NREMT-P)*

Calculation of the volume of fluid resuscitation or the dose of an IV medication for the pediatric patient depends on the patient's weight. In an emergency situation the age and weight of a child may not be known. The weight of a child is directly related to his length, and resuscitation tapes (Broselow tape or SPARC system) have been developed that estimate a child's weight by measuring his length. These tapes contain precalculated doses of IV fluids and emergency drugs for each weight range (Figure 9-6). They also include the correct sizes of emergency equipment and supplies for each weight range.

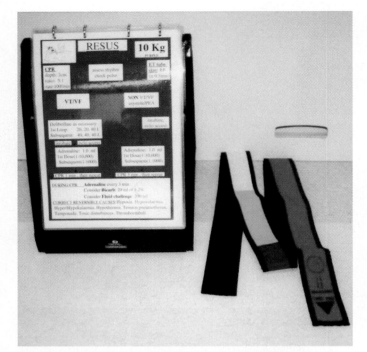

FIGURE 9-6 SPARC system has color-coded tape and booklet of precalculated doses of fluids and medications. *(Photo courtesy of Kyee Han, MD)*

PROCEDURE

❈ Estimating a Child's Weight with a Length-Based Resuscitation Tape

1. Place the patient in the supine position.

2. Using the tape, measure the patient from the crown to the heel. Place the red end with an arrow at the crown of the child's head, and stretch the tape to the child's heel (see Figure 9-7).

3. Note the box on the tape at which the child's heel falls. With the SPARC system, match the color of the tape at which the child's heel falls with the same colored area of the booklet.

4. If the measurement falls on a line, the box or colored panel proximal to the line is used to generate the fluid and drug doses and the size of equipment needed for resuscitation.

5. The tape may be disinfected if it becomes contaminated.

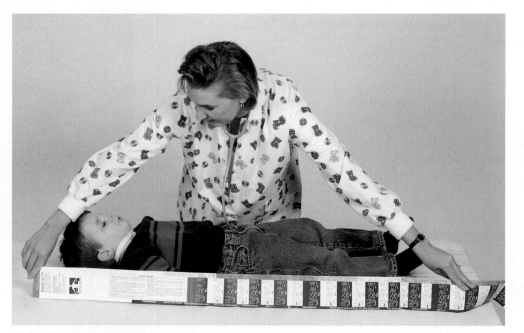

FIGURE 9-7 Measure the patient from crown to heel to read precalculated doses of fluids and medications.

Head Trauma

Roy L. Alson, PhD, MD, FACEP
John E. Campbell, MD, FACEP

OBJECTIVES

Upon completion of this chapter, you should be able to:

1. Describe the anatomy of the head and brain.
2. Describe the pathophysiology of traumatic brain injury.
3. Explain the difference between primary and secondary brain injury.
4. Describe the mechanisms for the development of secondary brain injury.
5. Describe the assessment of the patient with a head injury.
6. Describe the prehospital management of the patient with a head injury.
7. Recognize and describe the management of the cerebral herniation syndrome.
8. Identify potential problems in the management of the patient with a head injury.

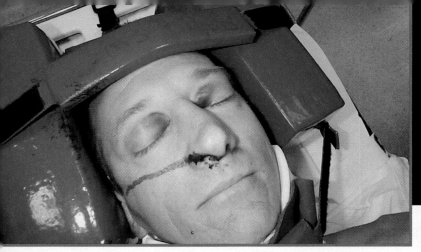

(Photo courtesy of
Roy Alson, MD)

Joyce, Dan, and Buddy have been dispatched to a private home where a man has fallen off of a ladder. As they respond, they decide that Joyce will be team leader. When they arrive, they find a small group of people huddled around a 40-year-old man who was taking down Christmas decorations and slipped off the ladder, landing on his head. The scene is safe and he is the only patient. His fall was witnessed by his wife who, with tears in her eyes (she insisted that he remove the decorations that day), says that when his foot slipped, it caught in the rung of the ladder and he swung like a pendulum, striking his head on the concrete driveway. He was unconscious for a few minutes and she was sure that he was dead. Now he cannot remember going up the ladder at all. She says he is in good health, takes no medications, and has no allergies. She prepared him lunch (hamburgers) about 2 hours ago. He complains of a headache and nausea and says his neck hurts. *What injuries would you suspect from a mechanism such as this?* Keep this question in mind as you read the chapter. Then, at the end of the chapter, find out how the rescuers completed this call.

INTRODUCTION

Head injuries or, more specifically, traumatic brain injury (TBI) is a major cause of death and disability in multiple trauma patients. Forty percent of multisystem trauma patients have a central nervous system (CNS) injury. These patients have a death rate twice as high (35 percent versus 17 percent) as that of patients without CNS injuries. Head injuries account for an estimated 25 percent of all trauma deaths and up to one-half of all motor-vehicle fatalities. Worldwide, the cost of TBI is staggering, in terms of lives lost, families destroyed, and money spent for care. Prevention remains the most effective treatment. You can help reduce this major epidemic by encouraging the use of helmets and restraint devices in vehicles.

You may be called upon to manage head injuries that can range from the trivial to the immediately life threatening. By recognizing those injuries that need immediate intervention and providing transport to the appropriate facility, you can significantly improve the chances for a patient having a good outcome. Because it is not possible to perform a field clearance of the cervical spine in a patient with altered mental status and because head injury often results in the alteration of consciousness, you must always assume that a serious head injury is accompanied by an injury to the cervical spine and spinal cord.

Beginning with the third edition of this text, material included in this chapter has been based upon the recommendations of the Brain Trauma Foundation (a multidisciplinary organization dedicated to improving care of TBI victims by use of evidence-based treatment).

ANATOMY OF THE HEAD

To most effectively manage the head-injured patient, you should have a working knowledge of the basic anatomy and physiology of the head and brain. The head (excluding the face and facial structures) includes the following (see Figure 10-1):

- Scalp
- Skull
- Fibrous coverings of the brain (meninges: dura mater, arachnoid mater, pia mater)
- Brain tissue
- Cerebrospinal fluid
- Vascular compartments

The scalp is a protective covering for the skull, but it is very vascular and bleeds freely when lacerated. The skull is a closed box; the rigid and unyielding bony skull protects the brain from injury. It also contributes to several injury mechanisms in head trauma. Just like the ankle, which swells when twisted, the brain, when injured, swells. The only significant opening through which the pressure can be released is the foramen magnum at the base, where the brain stem becomes the spinal cord. Because the brain "floats" inside the cerebrospinal fluid and is anchored at its base, there is greater movement at the top of the brain than at the base. On impact, the brain is able to move within the skull and can strike bony prominences within the cranial cavity. This is the "third collision" described in mechanisms of injury in Chapter 1. The temporal bone (temple) is quite thin and easily fractured as are portions of the base of the skull. The fibrous coverings of the brain include the dura mater ("tough mother"), which covers the entire brain; the thinner pia arachnoid

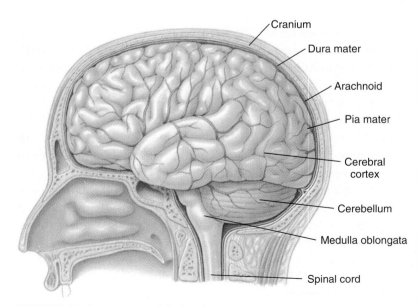

FIGURE 10-1 Anatomy of the head.

(called simply the *arachnoid*), which lies underneath the dura and in which are suspended both arteries and veins; and the very thin pia mater ("soft mother"), which lies underneath the arachnoid and is adherent to the surface of the brain. The cerebrospinal fluid (CSF) is found beneath the arachnoid and pia mater.

The intracranial volume is composed of the brain, the CSF, and the blood in the blood vessels. These three completely fill the cranial cavity. Thus the increase of any one of these is at the expense of the other two. This is of great importance in the pathophysiology of head trauma. Following injury, the brain, like all injured tissue, will swell. Because of the fixed space, as the tissue swells and the volume of fluid inside the skull increases, so does the pressure.

Cerebrospinal fluid (also called *spinal fluid*) is a nutrient fluid that bathes the brain and spinal cord. Spinal fluid is continually created within the ventricles of the brain at a rate of 0.33 mL/min. It is reabsorbed by the arachnoid membrane that covers the brain and spinal cord. Anything obstructing the flow of spinal fluid will cause an accumulation of spinal fluid within the brain (hydrocephalus) and an increase in intracerebral pressure (ICP).

PATHOPHYSIOLOGY OF HEAD TRAUMA
Primary and Secondary Brain Injuries

Head injuries are either open or closed, depending on whether the object responsible for the injury compromised the skull and exposed the brain. Brain injury can also be divided into two components, primary and secondary.

Primary brain injury is the immediate damage to the brain tissue that is the direct result of the injury force and is essentially fixed at the time of injury. Management of primary brain injury is best directed at prevention with such measures as better occupant restraint systems in autos, the use of helmets in sports and cycling, firearms education, and so forth.

While penetrating wounds to the brain always cause primary injury, most primary injuries occur either as a result of external forces applied against the exterior of the skull or from movement of the brain inside the skull. In deceleration injuries the head usually strikes an object such as the windshield of an automobile, which causes a sudden deceleration of the skull. The brain continues to move forward, impacting first against the skull in the original direction of motion and then rebounding to hit the opposite side of the inner surface of the skull (a "fourth" collision). Thus, injuries may occur to the brain in the area of original impact ("coup") or on the opposite side ("contracoup"). The interior base of the skull is rough (Figure 10-2), and movement of the brain over this area may cause various degrees of injury to the brain tissue or to blood vessels supporting the brain.

Good prehospital care can help prevent the development of secondary brain injury. Secondary brain injury is the result of hypoxia or decreased perfusion of brain tissue. Secondary injury is the result of the brain's response to the primary injury, with swelling causing a decrease in perfusion, or from complications of other injuries (hypoxia or hypotension). The initial response of the injured brain is to swell. Bruising or injury causes vasodilatation with increased blood flow to the injured area, and thus an accumulation of blood that takes up space and exerts pressure

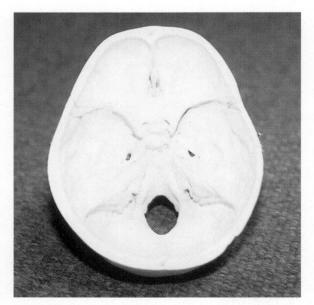

FIGURE 10-2 The rough inner base of the skull.

on surrounding brain tissue. There is no extra space inside the skull. Swelling of the injured area increases intracerebral pressure and eventually decreases blood flow to the brain that causes further brain injury. The increase in cerebral water (edema) does not occur immediately, but develops over hours. Early efforts to maintain perfusion of the brain can be life-saving.

The brain normally adjusts its own blood flow in response to metabolic needs. The autoregulation of blood flow is adjusted based on the level of carbon dioxide (CO_2) in the blood. The normal level of CO_2 is 35 to 40 mmHg. An increase in the level of CO_2 (hypoventilation) promotes cerebral vasodilatation and increases ICP, while lowering the level of CO_2 (hyperventilation) causes vasoconstriction and decreases blood flow. In the past, it was thought that hyperventilation (lowering of CO_2) in the head-injured patient would decrease brain swelling and thus improve cerebral blood flow. Research has shown that hyperventilation actually has only a slight effect on brain swelling, but causes a significant decrease in cerebral perfusion from vasoconstriction, which results in cerebral hypoxia. The injured brain does not tolerate hypoxia. Thus, both hyperventilation and hypoventilation can cause cerebral ischemia and increased mortality in the TBI patient. Maintaining good ventilation (not hyperventilation) at a rate of about one breath every 6 to 8 seconds (8 to 10 per minute) with high-flow oxygen is very important. Prophylactic hyperventilation for head injury is no longer recommended.

PEARLS
Hypoxia and Hypotension

- Patients with serious head injuries cannot tolerate hypoxia or hypotension. Give high-flow oxygen and monitor oxygenation with a pulse oximeter.

- Usually pediatric patients have a better recovery from TBI. If an adult and a child have the same injury, the child has a much better chance of recovery. However, hypoxia and hypotension appear to eliminate any neuroprotective mechanism normally afforded by age. If the child with a serious brain injury is allowed to become hypoxic or hypotensive, the chance of recovery is even worse than an adult with the same injury.

INTRACRANIAL PRESSURE

Within the skull and fibrous coverings of the brain are the brain tissue, cerebrospinal fluid, and blood. An increase in the volume of any one of these components must be at the expense of the other two because the adult skull (a rigid box) cannot expand. Although there is some give to the volume of cerebrospinal fluid, it accounts for little space and cannot offset rapid brain swelling. Blood supply cannot be compromised, for the brain requires a constant supply of blood (oxygen and glucose) to survive. Thus, since none of the supporting components of the brain can be compromised, brain swelling can be rapidly catastrophic.

The pressure of the brain and contents within the skull is termed *intracranial pressure (ICP)*. This pressure is usually very low. Intracranial pressure is considered dangerous when it rises above 15 mmHg; cerebral herniation may occur at pressures above 25 mmHg. The pressure of the blood flowing through the brain is termed the *cerebral perfusion pressure (CPP)*. Its value is obtained by subtracting the intracranial (intracerebral) pressure from the mean arterial blood pressure (MAP).

$$MAP = Diastolic\ BP + 1/3\ (Systolic\ BP - Diastolic\ BP)$$

$$CPP = MAP - ICP$$

If the brain swells or if bleeding occurs inside the skull, ICP increases and the perfusion pressure decreases, resulting in cerebral ischemia (hypoxia). If the swelling of the brain is severe enough, the ICP equals the MAP and blood flow to the brain ceases. The body has a protective reflex (Cushing's response or reflex) that attempts to maintain a constant perfusion pressure. When the ICP increases, the systemic blood pressure increases to try to preserve blood flow to the brain. The body senses the rise in systemic blood pressure and this triggers a drop in the pulse rate as the body tries to lower the blood pressure. With severe injury and/or ischemia, the pressure within the skull continues in an upward spiral until a critical point at which the ICP approaches the MAP and there is no cerebral perfusion. All vital signs deteriorate, and the patient dies. Because CPP depends on both the arterial pressure and the ICP, hypotension will also have a devastating effect if the ICP is high.

As stated above, the injured brain loses the ability to autoregulate blood flow. In this situation perfusion of the brain is directly dependent on the CPP. You must maintain a cerebral perfusion pressure of at least 60 mmHg (see earlier formula), which requires maintaining a systolic blood pressure of at least 110 to 120 mmHg in the patient with a severe head injury. This will rarely be a problem, as hypotension only occurs in about 5 percent of patients with severe TBI (GCS of < 9). Aggressive attempts to maintain CPP above 70 mmHg with fluids and pressors (dopamine, epinephrine) should be avoided because of the risk of adult respiratory distress syndrome (ARDS).

Cerebral Herniation Syndrome

When the brain swells, particularly after a blow to the head, a sudden rise in ICP may occur. This may force portions of the brain downward, obstructing the flow of cerebrospinal fluid and applying great pressure to the brain stem. The classic findings on exam, in this life-threatening situation, are a decreasing level of consciousness (LOC) that rapidly progresses to coma, dilation of the pupil and an outward–downward deviation of the eye on the side of the injury, paralysis of the arm and leg on the side opposite the injury, or decerebrate posturing (arms and legs extended). As the cerebral herniation is occurring, the vital signs frequently reveal increased blood pressure and bradycardia (Cushing's response). The patient may soon cease all movement, stop breathing, and die. This syndrome often follows an acute epidural or subdural hemorrhage.

If these signs are developing in a head-injury patient, cerebral herniation is imminent and aggressive therapy is needed. As noted earlier, hyperventilation will decrease the size of the blood vessels in the brain and briefly decrease ICP. In this situation the danger of immediate herniation outweighs the risk of cerebral ischemia that can follow hyperventilation. The cerebral herniation syndrome is the only situation in which hyperventilation is still indicated. (You must ventilate every 3 seconds [20/min] for adults, every 2½ seconds [25/min] for children, and every 2 seconds [30/min] for infants.)

To simplify knowing when to hyperventilate in the field, the clinical signs of cerebral herniation in the patient who has had hypoxemia and hypotension corrected are any one (or more) of the following:

- TBI patient with a GCS < 9 with extensor posturing (decerebrate posturing)
- TBI patient with a GCS < 9 with asymmetric (or bilateral), dilated, or nonreactive pupils
- TBI patient with an initial GCS < 9 who then drops his or her GCS by more than 2 points

For the above, "asymmetric pupils" means 1 mm (or more) difference in the size of one pupil, "fixed" means no response (< 1 mm) to bright light. Bilateral dilated and fixed pupils usually are a sign of brain stem injury and are associated with 91 percent mortality. A unilateral dilated and fixed pupil has been associated with good recovery in up to 54 percent

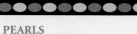

PEARLS
Brain Injury

A patient who, after correction of hypoxia and hypotension, shows rapid progression of brain injury (e.g., unresponsive with dilated pupil; decerebrate posturing; or drop in GCS score of >2 with an initial GCS score of < 9) should be transported rapidly to a trauma center capable of managing severe TBI patients. This is the only situation in which hyperventilation is still indicated (see Table 10-1). Hyperventilation, while known to cause ischemia, may decrease brain swelling temporarily. Although a desperate measure, this might buy enough time to get the patient to surgery that might be life-saving. Radio ahead so that a neurosurgeon can be available and the operating room prepared by the time you arrive at the hospital.

	TABLE 10-1 *Normal Ventilation Rates and Hyperventilation Rates*		
Age Group	**Normal Ventilation Rate**	**Hyperventilation Rate**
Adult	8–10 breaths/minute	20 breaths/minute
Children	15 breaths/minute	25 breaths/minute
Infants	20 breaths/minute	30 breaths/minute

of patients. Remember that hypoxemia, orbital trauma, drugs, lightning strike, and hypothermia also affect pupillary reaction, so take this into account before beginning hyperventilation. Flaccid paralysis usually means spinal injury. If the patient has signs of herniation as listed above and the signs resolve with hyperventilation, you should discontinue the hyperventilation.

HEAD INJURIES

Scalp Wounds

The scalp is highly vascular and often bleeds briskly when lacerated. Because many of the small blood vessels are suspended in an inelastic matrix of supporting tissue, the normal protective vasospasm that would limit bleeding is inhibited, which may lead to prolonged bleeding and significant blood loss. This can be very important in children who bleed as freely as adults but do not have the same blood volume. Though an uncommon cause of shock in an adult, a child may develop shock from a briskly bleeding scalp wound. As a general rule, if you have an adult patient with a scalp injury who is in shock, look for another cause for the shock (such as internal bleeding). However, do not underestimate the blood loss from a scalp wound. Most bleeding from the scalp can be easily controlled in the field with direct pressure if your exam reveals no unstable fractures under the wound.

PEARLS
Shock
Any unexplained shock in a patient with head injury is hypovolemic until proven otherwise. Treat hypotension.

Skull Injuries

Skull injuries can be linear nondisplaced fractures, depressed fractures, or compound fractures (Figure 10-3). Suspect an underlying skull fracture in adults who have a large contusion or darkened swelling of the scalp. There is very little that can be done for skull fractures in the field except to avoid placing direct pressure upon an obvious depressed or compound skull fracture. The real concern is forces that can cause a skull fracture can also cause a brain injury. Treat the brain injury with adequate oxygenation and maintain perfusion. Open skull fractures should have the wound dressed, but avoid excess pressure when controlling bleeding. Penetrating objects in the skull should be secured in place (not removed) and the patient transported immediately. If your patient has a gunshot wound to the head, unless there is a clear entrance and exit wound in a perfectly linear path, assume that the bullet may have ricocheted and is lodged in the neck near the spinal cord.

You should consider child abuse when you find a child with a head injury and no clear explanation of the cause. Suspect possible abuse if the story about the injury is inconsistent with the injury or the responsible adult suggests the child performed an activity that a child of this age is not physically capable of performing. Pay particular attention to the setting from which you rescued the child. Request police or social service assistance if the circumstances are suspicious for child abuse.

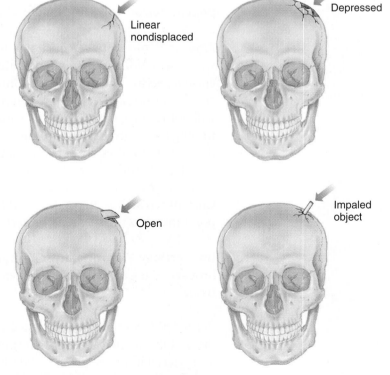

FIGURE 10-3 Types of skull fractures.

Brain Injuries

Concussion: A concussion implies no structural injury to the brain that can be demonstrated by current imaging techniques. There is a brief disruption of neural function that often results in loss of consciousness, but many people will have a concussion without a loss of consciousness. Classically there is a history of trauma to the head with a variable period of unconsciousness or confusion and then a return to normal consciousness. There may be amnesia following the injury. This amnesia usually extends to some point before the injury (retrograde short-term amnesia), so often the patient will not remember the events leading to the injury. Short-term memory is often affected, and the patient may repeat questions over and over as if he hasn't been paying attention to your answers. Patients may also report dizziness, headache, ringing in the ears, and/or nausea.

Cerebral Contusion: A patient with cerebral contusion (bruised brain tissue) will have a history of prolonged unconsciousness or serious alteration in level of consciousness (e.g., profound confusion, persistent amnesia, abnormal behavior). Brain swelling may be rapid and severe. The patient may have focal neurological signs (weakness, speech problems) and appear to have suffered a cerebrovascular accident (stroke). Depending upon the location of the cerebral contusion, the patient may have personality changes such as inappropriately rude behavior or agitation.

Subarachnoid Hemorrhage: Blood can enter the subarachnoid space as a result either of trauma or a spontaneous hemorrhage. The subarachnoid blood causes irritation that results in intravascular fluid "leaking" into the brain and causing more edema. Severe headache, coma, and vomiting from the irritation are common. These patients may have so much brain swelling that they develop the cerebral herniation syndrome.

Diffuse Axonal Injury: A diffuse axonal injury is the most common type of injury as a result of severe blunt head trauma. The brain is injured so diffusely that there is generalized edema. Usually, there is no evidence of a structural lesion. In most cases the patient presents unconscious, without focal deficits.

Anoxic Brain Injury: Injuries to the brain from lack of oxygen (e.g., cardiac arrest, airway obstruction, near-drowning) affect the brain in a serious fashion. Following an anoxic episode, perfusion of the cortex is interrupted because of spasm that develops in the small cerebral arteries. After 4 to 6 minutes of anoxia, restoring oxygenation and blood pressure will not restore perfusion of the cortex (no-reflow phenomenon), and there will be continuing anoxic injury to the brain cells. If the brain is without oxygen for a period greater than 4 to 6 minutes, irreversible damage almost always occurs.

Hypothermia seems to protect against this phenomenon, and there have been reported cases of hypothermic patients being resuscitated after almost an hour of anoxia. Current research is directed toward finding medications that either reverse the persistent postanoxic arterial spasm or protect against the anoxic injury to the cells.

Intracranial Hemorrhage: Hemorrhage can occur between the skull and dura (the fibrous covering of the brain), between the dura and the arachnoid, or directly into the brain tissue.

Acute Epidural Hematoma: An acute epidural hematoma is most often caused by a tear in the middle meningeal artery that runs along the inside of the skull in the temporal region. The arterial injury is often caused by a linear skull fracture in the temporal or parietal region (Figure 10-4). Because the bleeding is arterial (although it may be venous from one of the dural sinuses), the bleeding and rise in ICP can occur rapidly, and death may occur quickly.

Symptoms of an acute epidural hematoma include a history of head trauma with initial loss of consciousness often followed by a period during which the patient is conscious and coherent (the "lucid interval"). After a period of a few minutes to several hours, the patient will develop signs of increasing ICP (vomiting, headache, altered mental status), lapse into unconsciousness, and develop body paralysis on the side opposite of the head injury (see earlier section on cerebral herniation syndrome). There is often a dilated and fixed (no response to bright light) pupil on the side of the head injury. These signs are usually followed rapidly by death. The classic example is the boxer who is knocked unconscious, wakes up, and is allowed to go home, only to be found dead in bed the next morning. If the underlying brain tissue is not injured, surgical removal of the blood and ligation of the ruptured blood vessel often allows full recovery.

Acute Subdural Hematoma: This is the result of bleeding between the dura and the arachnoid and is associated with injury to the underlying brain tissue (Figure 10-5). Because the bleeding is venous, intracranial pressure increases more slowly, and the diagnosis often is not apparent until hours or days after the injury. The signs and symptoms include headache, fluctuations in the level of consciousness, and focal neurologic signs (e.g., weakness of one extremity or one side of the body, altered deep tendon reflexes, and slurred speech). Because of underlying brain tissue injury, prognosis is often poor. Mortality is very high (60 percent–90 percent) in patients who are comatose when found. Always suspect a subdural hematoma in an alcoholic with any degree of altered mental status following a fall. Elderly patients and those taking anticoagulants are also at high risk for this injury.

Intracerebral Hemorrhage: Intracerebral hemorrhage is bleeding within the brain tissue (Figure 10-6). Traumatic intracerebral hemorrhage may result from blunt or penetrating injuries of the head. Unfortunately, surgery is often not helpful. The signs and symptoms depend upon the regions involved and the degree of injury. They occur in

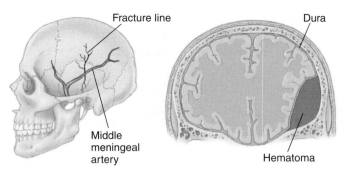

FIGURE 10-4 Acute epidural hematoma. This hemorrhage may follow injury to the extradural arteries. The blood collects between the fibrous dura and the periosteum.

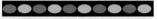

PEARLS
Altered Mental Status
Remember that hypoglycemia, hypoxia, cardiac dysrhythmias, and drugs can also cause altered mental status. When narcotic abuse is a possibility, administer naloxone (Narcan) to any patient with altered mental status. Monitor the heart and oxygenation and check the blood glucose level on all patients with altered mental status. If you cannot perform a glucose determination but suspect hypoglycemia (diabetics and alcoholics), give glucose or thiamine and glucose.

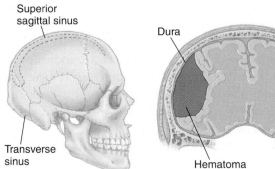

FIGURE 10-5 Acute subdural hematoma. This usually occurs following the rupture of dural veins. Blood collects and often severely compresses the brain.

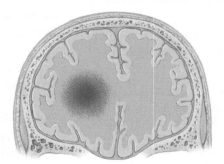

FIGURE 10-6 Intracerebral hemorrhage.

patterns similar to those that accompany a stroke; spontaneous hemorrhages of this type may be seen in patients with severe hypertension. Alteration in the level of consciousness is commonly seen, though awake patients may complain of headache and vomiting.

EVALUATION OF THE HEAD-TRAUMA PATIENT

Determining the exact type of TBI or hemorrhage cannot be done in the field, as it requires imaging techniques, such as a CAT scan. It is more important that you recognize the presence of a brain injury and be ready to provide supportive measures while transporting the patient. TBI patients may be difficult to manage because they are often uncooperative and may be under the influence of alcohol or drugs. As a rescuer, you must pay extraordinary attention to detail and never lose your patience with an uncooperative patient.

ITLS Primary Survey

Remember that every trauma patient is initially evaluated in the same sequence (Figure 10-7).

Scene Size-up: The results of the Scene Size-up will begin to determine if you have a load-and-go patient. Dangerous generalized mechanisms (MVC, fall from a height) will require a complete examination (Rapid Trauma Survey). Dangerous focused mechanisms (hit in head with baseball bat) will allow you to "focus" your exam (ABCs, with head and neurological exams) rather than having to perform a complete exam.

Initial Assessment: The goals of the Initial Assessment are to determine if this is a priority patient and to find immediate life-threats. The Initial Assessment in the head-trauma patient is to determine quickly if the patient is brain injured and, if so, if the patient's condition is deteriorating. Obviously, a patient with a history and physical examination that indicate a loss of consciousness following a lucid period postinjury (possible epidural hematoma) should be transported with more urgency than one who is alert and oriented after being knocked out (possible concussion). It is very important that all observations be recorded (but do not interrupt patient care to do this), because later treatment is often dictated by detection of the deterioration of clinical stability.

All patients with head or facial trauma and an altered level of consciousness should be assumed to have a cervical-spine injury until proven otherwise. Because of the alteration of LOC, it is often not possible, in this situation, to clear the cervical spine until after arrival at the hospital. Restriction of cervical-spine movement should accompany airway and breathing management. Evaluation for head injury is begun as you obtain your initial level of consciousness by speaking to the patient.

During the Initial Assessment your neurological exam is limited to level of consciousness and any obvious paralysis. Level of consciousness is the most sensitive indicator of brain function. Initially, the AVPU method is quite adequate (see Chapter 2). If there is a history of head trauma, or if the initial exam reveals an altered mental status, then the Rapid Trauma Survey will include a more complete neurological exam. A decrease in the level of consciousness is the first indicator of a brain injury or rising ICP.

Control of the airway cannot be overemphasized. The supine, restrained, and unconscious patient is prone to airway obstruction from the tongue, blood, vomit, or other secretions. Vomiting is very common within the first hour following a head injury.

Protect the airway of the unconscious patient with no gag reflex by endotracheal intubation or by placement of an oral or nasal airway and frequent suctioning. Perform endotracheal intubation of the unconscious head-injured patient as rapidly and

```
┌─────────────────────────────────────────────────────────┐
│                    ITLS PRIMARY SURVEY                    │
│                                                           │
│                      SCENE SIZE-UP                        │
│   Standard Precautions, Hazards, Number of Patients,      │
│      Need for Additional Help/Equipment,                  │
│              Mechanism of Injury                          │
│   - - - - - - - - - - - - - - -│- - - - - - - - - - - -   │
│                                ↓                          │
│                   INITIAL ASSESSMENT                      │
│                    General Impression                     │
│  (Age, Sex, Weight, General Appearance, Position,         │
│      Activity, Obvious Injuries/Bleeding)                 │
│                         LOC                               │
│                       (AVPU)                              │
│                 Control Cervical Spine                    │
│                        Airway                             │
│          (Snoring, Gurgling, Stridor, Silence)            │
│                      Breathing                            │
│            (Present? Rate, Depth, Effort)                 │
│                  Radial/Carotid Pulses                    │
│           (Present? Rate, Rhythm, Quality)                │
│   Skin Color, Temperature, Moisture; Capillary Refill     │
│            Uncontrolled External Hemorrhage?              │
│   - - - - - - - - - - - - - - -│- - - - - - - - - - - -   │
│                                ↓                          │
│                  RAPID TRAUMA SURVEY                       │
│                  Inspect Head and Neck                    │
│  (Major Facial Injuries, Bruising, Swelling,              │
│      Penetrations, Subcutaneous Emphysema)                │
│     (Neck Vein Distention? Tracheal Deviation?)           │
│                    Inspect Chest                          │
│  (Asymmetry, Contusions, Penetrations, Paradoxical        │
│          Motion, Instability, Crepitation)                │
│                    Breath Sounds                          │
│                  (Present? Equal?)                        │
│                (If unequal: Percussion)                   │
│                     Heart Tones                           │
│                      Abdomen                              │
│  (Bruising, Penetration/Evisceration, Tenderness,         │
│            Rigidity, Distention)                          │
│                      Pelvis                               │
│         (Tenderness, Instability, Crepitation)            │
│               Lower/Upper Extremities                     │
│  (Swelling, Deformity, Instability, Motor and Sensory)    │
│               Place Patient on Backboard                  │
│                     Posterior                             │
│     (Penetrations, Deformity, Presacral Edema)            │
│   If Critical Situation, Transfer to Ambulance to         │
│                  Complete Exam.                           │
│                 Baseline Vital Signs                      │
│   Measured Pulse, Respirations, Blood Pressure            │
│                       Pupils                              │
│             (Size? Reactive? Equal?)                      │
│             (If Altered Mental Status:)                   │
│               Glascow Coma Scale Score                    │
│     Eyes, Voice, Motor, Orientation, Emotional State      │
└─────────────────────────────────────────────────────────┘
```

FIGURE 10-7 The ITLS Primary Survey.

smoothly as possible in order to avoid patient agitation, straining, and breath-holding that may contribute to elevated intracranial pressure. Use of intravenous lidocaine when intubating head-injured patients is no longer recommended. Head-injured patients may seize from their injury (if hypoxic) or have their teeth and jaws clenched, making intubation difficult. Attempting to force an artificial airway into this patient may cause additional injury. Nasotracheal intubation or use of rapid sequence intubation (RSI) should be considered in this situation, if permitted under local protocols. Before beginning intubation, ventilate (do not hyperventilate) with high-flow oxygen. Do not allow the head-injured patient to become hypoxic. Even one brief episode of hypoxia can increase mortality. As stated above, it is important to note the patient's basic neurological status prior to RSI, as the medications given can prevent a complete neurological assessment in the hospital.

Rapid Trauma Survey: All patients with an abnormal level of consciousness get a Rapid Trauma Survey (see Chapter 2).

Head: Once the initial exam is completed, continue with the exam guided by the mechanism of injury. Begin with the scalp and quickly, but carefully, examine for obvious injuries such as lacerations or depressed or open skull fractures. The size of a laceration is often misjudged because of the difficulty in assessment through hair matted with blood. Feel the scalp gently for obvious unstable areas of the skull. If none are present, you may safely apply a pressure dressing or hold direct pressure upon a bandage to stop scalp bleeding.

A basilar skull fracture may be indicated by any of the following: bleeding from the ear or nose, clear or serosanguineous fluid running from the nose or ear, swelling and/or discoloration behind the ear (Battle's sign) (Figure 10-8a), and/or swelling and discoloration around both eyes (raccoon eyes) (Figure 10-8b). Raccoon eyes are a sign of anterior basilar skull fracture that may go through the thin cribriform plate in the upper nasal cavity and allow spinal fluid and/or blood to leak out. Raccoon eyes with or without drainage from the nose are an absolute contraindication to inserting a nasogastric tube or nasotracheal intubation. The tube can go through the fractured cribriform plate and into the brain.

Pupils: The pupils (Figure 10-9) are controlled in part by the third cranial nerve. This nerve takes a long course through the skull and is easily compressed by brain swelling, and thus may be affected by increasing ICP. Following a head injury, if both pupils are dilated and do not react to light, the patient probably has a brain stem injury and the prognosis is grim. If the pupils are dilated but still react to light, the injury is often still reversible, so every effort should be made to transport the patient quickly to a facility capable of treating a head injury. A unilaterally dilated pupil that remains reactive to light may be the earliest sign of increasing ICP. The development of a unilaterally dilated, nonreactive pupil ("blown pupil") while you are observing the comatose patient is an extreme emergency and mandates rapid transport and hyperventilation. Other causes of dilated pupils that may or may not react to light include hypothermia, light-

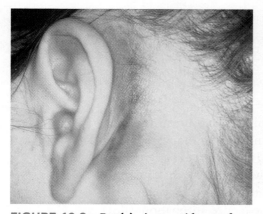

FIGURE 10-8a Battle's sign—evidence of a posterior basilar skull fracture. *(Photo courtesy of David Effron, MD, FACEP)*

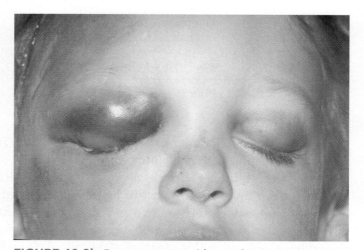

FIGURE 10-8b Raccoon eyes—evidence of an anterior basilar skull fracture. *(Photo courtesy of David Effron, MD, FACEP)*

ning strike, anoxia, optic nerve injury, drug effect (e.g., atropine), or direct trauma to the eye. Fixed and dilated pupils signify increased intracranial pressure only in patients with a decreased level of consciousness. If the patient has a normal level of consciousness, the dilated pupil is not from head injury (more likely due to eye trauma or drugs such as atropine).

Fluttering eyelids are often seen with hysteria. Slow lid closure (like a curtain falling) is rarely seen with hysteria. Testing for a blink response (corneal reflex) by touching the cornea with the edge of a gauze pad or cotton swab, or by applying overly noxious stimuli to a patient to test for response to pain, are techniques that are unreliable and do not contribute to prehospital assessment.

Extremities: Note sensation and motor function in the extremities. Can the patient feel you touch her hands and feet? Can she wiggle her fingers and toes? If the patient is unconscious, note her response to pain. If she withdraws or localizes to the pinching of her fingers and toes, she has grossly intact sensation and motor function. This usually indicates that there is normal or only minimally impaired cortical function.

Both decorticate posturing or rigidity (arms flexed, legs extended) and decerebrate posturing or rigidity (arms and legs extended) are ominous signs of deep cerebral hemispheric or upper brain stem injury (Figure 10-10). Decerebrate posturing is worse and usually signifies cerebral herniation. It is one of the indications for hyperventilation. Flaccid paralysis usually denotes spinal-cord injury.

Neurological Exam: To apply the Revised Trauma Score and other field triage scoring systems (see Appendix F), you should be familiar with the Glasgow Coma Scale score (GCS), which is simple, easy to use, and has good prognostic value for eventual outcome (Table 10-2). In the TBI patient, a Glasgow Coma Scale score of 8 or less is considered evidence of a severe brain injury. The GCS score that is determined in the field serves as the baseline for the patient; be sure to record it. Record the score for each part of the GCS, not just the total score. You should perform a finger-stick glucose on all patients with altered mental status.

Vital Signs: Vital signs should be obtained by another team member while you are performing the exam. They are extremely important in following the course of a patient with head trauma. Most important, they can indicate changes in ICP (Table 10-3). Observe and record vital signs at the end of the ITLS Primary Survey, during the Detailed Exam, and each time you perform the ITLS Ongoing Exam.

■ *Respiration.* Increasing intracranial pressure causes the respiratory rate to increase, decrease, and/or to become irregular. Unusual respiratory patterns may reflect the level of brain or brain stem injury. Just before death, the patient may develop a

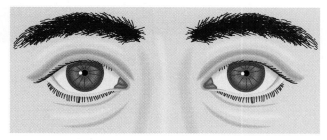
Constricted pupils

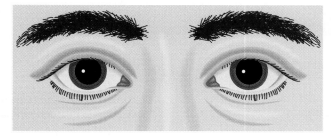
Dilated pupils

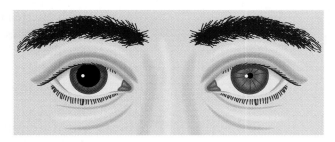
Unequal pupils

FIGURE 10-9 Examination of pupils.

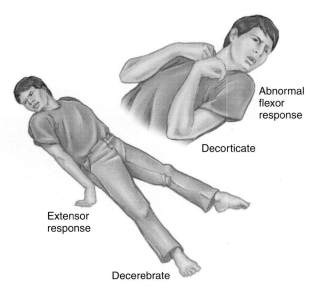
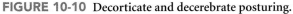
Abnormal flexor response

Decorticate

Extensor response

Decerebrate

FIGURE 10-10 Decorticate and decerebrate posturing.

TABLE 10-2 *Glasgow Coma Scale*

Eye Opening	Points	Verbal Response	Points	Motor Response	Points
Spontaneous	4	Oriented	5	Obeys commands	6
To voice	3	Confused	4	Localizes pain	5
To pain	2	Inappropriate words	3	Withdraws	4
None	1	Incomprehensible sounds	2	Abnormal flexion	3*
		Silent	1	Abnormal extension	2**
				No movement	1

*Decorticate posturing to pain
**Decerebrate posturing to pain

rapid, noisy respiratory pattern called central neurogenic hyperventilation. Because respiration is affected by so many factors (e.g., fear, hysteria, chest injuries, spinal-cord injuries, diabetes), it is not as useful an indicator as are the other vital signs in monitoring the course of head injury. Abnormal respiratory patterns may indicate a chest injury or other problem that could lead to hypoxia if untreated.

■ *Pulse.* Increasing ICP causes the pulse rate to decrease.

■ *Blood pressure.* Increasing ICP causes increased blood pressure. This hypertension is usually associated with a widening of the pulse pressure (systolic minus diastolic pressure). Other causes of hypertension include fear and pain. Hypotension in the presence of a head injury is usually caused by hemorrhagic or neurogenic shock and should be treated as if caused by hemorrhage. It is a rare (5 percent) finding in the patient with a severe TBI. The injured brain does not tolerate hypotension. A single instance of hypotension (BP 90 mmHg systolic) in an adult with a brain injury may increase the mortality rate by 150 percent. The increase in mortality rate for hypotension and a severe TBI is even worse in children. Give IV fluids to maintain a blood pressure of at least 110 to 120 mmHg systolic in the adult patient with a severe head injury (GCS 8 or less) even if the patient has associated penetrating trauma

TABLE 10-3 *Comparison of Vital Signs in Shock and Head Injury*

	Shock	Head Injury with Increased Intracranial Pressure
Level of consciousness	Decreased	Decreased
Respiration	Increased	Varies but frequently decreased
Pulse	Increased	Decreased
Blood pressure	Decreased	Increased
Pulse pressure	Narrows	Widens

with hemorrhage. As noted above, the goal is to maintain cerebral perfusion pressure (CPP) above 60 mmHg. Children with severe TBI should have their blood pressure maintained at the normal range for their age.

History: Begin obtaining the history before and during the exam. It is essential to obtain as thorough a history about the event as possible. The circumstances of the head injury may be extremely important for patient management and may be of prognostic importance to the ultimate outcome. Pay particular attention to reports of near-drowning, electrocution, lightning strike, drug abuse, smoke inhalation, hypothermia, and seizures. Always inquire about the patient's behavior from the time of the head injury until the time of your arrival. Try to obtain the past medical history; nontraumatic events can also cause an alteration in the LOC.

ITLS Secondary Survey

Head-trauma patients with altered mental status are load-and-go situations. The ITLS Secondary Survey (see Chapter 2) will be done during transport (or not at all, if a short transport).

ITLS Ongoing Exam

Each time you perform the ITLS Ongoing Exam, record the level of consciousness, the pupil size and reaction to light, the Glasgow Coma Scale score, and the development (or improvement) of focal weakness or paralysis. This, along with the vital signs, provides enough information to monitor the condition of the head-injured patient. Decisions on the management of the head-trauma patient are based on the changes in all the parameters of the physical and neurological examination. You are establishing the baseline from which later judgments must be made; record your observations.

PEARLS
Seizures

Seizures in TBI patients are usually caused by hypoxia. If the patient has an open airway and you are already ventilating with 100 percent oxygen, you may be ordered to administer IV medication to control the seizures. Seizures should always cause you to recheck the airway, ventilation, and oxygenation of your patient.

MANAGEMENT OF THE HEAD-TRAUMA PATIENT

Your job is to prevent secondary brain injury. It is extremely important to make a rapid assessment and then transport the patient to a facility capable of managing head trauma. Appropriate triage of the patient to facilities capable of managing TBI can have a significant impact on the outcome of the patient. The important points of management in the prehospital phase are listed here.

Brain Trauma Foundation Guidelines are classified as follows:

■ Level I recommendations, supported by Class I scientific evidence (formerly called Standards)

■ Level II recommendations, supported by Class II scientific evidence (formerly called Guidelines)

■ Level III recommendations, supported by Class III scientific evidence (formerly called Options)

PROCEDURE

❋ **Managing the Head-Trauma Patient**

1. Secure the airway and provide good oxygenation. The injured brain does not tolerate hypoxia, so every TBI patient should receive 100 percent oxygen. If possible, monitor the oxygen saturation with a pulse oximeter. Do not allow the SaO_2 to become less than 90 percent (Level II). It is best to maintain a level above 95 percent.

Maintain good ventilation (not hyperventilation) with high-flow oxygen at a rate of about one breath every 6 to 8 seconds (8 to 10 breaths per minute). Studies have found that we tend to hyperventilate the critical patient without realizing it. You can prevent this if you have an end-tidal CO_2 monitor. Try to keep the CO_2 between 35 and 40 mmHg.

Endotracheal intubation is still recommended for adults if the airway cannot be maintained or if you cannot maintain adequate oxygenation with supplemental oxygen. There is no reason to routinely intubate patient's who are maintaining their airway and have a normal oxygen saturation. Some studies have found a decreased survival rate for TBI patients who have been intubated in the field. Possible causes of this are unrecognized hyperventilation and/or unrecognized esophageal intubation. Use of capnography will prevent both of these problems (see Chapter 5). Brain Trauma Foundation guidelines recommend capnography, pulse oximetry, and BP monitoring as critical monitoring procedures for all intubated TBI patients (Level III).

There is no evidence to support out-of-hospital endotracheal intubation over bag-valve mask ventilation of pediatric patients with TBI (Level II).

Because head-injured patients are prone to vomiting, be prepared to log-roll the motion-restricted patient and to suction the oropharynx, particularly if an endotracheal tube has not been placed. Try to avoid use of antiemetics, as some may decrease the LOC.

2. Stabilize the patient on a backboard. Restrict motion of the neck in a rigid collar and a padded head motion-restriction device.

3. Agitated and combative patients fighting against restraints or ventilations can raise their ICP, as well as place themselves at risk for further cervical-spine injury. Consider sedation in this situation; though be aware that sedation will complicate the neurological evaluation of your patient. Careful use of benzodiazepines can decrease agitation without dropping blood pressure.

   An added benefit of the use of benzodiazepines is that they prevent seizures. Seizure prophylaxis in the head-injured patient should be initiated on the recommendation of medical direction. Other agents suitable for use include phenytoin. Do not use barbiturates, as they can cause hypotension.

4. Record baseline observations. Record vital signs (describe rate and pattern of breathing), the level of consciousness, the pupils (size and reaction to light), the Glasgow Coma Scale score, and the development (or improvement) of focal weakness or paralysis. If the patient develops hypotension, suspect hemorrhage or spinal injury. Every patient with altered mental status should have a finger-stick glucose checked and recorded.

5. Continuously monitor the observations listed in step 4. Record them every 5 minutes.

6. Insert two large-bore IV catheters. Fluid resuscitation (crystalloid) in patient with TBI should be administered to avoid hypotension and/or limit hypotension to the shortest duration possible (Level II). In the past it was thought that fluids should be limited in head-injured patients. It has been found that the danger of increasing brain swelling by giving fluids is much less than the danger of allowing the patient to be hypotensive.

   Hyperventilation is recommended for use in treating the patient with signs of cerebral herniation after correcting hypotension and/or hypoxia (Level III).

If you have capnography available, try to maintain the CO_2 level at about 25 mmHg during hyperventilation. Further research is needed on the utility of hypertonic saline solutions over current crystalloids for treatment of hypotension in TBI patients. Routine administration of steroids for TBI has not been shown to improve outcomes.

Case Study
continued

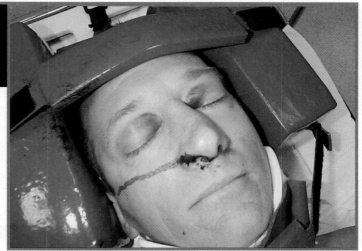

Joyce, Dan, and Buddy have been dispatched to a private home where a 40-year-old man has fallen off of a ladder. The man's wife tells Joyce, the team leader on this call, that when his foot slipped, it caught in the rung of the ladder and he swung like a pendulum, striking his head. He was unconscious for a few minutes. He is now awake but cannot remember going up the ladder. His wife says he is in good health, takes no medications, and has no allergies. She prepared him a hamburger at lunch about 2 hours ago. He complains of a headache and nausea and says his neck hurts.

Joyce introduces the team and cautions the patient not to move while they are examining him. Her initial impression is cautiously good, but she is worried by the drainage from his nose. Dan stabilizes the patient's neck while Joyce begins the exam and Buddy brings the backboard. The airway is open because the patient can speak normally. He responds appropriately to questions but has amnesia for the event. He has a strong, regular pulse and his respiration is normal.

Because of the mechanism, Joyce performs a Rapid Trauma Survey and finds a hematoma on the right side of the head in the temporal area. The pupils are 5 mm and equal and there are ecchymoses of both upper eyelids. There is dried blood in both nostrils and a thin, serosanguineous drainage from the right nostril. The face feels stable. There is tenderness and spasm of the neck but no palpable deformity. The neck veins are flat and trachea is in the midline. The chest is normal to inspection with no tenderness, and breath sounds are present and equal. Heart sounds are easily heard. The abdomen is nontender. The pelvis is stable and nontender. The extremities are nontender with normal PMS. A cervical collar is placed on the patient and he is log-rolled onto the backboard (the back is normal) and packaged. Joyce decides to transport immediately, so he is transferred to the ambulance. Buddy drives.

While Dan obtains the vital signs, Joyce does a neurological exam. The patient is awake and oriented with a retrograde amnesia. He has a GCS of 15 (E-4, V-5, M-6). His pupils are still 5 mm and react equally. He has good sensation and movement in his fingers and toes bilaterally. The vital signs are pulse 95, respiration 12, BP 140/80, and pulse oximeter 100 percent on oxygen by nasal cannula at 3 liters per minute. Joyce notifies medical direction that they have a patient with a probable anterior basilar skull fracture with a spinal fluid leak and are taking him directly to the local trauma center.

Joyce starts a saline lock IV while Dan attaches a cardiac monitor. The patient begins to get restless and becomes more confused. He tries to pull out his IV and then vomits the hamburger he had for lunch.

Joyce immediately performs an ITLS Ongoing Exam. Exam of the head reveals no change in the temporal hematoma, but the right pupil is now 8 mm and poorly reactive. The left pupil is still 5 mm. The neck, chest, and abdomen are unchanged. Noted now is a slight difference in strength on the left side compared to the right. The vital signs are pulse 70, respiration 8, BP 170/80, and pulse oximeter 95 percent on oxygen by nasal cannula at 3 liters per minute. Dan begins to assist respiration at a rate of 8 to 10 breaths per minute with 100 percent oxygen by bag-valve mask.

The patient is no longer restless but is now less reactive. He still localizes to pain. He opens his eyes to verbal stimuli but his speech is mostly unintelligible sounds and cursing. His GCS score is now 11 (E-3, V-3, M-5). Joyce notifies medical direction of the change, and she has the trauma team meet them at the ambulance. The patient is taken straight to CAT scan, where a right epidural hematoma is revealed. He is then taken directly to surgery, where the bleeding right middle meningeal artery is ligated and the hematoma evacuated. After surgery, x-rays reveal a nondisplaced fracture of the fifth cervical vertebra. He recovers completely from his injuries and returns home.

Case Study Wrap-up

The mechanism of injury, coupled with the spinal fluid draining from the nose, alerted Joyce that the patient had an anterior basilar skull fracture. The mechanism was also suspicious for spinal injury. The patient was packaged for transport. As is common with an injury of this type, the patient initially looked good but began to deteriorate soon afterwards. He developed symptoms of an epidural hematoma with increased ICP but never deteriorated enough to require hyperventilation. If endotracheal intubation had been needed, the nasotracheal route would have been contraindicated because of the basilar skull fracture. Joyce was wise in bypassing lower levels of care to go to a trauma center where he would receive immediate evaluation and life-saving surgery before he reached the point of cerebral herniation. He was in danger of developing meningitis from the basilar skull fracture from which the spinal fluid was leaking. He was lucky that it sealed and healed without any infection developing. He could easily have had a spinal-cord injury in this situation but his cervical-spinal fracture was stable and healed without further surgery.

SUMMARY

Head injury is a serious complication of trauma. In order to give your patient the best chance of recovery, you should be familiar with the important anatomy of the head and central nervous system and understand how trauma to the various areas presents clinically. The most important steps in the management of the head-injured patient are rapid assessment, good airway management, prevention of hypotension, rapid transport to a trauma center, and frequent ITLS Ongoing Exams. In no other area of trauma care is the recording of repeated assessments so important to future management decisions.

BIBLIOGRAPHY

1. The Brain Trauma Foundation. 2006. *Guidelines for prehospital management of traumatic brain injury.* 2nd ed. New York.

2. The Brain Trauma Foundation. The American Association of Neurological Surgeons. The Joint Section on Neurotrauma and Critical Care. 2000. Hyperventilation. *Journal of Neurotrauma* 17(6): 513–20.

3. Chestnut, R. M., L. F. Marshall, M. R. Klauber, and others.1993. The role of secondary brain injury in determining outcome from severe head injury. *Journal of Trauma* 34: 216–22.

4. Cruz, J., G. Minoja, K. Okuchi. 2001. Improving clinical outcomes from acute subdural hematomas with the emergency preoperative administration of high doses of mannitol: A randomized trial. *Neurosurgery* 49(4): 864–71.

5. Davis, D., D. Hoyt, M. Ochs, et al. 2003. The effect of paramedic rapid sequence intubation on outcome in patients with severe traumatic brain injury. *Journal of Trauma—Injury Infection & Critical Care* 54(3): 444–53.

6. Davis, D., J. Dunford, J. Poste, et al. 2004. The impact of hypoxia and hyperventilation on outcome after paramedic rapid sequence intubation of severely head-injured patients. *Journal of Trauma* 57(1): 1–8.

7. Davis, D., J. Dunford, M. Ochs, et al. 2004. The use of quantitative end-tidal capnometry to avoid inadvertent severe hyperventilation in patients with head injury after paramedic rapid sequence intubation. *Journal of Trauma—Injury Infection & Critical Care* 56(4): 808–14.

8. McKeag, D.B. 2003. Understanding sports-related concussion. Coming into focus but still fuzzy. *JAMA* 290: 2604–5.

9. Pigula, F. A., S. L. Wald, S. R. Shackford, and others. 1993. The effect of hypotension and hypoxia on children with severe head injuries. *Journal of Pediatric Surgery* 28: 310–16.

10. Wang, H., A. Peitzman, et al. 2004. Out-of-hospital endotracheal intubation and outcome after traumatic brain injury. *Annals of Emergency Medicine* 44: 439–50.

Spinal Trauma

James J. Augustine, MD, FACEP

OBJECTIVES

Upon completion of this chapter, you should be able to:

1. Explain the normal anatomy and physiology of the spinal column and spinal cord.

2. Define spinal motion restriction (SMR) and explain why this term is preferred to the term spinal immobilization.

3. Describe mechanisms of injury that indicate SMR may be required.

4. Describe the process of SMR from extrication through transportation, including airway maintenance.

5. Explain the difference between Emergency Rescue and Rapid Extrication techniques and give examples of when each would be appropriate.

6. Describe history and assessment criteria that identify patients who do not need SMR.

7. Give examples of special situations for which SMR techniques may need to be altered.

8. Using the clinical evaluation, differentiate neurogenic shock from hemorrhagic shock.

(Photo courtesy of Bob Page, NREMT-P)

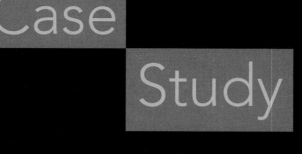

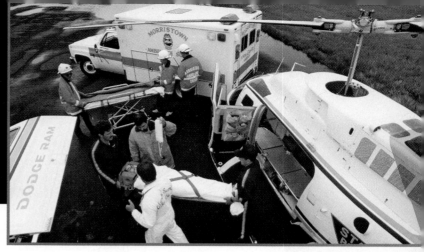

(Photo © Bob Krist/
CORBIS)

Dan, Joyce, and Buddy have been called to a
public swimming pool. They are told that there
has been a diving injury. *What injuries should they expect with a mechanism of this
type? Is a spinal injury likely? What other emergency may be associated with a
diving injury?* Keep these questions in mind as you read the chapter. Then, at the
end of the chapter, find out how the rescuers completed this call.

INTRODUCTION

Spinal-cord injury is a devastating and life-threatening result of modern trauma. If a patient with a spinal-cord injury survives, he could lose his independence and the cost of supporting him over a lifetime could be in the millions of dollars. The management of trauma patients requires continuous vigilance for spinal injuries.

Various terms have been used through the years to describe the process by which emergency personnel attempt to prevent spinal-cord injuries. It has been called *traction* and then *immobilization.* Now the preferred term is *spinal motion restriction (SMR).* It most accurately defines the process used in the field, because in certain patients, especially in the prehospital environment, the spine cannot be completely immobilized.

There have been no prospective randomized controlled clinical trials that compare methods of spinal motion restriction. Thus, there is no Class I evidence and no formal standards of care. Recommendations in this chapter are guidelines. Based on mechanism of injury and evaluation, some patients will require SMR, but this procedure is associated with complications for the patient and the EMS providers. The complications with the most potential danger are those related to the patient's ability to maintain an airway and breathe effectively.

Rescue personnel must skillfully assess the mechanism of injury and the patient to provide safe and appropriate SMR to trauma patients. This chapter reviews the process of evaluating the mechanism of injury, providing a structured assessment, and packaging, treating, and transporting patients with known or potential spinal-cord injuries.

THE NORMAL SPINAL COLUMN AND CORD

Spinal Column

It is important to differentiate the spinal column from the spinal cord. The spinal column is a bony tube composed of 33 vertebrae (Figure 11-1). It supports the body in an upright position, allows the use of our extremities, and protects the delicate spinal cord. The column's 33 vertebrae are identified by their location: 7 cervical (the C-spine), 12 thoracic

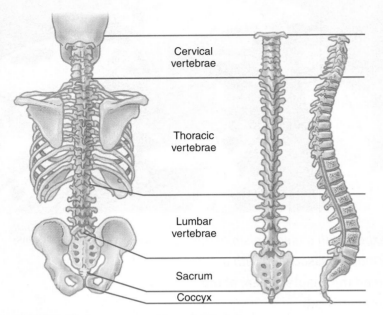

FIGURE 11-1 Anatomy of the spinal column.

(the T-spine), 5 lumbar (the L-spine), and the remainder fused together as the posterior portion of the pelvis (5 sacral and 4 coccygeal). The vertebrae are numbered in each section, from the head down to the pelvis. The third cervical vertebra from the head is designated C3, the sixth is called C6, and so forth. The thoracic vertebrae are T1 through T12, and each attaches to one of the 12 pairs of ribs. The lumbar vertebrae are numbered L1 through L5, with L5 being the last vertebra above the pelvis.

The vertebrae are each separated by a fibrous disc that acts as a shock absorber. The alignment is maintained by strong ligaments between the vertebrae and by muscles that run along the length of the bony column from head to pelvis. (These are the muscles strained when one lifts improperly.) The spinal column is aligned in a gentle S-curve that is most prominent at the C5–C6 and T12–L1 levels in adults, making these areas the most susceptible to injury.

Spinal Cord

The spinal cord is an electrical conduit that serves as an extension of the brain stem. It is continuous down to the level of the first lumbar vertebra and at that point separates into nerves. The cord is 10 to 13 mm in diameter and is suspended in the middle of the vertebral foramen (Figure 11-2). The cord is soft and flexible like a cotton rope, and is surrounded and bathed by cerebrospinal fluid along its entire length. The fluid and the flexibility provide some protection to the cord from injury.

The cord is composed of specific bundles of nerve tracts that are arranged in a predictable manner, much as a rope is composed of individual strands of fiber. The spinal cord passes down the vertebral canal and gives off pairs of nerve roots that exit at each vertebral

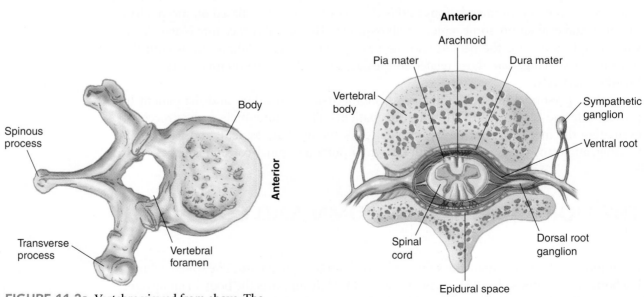

FIGURE 11-2a Vertebra viewed from above. The spinal cord passes through the vertebral foramen.

FIGURE 11-2b Vertebra with spinal cord in place.

level (Figure 11-3). The roots lie next to the intervertebral discs and the lateral part of the vertebrae, making the nerve roots susceptible to injury when trauma occurs in these areas (Figure 11-4). The nerve roots carry sensory signals from the body to the spinal cord and then to the brain.

The roots also carry signals from the brain to specific muscles, causing them to move. These signals pass back and forth rapidly, and some are strong enough to cause actions on their own, called *reflexes*. This reflex system can be demonstrated by tapping the patella tendon below the knee, causing the lower leg to jerk. If you accidentally put your finger on a hot burner, your reflex system causes your hand to move even before your brain receives the warning message. Strong signals also can overwhelm the spinal cord's ability to keep signals moving separately to the brain. This is why a trauma patient with a fractured hip may complain of knee pain or a patient with a ruptured spleen may complain of shoulder pain.

The integrity of spinal-cord function is tested by motor, sensory, and reflex functions. The level of sensory loss is most accurate for predicting the level of spinal-cord injury. Muscle strength is another function that is easy to assess in the conscious patient. Reflexes are helpful for distinguishing complete from partial spinal-cord injuries, but are best left for hospital assessment. The spinal cord is also an integrating center for the autonomic nervous system, which assists in controlling heart rate, blood vessel tone, and blood flow to the skin. Injury to this component of the spinal cord results in neurogenic shock (commonly called *spinal shock*), which is discussed later.

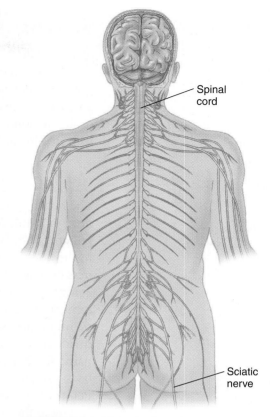

FIGURE 11-3 The spinal cord is a continuation of the central nervous system outside the skull.

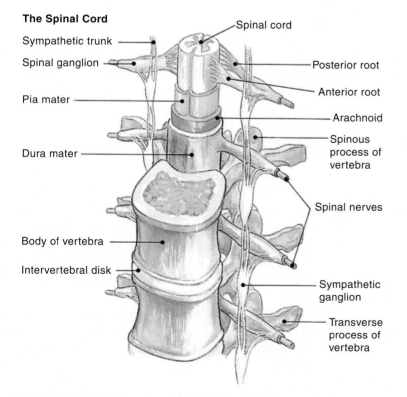

FIGURE 11-4 Relationship of the spinal cord to the vertebrae. Note how the nerve roots exit between the vertebrae.

SPINAL INJURY

A normal healthy spinal column can be severely stressed and maintain its integrity without damage to the spinal cord. However, certain mechanisms of trauma can overcome the protective defenses, injuring the spinal column and cord. The most common mechanisms are hyperextension, hyperflexion, compression, and rotation. Less commonly, lateral stress or distraction will injure the cord. These mechanisms and their subsequent injuries are illustrated in Table 11-1.

Mechanisms of Blunt Spinal-Column Injury

The head is a relatively large ball perched on top of the neck. Sudden movement of the head or trunk will produce stresses that may damage the bony or connective tissue components of the spinal column. Injury to the spinal column is like injury to any other bone in the body. It requires a significant amount of force, unless there is a preexisting weakness or defect in the bone. For that reason, the elderly and those with severe arthritis are at higher risk for spinal injuries. Like other bone injuries, pain is the most common symptom, but it may be unnoticed by the patient. This is especially true if the patient has other painful injuries. At the site of a bone injury, local muscle spasm may occur. Injury to individual nerve roots can result from bony spinal-column injury, with resulting localized pain, paralysis, or sensory loss. Therefore, signs that may indicate spinal injury include back pain, tenderness along the spinal column, pain with movement of the back, obvious deformity or wounds of the back, paralysis, weakness, or paresthesia (tingling or burning feeling to the skin).

Fortunately, spinal column injury can occur without injuring the spinal cord. Statistically, only 14 percent of all column injuries have evidence of spinal-cord damage. In the cervical spine region it is much more common to have cord injury, with almost 40 percent of column injuries having cord damage. The converse is also possible, in that cord injuries can occur in the absence of obvious spinal-column damage. This is particularly true in children. Only 63 percent of spinal-cord injuries have evidence of spinal-column damage. The unconscious trauma patient carries a high risk (15–20 percent) of spinal column injury. The injuries are frequently in more than one place, and therefore SMR should be performed immediately on the unconscious trauma patient.

Mechanisms of Blunt Spinal-Cord Injury

Spinal-cord injury is devastating and occurs most commonly in young adults. As the population ages, so has the median age of the victims. Currently about 11 percent of spinal-cord injuries occur in patients over age 50. There are approximately 11,000 new spinal-cord injuries in the United States each year—48 percent involve MVCs (including pedestrians), 23 percent falls, 14 percent penetrating wounds, 9 percent recreational activities, and the remaining 6 percent are from all other causes. Under age 8, the relatively large size of the head makes the upper end of the cervical cord the most common site of injury, which can be extremely devastating.

Spinal-cord injury results in a defective signal-conducting function, presenting as a loss of motor function and reflexes, loss or change in sensation, and/or neurogenic shock. The delicate structure of the spinal cord's nerve tracts makes it very sensitive to any form of trauma. What is termed *primary damage* occurs at the time of the trauma itself. Primary damage results from the cord being cut, torn, or crushed or by its blood supply being cut off. This damage is usually irreversible despite the best trauma care. *Secondary damage* occurs from hypotension, generalized hypoxia, injury to blood vessels, swelling,

TABLE 11-1 *Mechanisms of Blunt Spinal Injury*

Description	Diagram	Examples
Hyperextension Excessive posterior movement of the head or neck		Face into windshield in MVC Elderly person falling to the floor Football tackler Dive into shallow water
Hyperflexion Excessive anterior movement of head onto chest		Rider thrown off horse or motorcycle Dive into shallow water
Compression Weight of head or pelvis driven into stationary neck or torso		Dive into shallow water Fall of greater than 10 to 20 feet onto head or legs
Rotation Excessive rotation of the torso or head and neck, moving one side of the spinal column against the other		Rollover MVC Motorcycle crash
Lateral Stress Direct lateral force on spinal column, typically shearing one level of cord from another		"T-bone" MVC Fall
Distraction Excessive stretching of column and cord		Hanging Child inappropriately wearing shoulder belt around neck Snowmobile or motorcycle under rope or wire

or compression of the cord from surrounding hemorrhage. Emergency efforts are directed at preventing secondary damage through attention to the ABCs, medications, and careful packaging of the patient.

Neurogenic Shock

Injury to the cervical or thoracic spinal cord can produce high-space shock (see Chapter 8). Neurogenic shock results from the malfunction of the autonomic nervous system in regulating blood vessel tone and cardiac output. Classically, neurogenic shock in the injured patient results in hypotension, with normal skin color and temperature and an inappropriately slow heart rate that contrasts with hypovolemic shock.

In the healthy patient, blood pressure is maintained by the controlled release of catecholamines (epinephrine and norepinephrine) from the adrenal glands. Sensors in the aortic and carotid arteries monitor the blood pressure. Catecholamines cause constriction of the blood vessels, increase the heart rate and the strength of heart contraction, and stimulate sweat glands. The brain and spinal cord signal the adrenal glands to release catecholamines to keep the blood pressure in the normal range. In pure hemorrhagic shock, these sensors detect the hypovolemic state and compensate by constricting the blood vessels and speeding the heart rate. The high levels of catecholamines cause pale skin, tachycardia, and sweating.

The mechanism of shock from spinal-cord injury is just the opposite. There is no significant blood loss, but the injury to the spinal cord destroys the ability of the brain to regulate the release of catecholamines from the adrenals (the spinal cord cable is out), so no catecholamines are released. When the levels of catecholamines drop, the blood vessels dilate causing the blood to pool. This drop in preload causes the blood pressure to fall. The brain cannot correct this because it cannot get the message to the adrenal glands.

The patient with neurogenic shock cannot show the signs of pale skin, tachycardia, and sweating because the cord injury prevents release of catecholamines. Intra-abdominal injury is difficult to evaluate because the patient with neurogenic shock usually has no sensation in the abdomen. The multiple-trauma patient may have both neurogenic shock and hemorrhagic shock. Neurogenic shock is a diagnosis of exclusion, after all other potential causes of shock have been ruled out. In the prehospital setting, neurogenic shock is treated in the same way as hemorrhagic shock (see Chapter 8).

ASSESSMENT AND MANAGEMENT OF THE TRAUMA PATIENT

Assessing for Possible Spine Injury

All trauma patients are evaluated in the same manner using the ITLS Primary Survey, of which evaluation of spinal-cord function is a part. Clues to spinal-cord injury are given in Table 11-2. Parts of the neurological exam are performed during the ITLS Primary Survey and the remainder of the neurological exam is performed during the ITLS Secondary Survey. This is frequently done after the patient is loaded into the ambulance.

The patient who requires extrication is a special situation. Before beginning extrication, you should check sensory and motor function in the hands and feet, and document these findings later in the written report. Not only does this pre-extrication neurological exam alert you to any spinal injury, it also provides documentation on whether or not there was loss of function before extrication was begun. Sadly, there are a few reports of patients who have claimed that their spinal injuries were caused by their rescuers. You will not have time to perform the pre-extrication neurological exam on the patient who requires Emergency Rescue and you may not have time on those requiring Rapid Extrication.

PEARLS
High-Space Shock

Injury to the spinal cord can produce high-space shock, with the patient experiencing hypotension, normal skin color and temperature, and an inappropriately slow heart rate.

PEARLS
Motor and Sensory Function

Perform brief motor and sensory checks in the upper and lower extremities before and after moving any patient.

TABLE 11-2 *Clues to Spinal-Cord Injury Revealed During Patient Assessment**

Mechanism of Injury
- Blunt trauma above the clavicle
- Diving accident
- Motor vehicle or bicycle accident
- Fall
- Stabbing or impalement anywhere near the spinal column
- Shooting or blast injury to the torso
- Any violent injury with forces that could act on the spinal column or cord

Patient Complaints
- Neck or back pain
- Numbness or tingling
- Loss of movement or weakness

Signs Revealed During Assessment
- Pain on movement of back or spinal column
- Obvious deformity of back or spinal column
- Guarding against movement of back
- Loss of sensation
- Weak or flaccid muscles
- Loss of control of bladder or bowels
- Erection of the penis (priapism)
- Neurogenic shock

*The "clues" listed are indicators that the spine may have been injured. These patients may require SMR. (Please refer to Figure 11-8.)

The neurological exam is described in more detail in Chapters 2 and 10, but we will review the exam of the peripheral nervous system here. The ITLS Primary Survey must be time efficient. If the conscious patient can move his fingers and toes, the motor nerves are intact. Anything less than normal sensation (tingling or decreased sensation) is suspicious for cord injury. The unconscious patient may withdraw if you pinch his fingers and toes. If so, you have demonstrated intact motor and sensory nerves and thus an intact cord. However, this does not mean SMR is not needed. All unconscious trauma patients should have SMR. Flaccid paralysis and no reflexes or withdrawal, even in the unconscious head-injury patient, usually means spinal-cord injury. Document these important findings.

Managing the Trauma Patient

Minimizing Spinal Movement: Based on the mechanism of injury, it is appropriate to place the head and neck in a neutral position as you first evaluate the patient. The purpose of SMR is to minimize spinal movement to avoid aggravating any spinal-cord or column injury. Preparation for managing spinal-cord or column injury can begin when you are dispatched to the scene of a motor-vehicle collision, fall, explosion, head injury, or neck injury.

There are two types of situations that require modification of the usual SMR. The patient who is in immediate danger of death in a hostile environment or in an immediate life-threatening position in a structure or vehicle may require emergency rescue. An example would be the patient who is in an MVC and, when you arrive, the auto is on fire. In cases where even a few seconds may mean the difference between life and death, you are justified in saving the patient in any way possible. Anytime this manner of rescue is used, you should document the reason and request a review of the chart by medical direction. Some examples of situations that might require emergency rescue are when Scene Size-up identifies a condition that may immediately endanger you or the patient, such as:

■ Fire or immediate danger of fire or explosion
■ Hostile environment, gunfire or other weapons
■ Danger of being carried away by rapidly moving water
■ Structure in immediate danger of collapse
■ Continuing immediately life-threatening toxic exposure

The second situation that requires modification of usual SMR is for patients whose ITLS Primary Survey indicates a critical degree of ongoing danger that requires an intervention within 1 or 2 minutes. Indications for rapid extrication are the following:

■ Airway obstruction that cannot be relieved by modified jaw thrust or finger sweep
■ Cardiac or respiratory arrest
■ Chest or airway injuries requiring ventilation or assisted ventilation
■ Deep shock or bleeding that cannot be controlled

Rapid extrication requires multiple rescuers who remove the patient along the long axis of the body, using their hands to minimize spinal movement (see skills in Chapter 12). When the rapid extrication technique is used, the written report should also be carefully reviewed to ensure appropriate documentation of the technique and its indication.

The most easily applied and readily available method of cervical-motion restriction is with your hands or knees. Your hands should be placed to stabilize the neck in relation to the long axis of the spinal column (Figure 11-5). "Pulling traction" is not a prehospital option, and the term *traction* is not an appropriate description for motion restriction of the spine. Traction will usually result in further instability of any spinal-column injury. The correct approach is stabilization, without pulling on the neck. When packaging the body on a backboard, the neutral in-line position allows the most room for the spinal cord, so that is the optimal position for SMR.

You can place an appropriately sized cervical-spine extrication collar on the patient as airway assessment is being done. Commercial cervical motion-restriction devices may be left in place on the backboard. These one- or two-piece collars are not definitive devices for restricting cervical-spine motion, but should be used only as a reminder that SMR is necessary and to prevent gross neck movement. The rescuer's hands can be removed only when the patient (head and body) has been strapped on a backboard with an attached head motion-restriction device. For the conscious patient, positioning the head and neck in a position of comfort is a good guideline. Adequate strapping must secure the head, torso, and upper legs to the backboard. Inadequate strapping will torque the neck against the body if the patient moves, rolls, is dropped, or is rotated.

Placing and strapping a patient on the board effectively eliminates the patient's ability to protect the airway; therefore, the rescuer is responsible. Once the patient is secured to the board, a rescuer must be present and capable of rolling the board if the patient begins to vomit or loses his airway. This rule continues in effect in the emergency department, where an emergency department staff person must assume responsibility for airway protection.

Definitive SMR occurs when the body is strapped securely to the board with cushions, blanket, or towel rolls, maintaining the head, cervical spine, torso, and pelvis in line. In the past, sandbags have been used for motion restriction of the head and perform well when the patient is kept supine. However, if the board is tilted or the patient and the board are

PEARLS
Emergency Rescue

• Emergency Rescue is reserved for those situations where there is immediate (within seconds) environmental threat to the life of the victim and/or rescuer. Patients should be moved to a safe area in a manner that places the rescuer at the least risk.

• Rapid Extrication should be considered for patients whose medical conditions or situations require fast intervention (one or two minutes—but not seconds) to prevent death.

PEARLS
Traction

Do not apply traction to the head and neck. Maintain in-line stabilization of the head, neck, and spine.

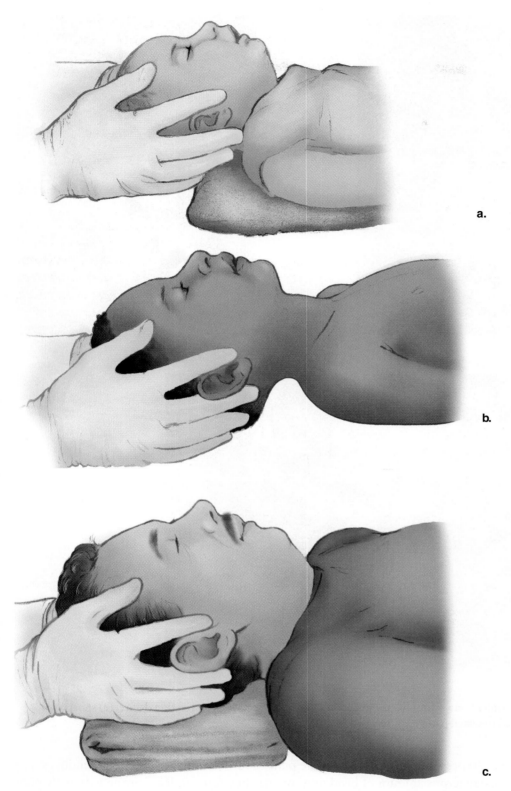

FIGURE 11-5 Neutral spinal positioning for infant, child, and adult patients. (a) Due to the large heads of younger children, you may need to raise the shoulders with padding. (b) In older children, obtain neutral positioning with shoulders and head on a flat surface. (c) With adults, elevate the head 1 to 2 inches.

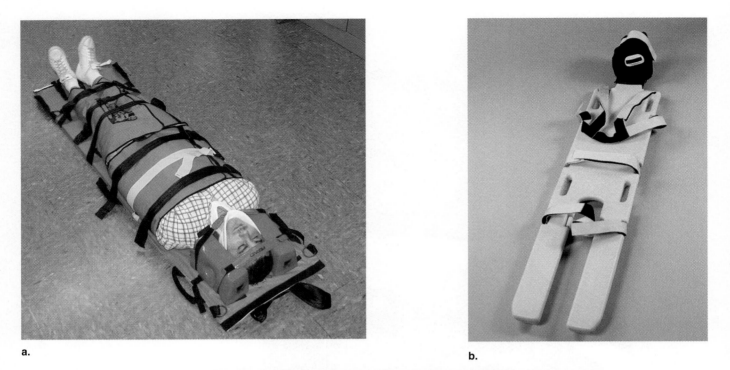

a.

b.

c.

FIGURE 11-6 (a) Reeves sleeve; (b) Miller body splint; (c) pediatric SMR device; (d) Kendrick extrication device; (e) short backboard; (f) short backboard applied to seated patient.

rotated (to prevent aspiration when the patient vomits), the weight of the sandbags may cause a dangerous amount of head movement. Therefore sandbags are an extremely poor option for prehospital SMR. Lighter-weight bulky objects, such as towel rolls, blanket rolls, or head cushions, are better tools for this job. When applied properly, these devices allow removal of the front portion of the cervical collar and observation of the neck, as in the patient with open neck wounds.

There are some patients (frightened children and patients with altered mental status) who will struggle so violently that they defeat your attempts to eliminate spinal movement. There may be no good solution to this. The Reeves sleeve (Figure 11-6) may be the best de-

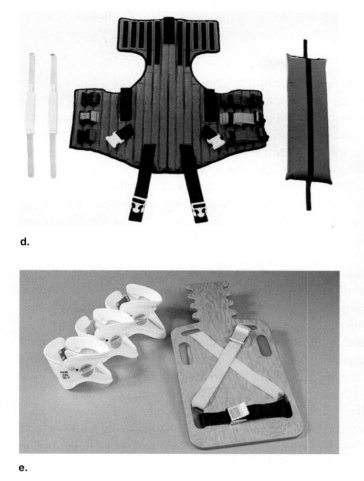

d.

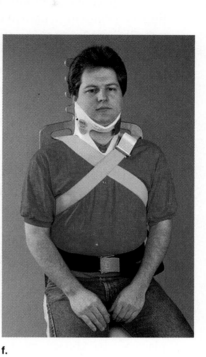

e.   f.

FIGURE 11-6 (continued)

vice to restrict spinal motion in the combative adult patient. You should always carefully document those situations in which the patient refuses to cooperate with SMR.

A truly neutral cervical-spine position for an adult is usually obtained with the use of 1 to 2 inches of occipital padding on a long backboard. This slightly elevates the head and brings the neck into a neutral position that tends to make the patient more comfortable and also makes endotracheal intubation easier if needed. This is accomplished with the head pad on a cervical motion-restriction device or the padding that is used with many backboard devices. Elderly patients whose necks have a natural flexed posture will require more padding. Children, because their heads are proportionately larger, usually require padding under the shoulders to prevent neck flexion on the backboard.

In certain situations, once the patient is packaged onto the backboard, the board and patient may have to be rolled up onto his side (Figure 11-7). Careful strapping can prevent lateral movement of the spine in this situation, but use of the vacuum backboard is far superior for this. Women who are more than 20 weeks pregnant should always be transported with the backboard tilted 20 to 30 degrees to the patient's left side in order to keep the uterus off the inferior vena cava.

Patients with airway problems who are not intubated are better transported on their side. This is especially critical when there is uncontrolled bleeding into the airway or if there is massive face or neck trauma. In these situations gravity helps drain fluids out of the

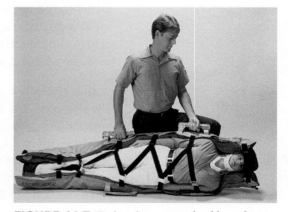

FIGURE 11-7 Patient in vacuum backboard turned on side. Notice that the body is maintained in a straight line.

airway and may prevent aspiration if the patient vomits. Because of the danger of vomiting and aspiration, unconscious patients who are not intubated should be transported rolled to the side.

The Log Roll: The log-roll technique is used for moving a patient onto a backboard. It is commonly used because it is easy to perform with a minimum number of rescuers. As yet no movement technique has been devised that maintains complete spinal immobilization while moving a patient onto a backboard. Properly performed, the log-roll technique will minimize movement of the spinal column as well as any other technique.

The log-roll technique moves the spinal column as a single unit with the head and pelvis. It can be performed on patients lying prone or supine. Using three or more rescuers—controlled by the rescuer at the patient's head—the patient (with her arms at her side) is rolled onto her uninjured side, a board is slid underneath, and the patient is rolled face up onto the board. The log-roll technique is then completed when the patient's chest, pelvis, and head are secured to the board.

The log roll may be modified for patients with painful arm, leg, and chest wounds who need to be rolled onto their uninjured side. The side to which you turn the patient during the log-roll procedure is not critical and can be changed in situations in which you can only place the backboard on one side of the patient.

The log-roll technique is useful for most trauma patients, but for patients with an unstable fractured pelvis, it may aggravate the injury to roll their weight onto the pelvis. If the pelvic fracture appears stable, the log roll should be carefully performed, turning the patient onto the uninjured side (if it can be identified). Patients with obviously unstable pelvic fractures should not be log rolled, but should be lifted carefully onto a board by four or more rescuers. The scoop stretcher could also be used to move patients with unstable pelvic fractures onto the backboard. At least one model of scoop stretcher can be used in place of a backboard (see 13 in the Bibliography at the end of this chapter).

Spinal Motion-Restriction Devices: There is a wide range of devices currently marketed to provide SMR for injured patients (see Figure 11-6). No device has yet been proven to excel over all others, and no device will ever be produced that can be used to provide SMR for all patients. No device is better than the crew using it; training with the available tools is the most critical factor in providing good patient care.

Complications of SMR: There are complications of strapping a patient to a board. The patient will be uncomfortable and will often complain of head and low back pain that is directly related to being strapped onto the hard backboard. The head and airway are in a fixed position, which can produce airway compromise and aspiration if the patient vomits. Obese patients and those with congestive heart failure can suffer life-threatening hypoxia. On a rigid board there is uneven skin pressure that can result in pressure sores. Lifting the patient and the board can cause injuries to rescue personnel. SMR should be applied appropriately to those who will most likely benefit, and it should be avoided if not necessary.

Indications for SMR: Worldwide controversy exists regarding when and how to stabilize the spine. The widely held belief is that injured patients must have SMR performed until an injury can be ruled out. However, as mentioned above, there are no Class I studies to confirm this and some countries do not perform SMR. They report no difference in spinal injury occurrence or outcome. At least one study has been done comparing the EMS systems of a country that performs no SMR (Malaysia) and one that consistently performs SMR (the United States). The study concluded that prehospital SMR had little or no effect on neurological outcome in patients with blunt spinal trauma. This is not to condemn SMR, but to remind us that what we are doing is based on logic and not actually based on scientific evidence.

Recent studies have documented circumstances under which spinal-column or cord injury is very unlikely, and therefore the patient can be managed without SMR. These studies have resulted in a clinical pathway referred to as the *Maine Protocol for Spinal Motion Restriction* and was written by Peter Goth, MD (Figure 11-8). This protocol is supported by the National Association of EMS Physicians (see Table 11-3 for NAEMSP's position paper on spinal motion restriction). You must assess the mechanism of injury, interview and examine the patient, then use this information to determine which patients need SMR. From the Scene Size-up, history, and assessment come the clues that identify those patients who do not need SMR.

Under the Maine protocol, the rescuer first assesses the mechanism of injury. SMR is not required if there is no mechanism of injury that would damage the spine (foot crushed by a car). If the mechanism is a high-risk event, SMR is performed regardless of other clinical findings. These high-risk situations include high-speed MVCs, falls of greater than three times the patient's height, penetrating wounds into or near the spinal column, sports injuries to the head or neck, diving accidents, and any trauma situation in which the patient remains unconscious.

If the danger of spinal injury is uncertain (ground-level fall, low-speed "fender bender"), the rescuer should manually stabilize the spine and then assess the patient for signs of spinal injury. The patient must be reliable enough to understand the EMS provider and answer the questions accurately, so children and patients with altered mental status or acute stress reactions are excluded. The patient is assessed for evidence of intoxication or distracting injuries that may not allow the patient to clearly feel the pain associated with a spinal injury. The patient is asked if he has pain in the area of the spinal column. If no pain is present in the neck or back, and no other injuries are so painful as to distract the patient from comprehending back or neck pain, the rescuer then carefully examines the spinal column and performs a neurological exam. If there is any tenderness on palpation of the spinal column area or if the patient complains of midline pain when asked to move his back, SMR is performed. SMR is also performed if there are alterations in the motor or sensory exam.

If the patient has no high-risk mechanism of injury, no alteration of mental status, no distracting injuries, is not intoxicated, has no pain or tenderness along the spine, and has no neurological deficits, the patient may be treated and transported without SMR. This protocol has proven effective in research studies but, like all medical protocols, must be approved for local use by medical direction and followed up with a quality assurance program.

PEARLS
Spinal Motion Restriction

- Spinal clearance is not a priority in the patient suffering from multiple trauma; spinal motion restriction is.
- Protocols have been developed to allow you to properly choose which trauma patients need SMR, using mechanism of injury and careful evaluation.

TABLE 11-3 *Position Paper on Spinal Motion Restriction by the National Association of EMS Physicians**

Spinal motion restriction is indicated in prehospital trauma patients who sustain an injury with a mechanism having the potential for causing spinal injury and who have at least one of the following clinical criteria.

- Altered mental status
- Evidence of intoxication
- A distracting painful injury (e.g., long bone extremity fracture)
- Neurologic deficit
- Spinal pain or tenderness

*See reference 6 in this chapter's Bibliography.

Initial Assessment of Spinal Injury Clinical Criteria

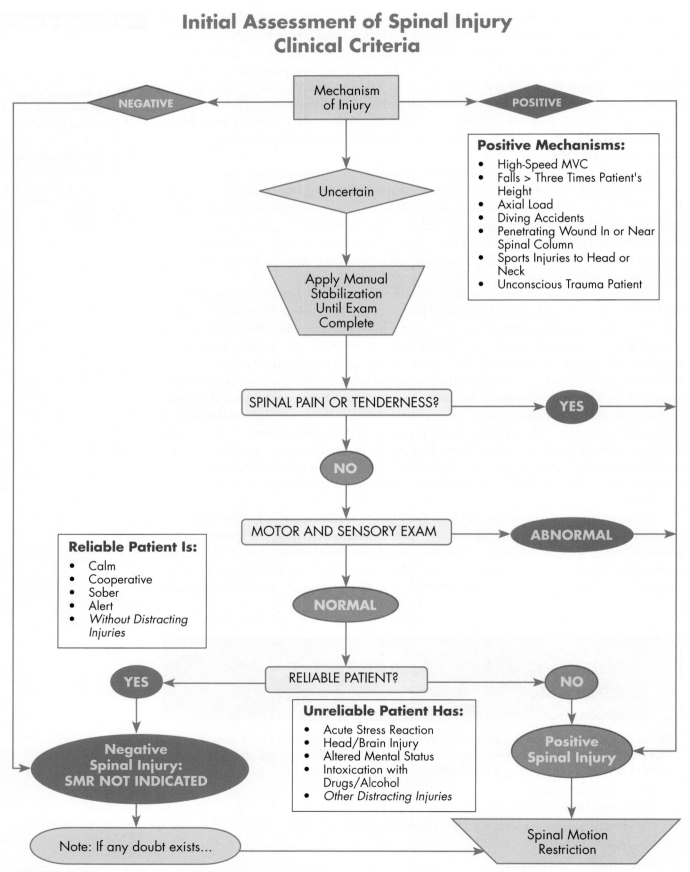

FIGURE 11-8 Decision tree for spinal motion restriction. *(Reprinted by permission of Peter Goth, MD)*

Airway Intervention

When the rescuer performs SMR in any manner, the patient loses some of her ability to maintain her own airway. As mentioned earlier, the rescuer must then assume this responsibility until the patient has a controlled airway or has the spinal column cleared in the emergency department and is released from the motion-restricting equipment (Figure 11-9). This is particularly critical in children, who have a greater potential for vomiting and aspiration after a traumatic injury.

Airway manipulations in the trauma patient require careful application. Current research indicates that any airway intervention will cause some movement of the spinal column. In-line manual stabilization is the most effective manner for minimizing this movement. Nasotracheal, orotracheal, or cricothyroid intubations all induce some bony movement. Your ITLS Primary Survey should include manual stabilization, then the use of the airway control method that you are most skilled at performing. When weighing the risks and benefits of each airway procedure, recall that the risk of dying with an uncontrolled airway is greater than the risk of inducing spinal-cord damage using a careful approach to intubation.

Special SMR Situations

You must be prepared to stabilize the spinal column of all patients who sustain major trauma. In some patients (see below), traditional techniques must be modified to provide safe and effective SMR.

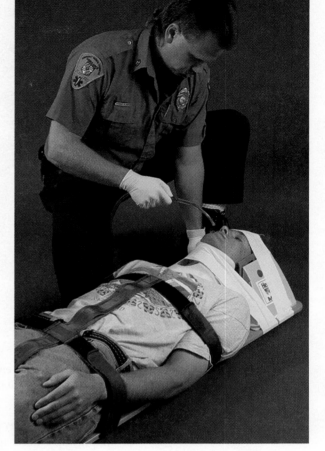

FIGURE 11-9 You are responsible for the patient's airway once the patient is strapped to a backboard.

Closed-Space Rescues: Closed-space rescues are performed in a manner appropriate for the clinical condition of the patient. The only general rules that can be applied to these rescues are to prevent gross cervical-spine movement and to move patients in line with the long axis of the body (Figure 11-10). Safety of the rescuer is of prime importance in all closed-space rescues. Asphyxia, toxic gases, and structure collapse are dangers of closed-space rescue and may require the use of emergency rescue. Never enter a closed space unless you are properly trained, equipped (air pack, safety line, and so on), and sure of scene safety.

Water Emergencies: You can perform water rescues by moving the patient in line, thereby preventing gross cervical movement. When the rescuers are in a stable position for performing SMR, the backboard is floated under the patient, and the patient is then secured and removed from the water (Scan 11.1). Safety of both rescuers and patients is of paramount importance. If you are not trained in water rescue, do not attempt to rescue victims in hazardous situations such as deep or swift water.

Prone, Seated, and Standing Patients: Prone, seated, and standing patients are stabilized in a manner that minimizes spinal column movement, ending with the patient in the conventional supine position.

■ *Prone patients* are log-rolled onto a backboard, with the careful coordination of head and chest rescuers.

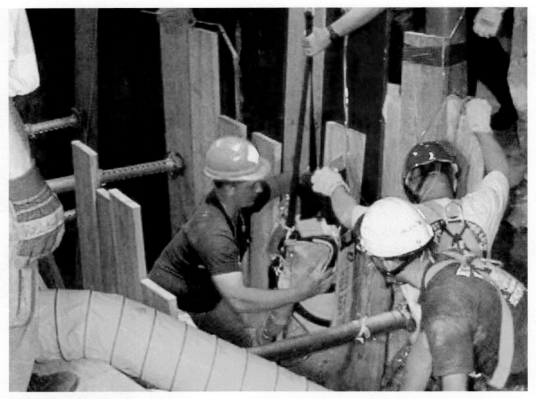

FIGURE 11-10 Patient entrapped in trench cave-in being lifted out along the long axis of the body. *(Photo courtesy of Roy Alson, MD)*

■ *Seated patients* may be stabilized using short backboards or their commercial adaptations. Used appropriately, short backboards provide initial stabilization of the cervical and thoracic spine and then facilitate the movement of the patient onto a long backboard.

■ *Standing patients* may be placed against the long board while upright and then strapped in place. The board is then gently lowered to the supine position.

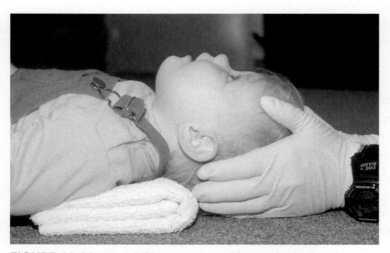

FIGURE 11-11 Most children require padding under back and shoulders to keep the cervical spine in a neutral position. *(Courtesy of Bob Page, NREMT-P)*

Pediatric Patients: It is best to provide initial SMR of the pediatric patient with your hands, and then use cushions or towel rolls to help secure the child on an appropriate board or device. Some pediatric trauma specialists suggest padding beneath the back and shoulders on the board in a child under the age of 3 years (see Figures 11-5 and 11-11). These children normally have a relatively large head that flexes the neck when placed on a straight board. Padding under the back and shoulders will prevent this flexion and also make the child more comfortable.

Children who are involved in an MVC while restrained in a child safety seat but have no apparent injuries may be packaged in the safety seat for transport to the hospital. Using towel or blanket rolls, cloth tape, and a little reassurance, you can secure the child in the safety seat and then belt the seat into the ambulance (Figure 11-12).

WATER RESCUE

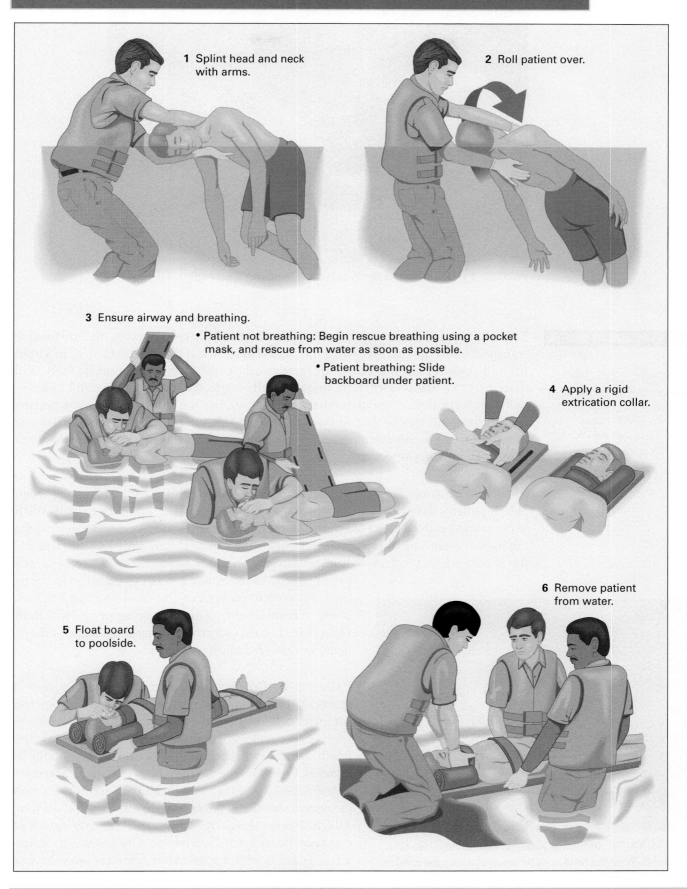

1 Splint head and neck with arms.

2 Roll patient over.

3 Ensure airway and breathing.

- Patient not breathing: Begin rescue breathing using a pocket mask, and rescue from water as soon as possible.
- Patient breathing: Slide backboard under patient.

4 Apply a rigid extrication collar.

5 Float board to poolside.

6 Remove patient from water.

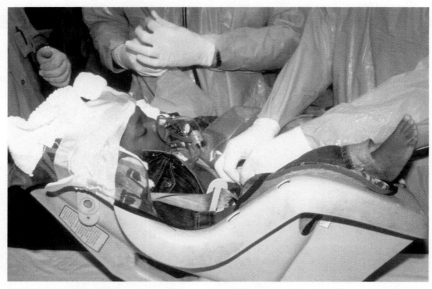

FIGURE 11-12 Infant secured in car seat. *(Courtesy of David Effron, MD, FACEP)*

This technique minimizes movement of the child and provides a secure method for child transport in the ambulance. When the child is in a car seat that is damaged, or in a built-in child-restraint seat that cannot be removed, the child must be removed for SMR. Children in such situations will have to be carefully extricated onto a backboard or another pediatric SMR device, using manual stabilization. For the child who is frightened and struggling, there may be no good way to obtain SMR. Careful reassurance, the presence of a comforting family member, and gentle management will help prevent more complications and further struggling.

Elderly Patients: Elderly patients require flexibility in packaging techniques. Many elderly patients have arthritic changes of the spine and very thin skin. Such patients will be very uncomfortable when placed on a backboard. Some arthritic spines are so rigid that the patient cannot be laid straight on the board, and some elderly patients have rigid flexion of the neck that will result in a large gap between the head and the board. You can make use of towels, blankets, and pillows to pad the elderly patient and prevent movement and discomfort on the backboard (Figure 11-13). This is a situation in which the vacuum backboard (which conforms to the shape of the patient) works very well (see Figure 11-7).

Patients in Protective Gear: Large helmets used in sports and cycling must be removed at some point to permit complete assessment and care. Helmets used in different sports present different management problems for rescuers. Football and ice hockey helmets are custom fitted to the individual. Unless special circumstances exist, such as respiratory distress coupled with an inability to access the airway, the helmet should not be removed in the prehospital setting. Athletic helmet design will generally allow easy airway access once the face guard is removed. The best way to remove a face guard is with a screwdriver (cordless screwdriver is best) and one should be on every response vehicle, but

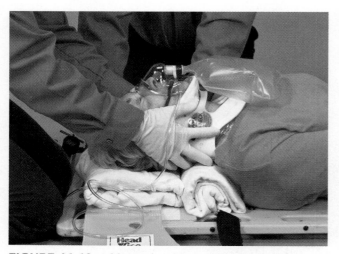

FIGURE 11-13 Additional padding, such as rolled blankets or towels behind the head, may be needed to keep the head in a neutral, in-line position.

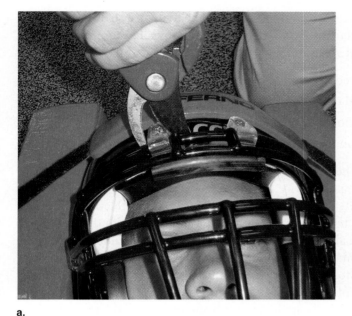

a.

FIGURE 11-14a The face guard of football helmets can be removed with a screwdriver or pruning shears. *(Photo courtesy of Jeff Hinshaw, MS, PA-C, NREMT-P)*

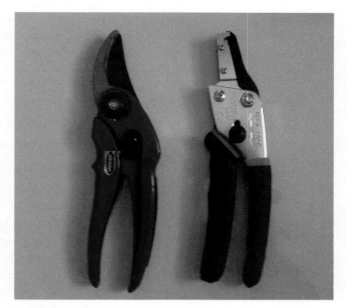

b.

FIGURE 11-14b Anvil pruning shears (left) or a face mask extractor (right) can be used to remove a football helmet face guard. *(Photo courtesy of Jeff Hinshaw, MS, PA-C, NREMT-P)*

sometimes the screw slot strips out and the face guard will have to be cut off. There is an excellent device made specifically for cutting off the four face guard mounting strips (face mask extractor by Collins Sports Medicine), but at this time it is extremely expensive. The next best choice is to use anvil pruning shears (Figure 11-14). Pick one of these devices, train with it, and know how to use it appropriately when the time comes. Rescue scissors have been advocated in the past but studies have found them to be unsuitable for this task.

The athlete wearing shoulder pads has his neck in a neutral position when on the backboard with the helmet in place. If the helmet is removed, padding must be inserted under the head to keep the neck from extending (Figure 11-15). After arrival at the emergency facility, the cervical spine can be x-rayed with the helmet in place. Once the spine is evaluated, the helmet can be removed by stabilizing the head and neck, removing the cheek pads, releasing the air inflation system, and then sliding the helmet off in the usual manner.

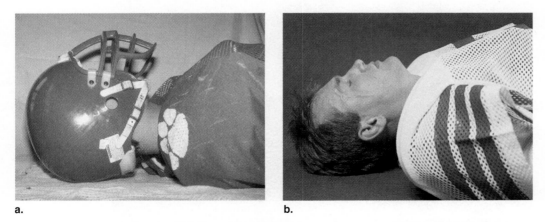

a.

b.

FIGURE 11-15 (a) Patients with shoulder pads and helmets are usually best immobilized with the helmet in place. The spine is maintained in a neutral position with a minimum of movement. *(Photo courtesy of Bob Page, NREMT-P)* (b) Patients with shoulder pads must have padding under the head to maintain a neutral position if the helmet is removed.

For prehospital providers, field removal of an athletic helmet is a last-ditch procedure but it must be entertained in certain unique patient-care situations. The four main reasons to consider field helmet removal are as follows:

- Face mask cannot be removed in a timely fashion
- Airway cannot be controlled due to the design of the helmet and chin strap
- Helmet and chin straps do not hold the head securely
- Helmet prevents stabilization for transport in an appropriate position

When removing an athletic helmet, it is imperative to cut the chin strap and not to attempt unsnapping or unbuckling the device.

Shoulder pad removal is often linked to helmet removal in the athletic setting. Not only is this done routinely with helmet removal, but also when faced with the inability to maintain neutral cervical-spine alignment (often due to ill-fitting shoulder pads), when you are unable to secure the athlete to the spine board, and when you need access to the chest for resuscitation efforts. Most shoulder pads can be removed by cutting the axillary straps and the laces on the front of the appliance, opening the appliance from the core outward (like a clam shell), and sliding the appliance out from under the athlete.

In contrast, motorcycle helmets often must be removed in the prehospital setting. The removal technique is modified to accommodate the different design. Motorcycle helmets are often designed with a continuous solid face guard that limits airway access. These helmets are not custom designed and frequently are poorly fitted to the patient. Their large size will usually produce significant neck flexion if left in place when the patient is positioned on a backboard (Figure 11-16). The motorcycle helmet will make it difficult to stabilize the neck in a neutral position, may obstruct access to the airway, and may hide injuries to the head or neck. It should be removed in the prehospital setting, using the techniques described in Chapter 12.

Very Large or Obese Patients: Very large or obese patients may not fit appropriately in standard equipment. You must be flexible, even using sheets of plywood and head cush-

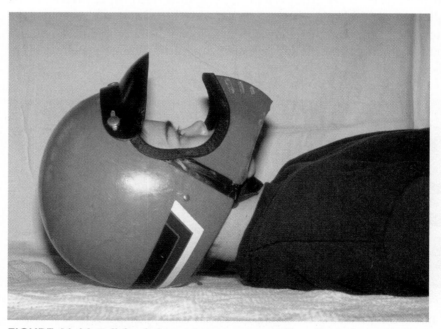

FIGURE 11-16 Full-face helmets obstruct access to the patient's airway. Notice that the helmet flexes the neck in a patient who is not wearing shoulder pads. *(Courtesy of Bob Page, NREMT-P)*

ions or towel rolls to stabilize the spine. In cold-weather climates, patients in bulky warm clothing will need to be snugly secured to prevent excessive movement.

Patients with Neck Wounds: Patients with penetrating or disfiguring wounds of the neck or lower face must be continually observed. Cervical collars will prevent continued examination of the wound site and may compromise the airway in wounds with expanding hematomas or subcutaneous air. If the mandible is fractured, the collar may again cause airway compromise. Therefore, for patients with these injuries, it may be wise to avoid collars, and use instead manual stabilization and head cushion devices or blanket rolls for cervical motion restriction.

Trauma patients with paralysis or neurogenic shock have lost vascular control and thus cannot control blood flow to the skin. They may lose heat rapidly, so it is important for you to prevent hypothermia.

Case Study continued

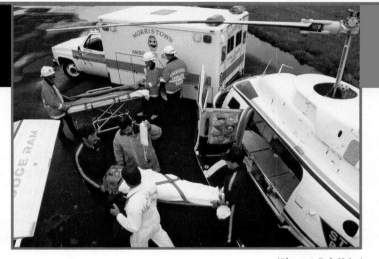

(Photo © Bob Krist/ CORBIS)

Dan, Joyce, and Buddy have been called to a public swimming pool for a diving injury. Dan is the team leader on this call. When they arrive on scene, they are told the patient had been chasing some friends and dived into the shallow end of the pool, striking his head on the bottom. He was briefly dazed but not unconscious and did not suffer near-drowning because his friends immediately pulled him from the shallow water. However, it is clear that they did not take spinal precautions while doing so.

The patient complains of severe pain in his neck with weakness in both arms and inability to move his legs. A Rapid Trauma Survey reveals tenderness along the cervical spine with spasm of the cervical spinal muscles and he is breathing with his diaphragm only. The patient is managed gently, meticulously packaged on a long backboard, given 100 percent oxygen to breathe, and transported to the level I trauma center. Vital signs just before lift-off are normal.

On arrival at the emergency department, he is found to be able to flex his arms at the elbow but cannot move his trunk or legs. His blood pressure has dropped to 80/50 with a pulse of 72. He is treated for neurogenic shock. A CAT scan reveals a compression fracture of the fifth cervical vertebra, causing cord compression. The patient will require spinal decompression and stabilization surgery and months of physical therapy in order to regain some use of his arms and legs. He eventually is able to walk with a cane and is able to return to school.

Case Study Wrap-up

Diving injuries or falls in which the victim lands on his head cause axial loading of the spinal column and can cause compression fractures of the cervical spine and cervical spinal-cord injury. In most trauma cases bystanders have learned to wait for EMS personnel to move the victim, but in the case of diving accidents there is such a concern for the person drowning that bystanders will usually immediately pull the victim from the water. People untrained in EMS rarely think of spinal injury in this situation and most do not know how to protect the spine when getting someone out of the water (see Scan 11.1). As in this case, even if there are already signs of spinal injury, you should carefully package the patient to prevent secondary injuries and give the patient the best chance at a good recovery. There are profound lifelong implications of spinal-cord injuries.

SUMMARY

Spinal-cord injury is a devastating consequence of modern-day trauma. Unstable or incomplete damage to the spinal column or cord is not completely predictable; therefore, trauma patients who are unconscious or have any dangerous mechanism of injury affecting the head, neck, or trunk should have SMR. Those trauma patients with uncertain mechanisms may not require SMR if they meet the physical exam criteria. Special trauma cases may require special SMR techniques. Once SMR is performed, the patient loses some ability to control his airway; so, you must be prepared at all times to intervene should the patient vomit or have evidence of airway compromise.

BIBLIOGRAPHY

1. Aprahamian, L. 1994. Experimental cervical spine injury model: Evaluation of airway management and splinting techniques. *Annals of Emergency Medicine* 23: 584.
2. Augustine, J. 2004. Failure on the board. *EMS* 33: 52–53.
3. British Trauma Society. 2003. Guidelines for initial management and assessment of spinal injury. *Injury, International Journal of the Injured* 34: 405–25.
4. Cordell, W. H., J. Hollingsworth, et al. 1995. Pain and tissue-interface pressures during spineboard immobilization. *Annals of Emergency Medicine* 26: 31–36.
5. Cross, D. A., J. Baskerville. 2001. Comparison of perceived pain with different immobilization techniques. *Prehospital Emergency Care* 5: 270–74.
6. Domeier, R. M. 1999. The National Association of EMS Physicians Standards and Clinical Practice Committee. *Prehospital Emergency Care* 3: 251–53.
7. Domeier, R. M., R. Evans, et al. 1999. The reliability of prehospital clinical evaluation for potential spinal injury is not affected by the mechanism of injury. *Prehospital Emergency Care* 3: 332–37.
8. Dunn, T. M., A. Dalton, T. Dorfman, W. Dunn. 2004. Are emergency medical technician-basics able to use a selective immobilization of the cervical spine protocol?: A preliminary report. *Prehospital Emergency Care* 8: 207–11.
9. Goth, P. C. 1994. Spine injury, clinical criteria for assessment and management. Augusta, ME: Medical Care Development, 1–36.
10. Hauswald, M., G. Ong, D. Tandberg, Z. Omar. 1998. Out-of-hospital spinal immobilization: Its effect on neurologic injury. *Academic Emergency Medicine* 5: 214–19.
11. Johnson, D. R., M. Hauswald, C. Stockhoff. 1996. Comparison of a vacuum splint device to rigid backboard for spinal immobilization. *American Journal of Emergency Medicine* 14: 369–72.
12. Kleiner, D. M., A. Pollak, C. McAdam. 2001. Helmet hazards. Do's and don'ts of football helmet removal. *JEMS* 26: 36–44, 46–48.
13. Krell, J. M., et al. 2006. Comparison of the Ferno scoop stretcher with the long backboard for spinal immobilization. *Prehospital Emergency Care* 10: 46–51.
14. Majernick, T. G. 1986. Cervical spine movement during orotracheal intubation. *Annals of Emergency Medicine* 15: 417.

Spine Management Skills

Donna Hastings, EMT-P

OBJECTIVES

Upon completion of this chapter, you should be able to:

1. Describe the essential components of a spinal motion-restriction (SMR) system.

2. Explain when to use SMR.

3. Perform SMR with a short backboard.

4. Perform log-rolling of a patient onto a long backboard.

5. Properly secure a patient to a long backboard.

6. Perform SMR on a patient in a standing position.

7. Stabilize the head and neck when a neutral position cannot be safely attained.

8. Perform rapid extrication.

9. Explain when helmets should and should not be removed from injured patients.

10. Properly remove a motorcycle helmet.

11. Demonstrate proper stabilization of the neck in patients who are wearing shoulder pads and helmets.

(Photo courtesy of Bob Page, NREMT-P)

ESSENTIAL COMPONENTS OF AN SMR SYSTEM

The five essential components of a full spinal motion-restriction (SMR) system are:

- *Backboard.* The purpose of the backboard is to keep the spinal column from moving. Several types are available.
- *Cervical collar.* Though cervical collars do not immobilize the neck, they provide some support and can serve to remind the patient to keep the neck still. Several types are available.
- *Head motion-restriction device.* These devices attach to the backboard and are used to restrict movement of the patient's head after the patient's body has been strapped to the backboard. When the head motion-restriction device has been applied, the cervical collar may be removed if necessary. There are several different types of these devices.
- *Straps.* Strapping systems are used to bind the patient's body to the backboard in order to restrict movement of the spinal column. The straps should be positioned to decrease patient movement from side to side and from sliding up and down on the backboard. Several different systems are available.
- *Airway management kit.* When you strap someone's body and head to a board, you must assume responsibility for his or her airway. You must have the airway kit immediately available and you must have the skills to use it. Airway management is a priority consideration within SMR; thus airway management skills and equipment are necessary components.

APPLYING SPINAL MOTION RESTRICTIONS (SMR)

Patients Requiring SMR

> **PEARLS**
> *The Short Backboard*
>
> - When placing the straps around the legs on a male patient, do not catch the genitals in the straps.
> - Do not use the short backboard as a "handle" to move the patient. Move patient and board as a unit. Many short backboard devices come with built-in handles. These are not to be used ALONE to move a patient.
> - You may need to modify your strapping techniques, depending on injuries.

The goal of spinal motion restriction (SMR) is to limit movement of the spine and thus prevent further harm. See Figure 12-1 for indications for SMR. Patients requiring SMR must have it done before they are moved at all. In the case of an automobile collision, you must stabilize the spine before removing the patient from the wreckage. More patient movement is involved in extrication than at any other time, so you must carefully stabilize the neck and spine before beginning extrication. Remember: Traction can cause permanent paralysis. You are stabilizing the spine, not pulling on it. Except in situations requiring Emergency Rescue and sometimes Rapid Extrication, always try to document sensation and motor function in the extremities before you move the patient.

SMR with a Short Backboard

The short backboard is used for patients who are in a position that does not permit use of the long backboard (such as in a motor vehicle). There are several different devices of this type. Some have strapping mechanisms different from the one explained here. Become familiar with your equipment (practice, practice, practice) before employing it in an emergency.

PROCEDURE

✚ Applying a Short Backboard

Remember that the priorities of evaluation and management are done before an SMR device is applied. To apply a short backboard, follow the steps listed on the next pages (Scan 12.1 and Scan 12.2).

Initial Assessment of Spinal Injury
Clinical Criteria

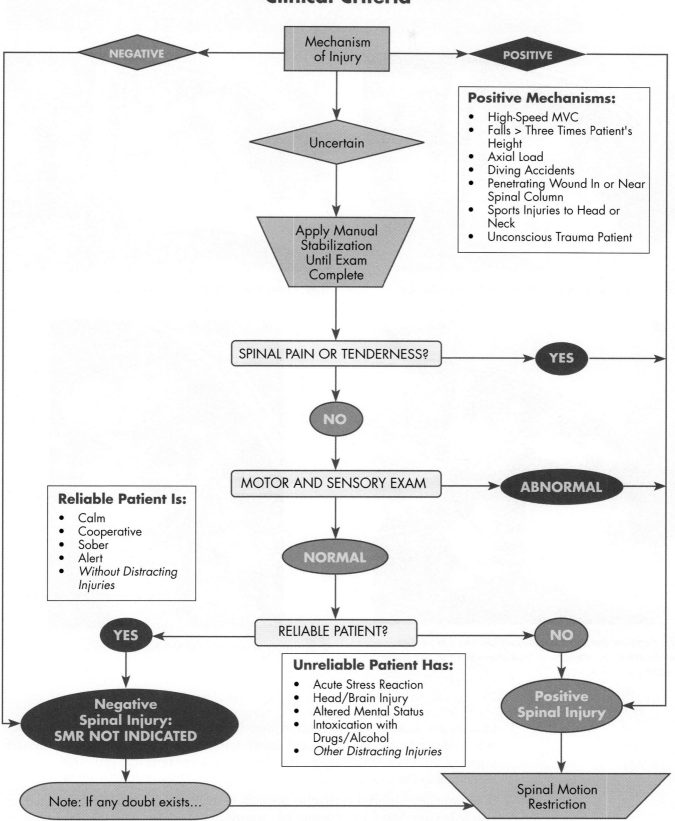

Mechanism of Injury

NEGATIVE

POSITIVE

Uncertain

Positive Mechanisms:
- High-Speed MVC
- Falls > Three Times Patient's Height
- Axial Load
- Diving Accidents
- Penetrating Wound In or Near Spinal Column
- Sports Injuries to Head or Neck
- Unconscious Trauma Patient

Apply Manual Stabilization Until Exam Complete

SPINAL PAIN OR TENDERNESS? → **YES**

NO

MOTOR AND SENSORY EXAM → **ABNORMAL**

NORMAL

Reliable Patient Is:
- Calm
- Cooperative
- Sober
- Alert
- *Without Distracting Injuries*

RELIABLE PATIENT?

YES

NO

Unreliable Patient Has:
- Acute Stress Reaction
- Head/Brain Injury
- Altered Mental Status
- Intoxication with Drugs/Alcohol
- *Other Distracting Injuries*

Negative Spinal Injury: SMR NOT INDICATED

Positive Spinal Injury

Note: If any doubt exists...

Spinal Motion Restriction

FIGURE 12-1 Decision tree for spinal motion restriction. *(Reprinted by permission of Peter Goth, MD)*

SCAN 12.1

Applying a Standard Short Backboard

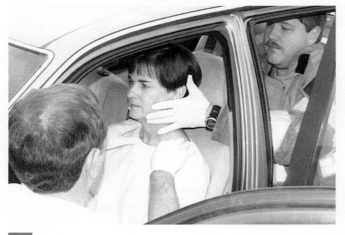

1 Stabilize neck and perform ITLS Primary Survey.

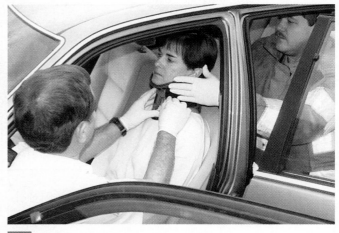

2 Apply a semirigid extrication collar.

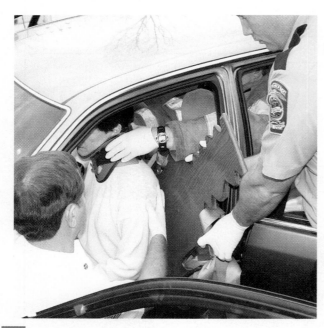

3 Position the short backboard behind the patient. Coordinate all movement so that movement of the spine is kept to a minimum.

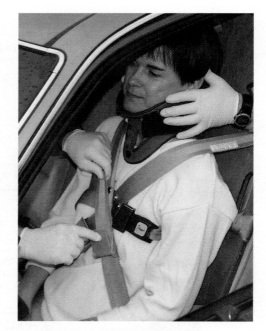

4 Apply straps and tighten securely.

1. One rescuer must, if possible, station himself behind the patient, place his hands on either side of the patient's head, and stabilize the neck in a neutral position. This step is part of the ABCs of evaluation. It is done at the same time that you begin evaluation of the airway.

2. When you have finished evaluating the neck in the Rapid Trauma Survey and have checked extremities for movement (document findings later), you should apply a semirigid extrication collar. If you have enough people, this can be done while someone else is doing the ABCs of evaluation and management. If you have limited

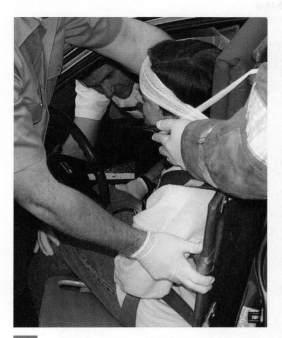

5 Turn the patient carefully. Then lower the patient onto the backboard.

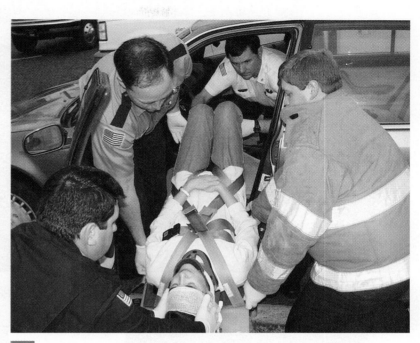

6 Slide the patient on the short backboard up into position on the long backboard. Loosen the straps and allow the legs to extend out flat. Then retighten the straps. Secure the patient and the short backboard to the long backboard. Apply a padded SMR device to secure the patient's head and neck.

help, apply the collar after finishing the Rapid Trauma Survey, but before transferring the patient to the backboard.

3. Position the short backboard behind the patient. The first rescuer continues to stabilize the neck while the short backboard is being maneuvered into place. The patient may have to be moved forward to get the backboard in position; great care must be taken so that moves are coordinated to support the neck and back.

4. Secure the patient to the board. There are usually three straps for this. Place the short strap under the armpits and across the upper chest as an anchor. Bring each long strap over a leg, down between both legs, back around the outside of the same leg, and across the chest. Then attach them to the upper strap opposite that which was brought across the shoulders at the midclavicular position.

5. Tighten the straps until the patient is held securely. If the patient is conscious, ask her to take a deep breath while placing your fingers under the straps to ensure that the straps have not been tightened to the point that it impedes breathing.

6. Secure the patient's head to the board by wide tape or elastic wraps around the forehead. Apply padding under the neck and head as needed to maintain a neutral position.

7. Transfer the patient to a long backboard. To do so, turn the patient so that her back is to the opening through which she is to be removed. Someone must support her legs so that the upper legs remain at a 90-degree angle to her torso. Position the long backboard through the opening until it is under the patient. Lower the patient's back onto the long backboard and slide her and the short backboard up into position on

Applying a Kendrick Extrication Device

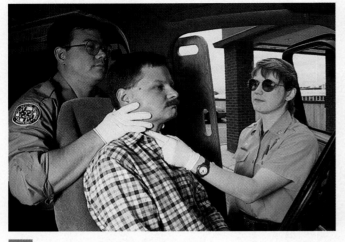

1 Stabilize the neck and perform the ITLS Primary Survey.

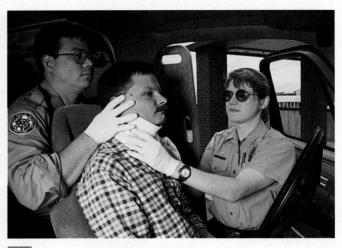

2 Apply semirigid extrication collar.

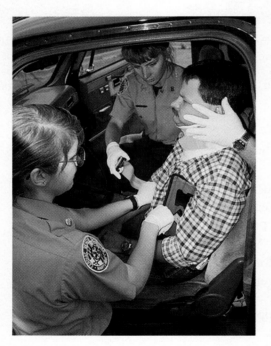

3 Position the device behind the patient. Coordinate all movements to restrict spinal motion. Position the chest panels up well into the armpits.

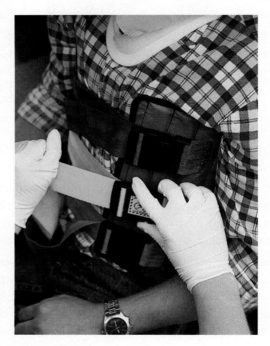

4 Tighten the chest straps.

the long backboard. Loosen the straps on the short board and allow the patient's legs to extend out flat, and then retighten the straps. Now secure her to the long backboard with straps, and secure her head with a padded motion-restriction device. When she is secured in this way, it is possible to turn the whole board up on its side if the patient has to vomit. The patient should remain securely strapped, with little or no movement.

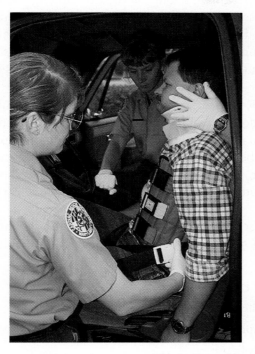

5 Loosen each leg strap around the ipsilateral (same side) leg and back to the buckle on the same side. Fasten snugly.

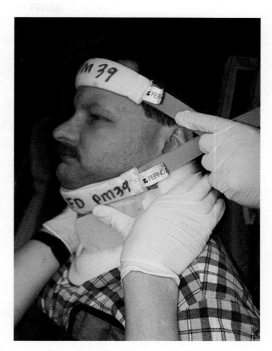

6 Apply firm padding as needed between the head and the headpiece to keep the head in a neutral position. Bring the head flaps around to the side of the head and secure firmly with straps, tape, or elastic wrap.

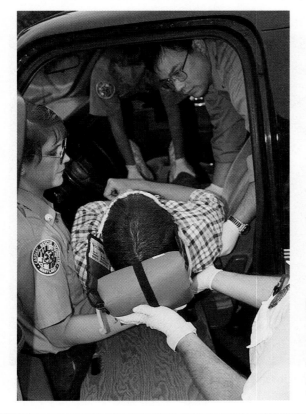

7 Turn the patient and the device as a unit. Then lower the patient onto a long backboard. Slide the patient and the device up into position on the board. Loosen the leg straps and allow the legs to extend out flat. Finally, retighten the straps and secure the patient and the device to the backboard.

Emergency Rescue and Rapid Extrication

Patients left inside vehicles following a collision are usually stabilized on a short backboard (or extrication device) and then transferred onto a long backboard. Although this is the best way to extricate anyone with a possible spinal injury, there are certain situations in which a more rapid method must be used. Note: International Trauma Life Support (ITLS) offers a one-day course called "Access" on basic extrication from motor vehicles using basic hand tools. Call 888-495-4857 for information (international calls: 630-495-6442).

Situations Requiring Emergency Rescue: This procedure is used only in situations in which the patient's life is in immediate danger. In some of these situations you may not have time to use any technique other than pulling the patient to safety. This is an example of "desperate situations demanding desperate measures." Use good judgment. Do not sacrifice your life in a dangerous situation. Whenever you use this procedure, it should be noted in the written report, and you should be prepared to defend your actions at a review by your medical director.

Perform Emergency Rescue if the Scene Size-up identifies a condition that may immediately (within seconds) endanger you and/or the patient, such as the following (Figure 12-2):

- Fire or immediate danger of fire or explosion
- Hostile environment, gunfire or other weapons
- Danger of being carried away by rapidly moving water
- Structure in immediate danger of collapse
- Continuing immediately life-threatening toxic exposure

Situations Requiring Rapid Extrication: You should perform Rapid Extrication if your ITLS Primary Survey of a patient identifies a critical degree of ongoing danger that

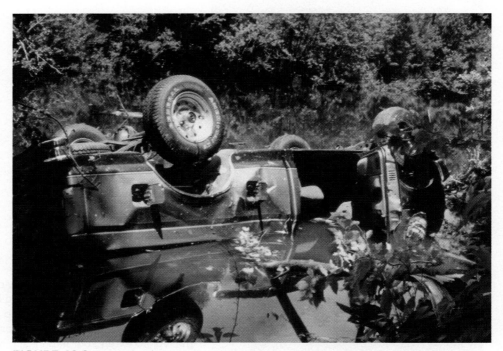

FIGURE 12-2 Example of a situation in which you may have to perform emergency rescue.
(Courtesy of Bonnie Meneely, EMT-P)

requires an intervention within 1 to 2 minutes. You must act immediately and rapidly, but you have time to stabilize the patient to some degree as you extricate him. Example situations that may require rapid extrication are as follows:

- Airway obstruction that you cannot relieve by jaw thrust or finger sweep
- Cardiac or respiratory arrest
- Chest or airway injuries requiring ventilation or assisted ventilation
- Deep shock or bleeding that you cannot control

PROCEDURE

❊ Performing a Rapid Extrication

The following steps are illustrated in Scan 12.3.

1. One rescuer must, if possible, station himself behind the patient, place his hands on either side of the patient's head, and stabilize the neck in a neutral position. This step is part of the ABCs. It is done at the same time that you begin evaluation of the airway.
2. Do a Rapid Trauma Survey. Then quickly apply a cervical collar. (You should have the collar with you when you begin.)
3. If your ITLS Primary Survey of the patient reveals one of the situations listed above, go to the Rapid Extrication technique. This requires at least four, and preferably five or six, persons to perform well.
4. Immediately slide the long backboard onto the seat and, if possible, at least slightly under the patient's buttocks.
5. A second rescuer stands close beside the open door of the vehicle and takes over control of the cervical spine.
6. Rescuer 1 or another rescuer is positioned on the other side of the front seat ready to rotate the patient's legs around.
7. Another rescuer is also positioned at the open door by the patient. By holding the upper torso, he works together with the rescuer holding the legs to turn the patient carefully.
8. The patient is turned so that his back is toward the backboard. His legs are lifted and his back is lowered to the backboard. The neck and back are not allowed to bend during this maneuver.
9. Using teamwork, the patient is carefully slid to the full length of the backboard and his legs are carefully straightened.
10. The patient is then moved immediately away from the vehicle (to the ambulance if available), and resuscitation is begun. He is secured to the backboard as soon as possible.

SMR Using the Long Backboard

One of the most important ways to apply SMR to a suspected spine-injured patient is to secure him from head to toe to a long backboard. But moving the patient onto the backboard must be accomplished in a careful, coordinated way that protects him from any further injury. That procedure is called a *log roll.*

PEARLS
The Long Backboard

- When you are applying the upper horizontal strap around a woman, place the upper strap above her breasts and under her arms, not across the breasts.
- When you are applying the lower horizontal strap on a pregnant woman, place it across the pelvis and not across the uterus.
- You may need to modify your strapping techniques, depending on injuries.
- Secure the patient well enough so that little or no motion of the spine will occur if the board is turned on its side. Do not make straps so tight that they interfere with breathing.

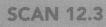

Performing a Rapid Extrication

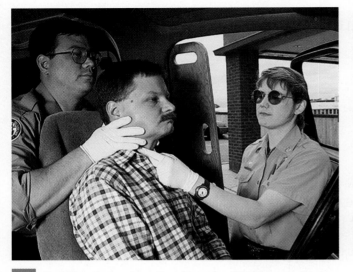

1 Stabilize the neck and perform the ITLS Primary Survey.

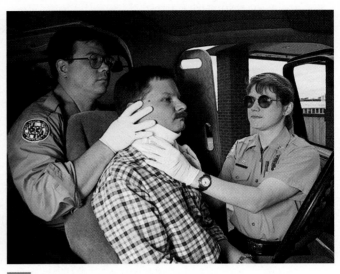

2 Apply a semirigid extrication collar.

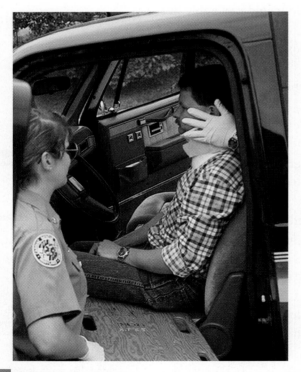

3 Slide the longboard onto the seat and slightly under the patient.

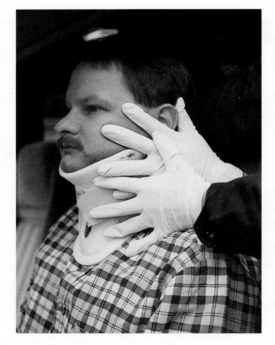

4 A second rescuer stands beside the open door of the vehicle and takes over control of the cervical spine.

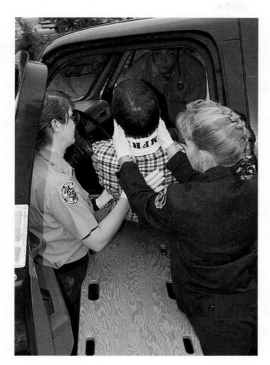

5 Carefully supporting the neck, torso, and legs, the rescuers turn the patient.

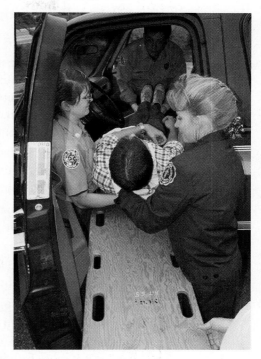

6 The legs are lifted and the back is lowered to the backboard.

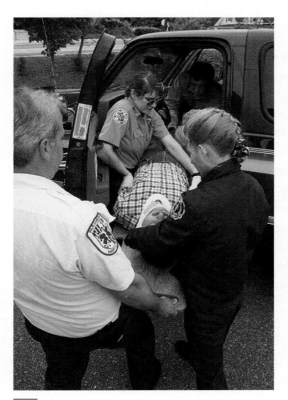

7 Carefully slide the patient to the full length of the backboard.

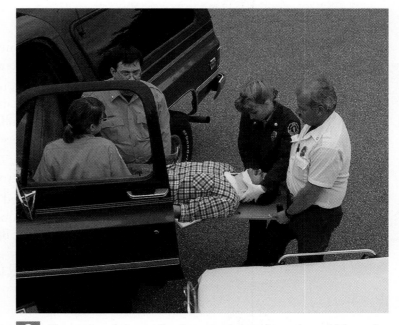

8 The patient is immediately moved away from the vehicle and into the ambulance, if available. Secure the patient to the backboard as soon as possible.

The Supine Patient

PROCEDURE

❖ Log-Rolling the Supine Patient onto a Long Backboard

The following steps are illustrated in Scan 12.4.

1. Rescuer 1 stabilizes the head and neck in a neutral position, but does *not* apply traction. He should grasp the patient's shoulders at the neck and gently position the patient's head between your forearms. Another rescuer should apply a semirigid extrication collar. Even with the collar in place, Rescuer 1 must maintain the head and neck in a neutral position until the log-rolling maneuver is completed.

2. The patient is placed with her legs extended in the normal manner and her arms (palms inward) extended by her sides. The patient will be rolled up on one arm with that arm providing proper spacing and acting as a splint for the body.

3. The long backboard is positioned next to the body. If one of the patient's arms is injured, place the backboard on the injured side so that the patient will roll upon the uninjured arm.

4. Rescuers 2 and 3 kneel at the patient's side opposite the board.

5. Rescuer 2 is positioned at the midchest area and Rescuer 3 is by the upper legs.

6. With his knees, Rescuer 2 holds the patient's near arm in place. He then reaches across the patient and grasps the shoulder and the hip, holding the patient's far arm in place. Usually, it is possible to grasp the patient's clothing to help with the roll if it is not loose fitting.

7. With one hand, Rescuer 3 reaches across the patient and grasps the hip. With his other hand, he holds the feet together at the lower legs.

8. When everyone is ready, the rescuer at the head (Rescuer 1) gives the order to log-roll the patient.

9. Rescuer 1 carefully maintains a neutral position of the head and neck (anteroposteriorly as well as laterally) during the roll.

10. Rescuers 2 and 3 roll the patient up on her side toward them. The patient's arms are kept locked to her side to maintain a splinting effect. The head, shoulders, and pelvis are kept in line during the log roll. Additional support may be provided by bracing the patient against the legs of Rescuers 2 and 3.

11. When the patient is on her side, Rescuer 2 (or Rescuer 4, if available) quickly examines the posterior surface from occiput to heels for injuries.

12. The backboard is now positioned next to the patient and held at a 30- to 45-degree angle by Rescuer 4. If there are only three rescuers, the board is pulled into place by Rescuer 2 or 3. The board is left flat in this case.

13. When everybody is ready, Rescuer 1 gives the order to log-roll the patient onto the backboard. This is accomplished by keeping head, shoulders, and pelvis in line.

Log-Rolling a Supine Patient

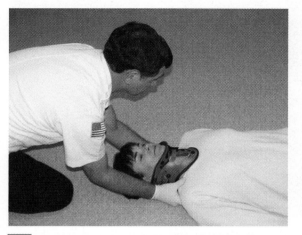

1 Rescuer 1 maintains the neck stabilized in a neutral position.

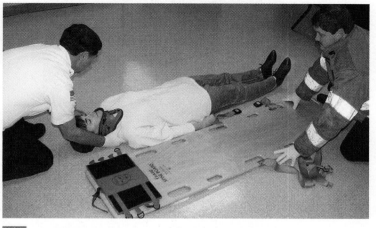

2 The long board is positioned beside the patient.

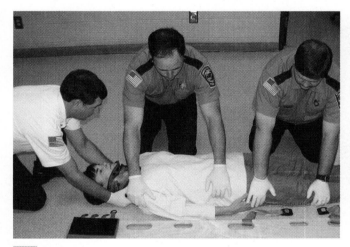

3 Rescuers 2 and 3 assume their positions at the patient's side opposite the board.

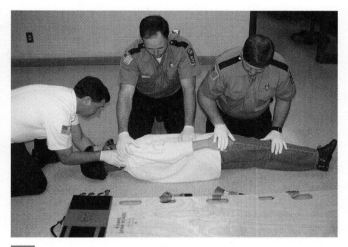

4 The patient is carefully rolled upon her side.

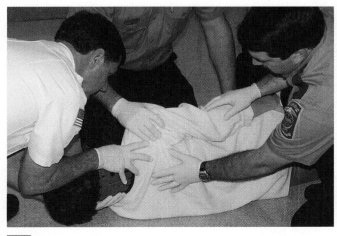

5 Quickly examine the patient's posterior surface for injuries.

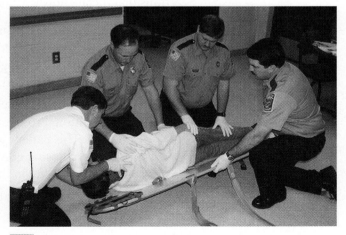

6 If another person is available, he positions the backboard next to the patient at a 30- to 45-degree angle.

(continued next page)

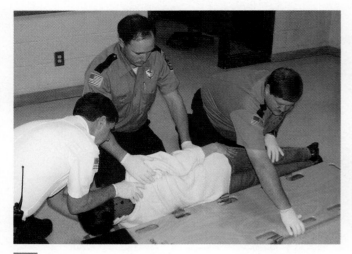

7 If no other help is available, Rescuer 2 or 3 positions the backboard and leaves it flat.

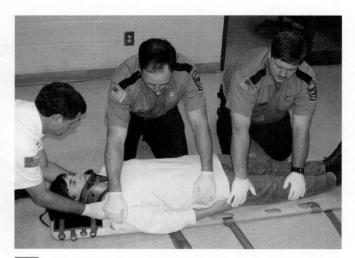

8 At Rescuer 1's order, the patient is rolled onto the backboard. All movements are coordinated so that the spine is kept straight at all times.

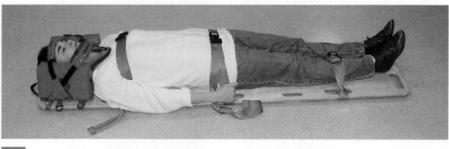

9 Log roll completed.

The Prone Patient: The status of the airway in a prone patient is critical for decisions about the order in which the log-rolling procedure is done. There are three clinical situations that dictate how you should proceed.

■ The patient who is not breathing or who is in severe respiratory difficulty must be log-rolled immediately to manage the airway. Unless the backboard is already positioned, you must log-roll the patient, manage the airway, and then transfer the patient to the backboard (in a second log-rolling step) when ready to transport.

■ The patient with profuse bleeding of the mouth or nose must not be turned to the supine position. Profuse upper airway bleeding in a supine patient is a guarantee of aspiration. This patient will have to have careful SMR and be transported prone or on his side, allowing gravity to help keep the airway clear. The vacuum backboard could be very useful in this situation (see Chapter 11, Figure 11-7).

■ The patient with an adequate airway and respiration should be log-rolled directly onto a backboard.

PROCEDURE

❋ Log-Rolling the Prone Patient with an Adequate Airway onto a Long Backboard

1. Rescuer 1 stabilizes the neck in a neutral position. When placing the hands on the head and neck, the rescuer's thumbs always point toward the patient's face (Figure 12-3). This prevents having the rescuer's arms crossed when the patient is log-rolled. Initial assessment and exam of the backside is done, and a semirigid extrication collar is applied.

2. The patient is placed with his legs extended in the normal manner and his arms (palms inward) extended by his sides. The patient will be rolled up on one arm, with that arm acting as a splint for the body.

3. The long backboard is positioned next to the body on the side of the first rescuer's lower hand. (If the first rescuer's lower hand is on the patient's right side, the backboard is placed on the patient's right side.) If the arm next to the backboard is injured, carefully raise the arm above the patient's head so he does not roll on the injured arm.

4. Rescuers 2 and 3 kneel at the patient's side opposite the board.

5. Rescuer 2 is positioned at the midchest area, and Rescuer 3 is by the upper legs.

6. Rescuer 2 grasps the shoulder and the hip. Usually, it is possible to grasp the patient's clothing (if not too loose) to help with the roll.

7. Rescuer 3 grasps the hip (holding the near arm in place) and the lower legs (holding them together).

8. When everyone is ready, Rescuer 1 gives the order to log-roll the patient.

9. Rescuer 1 carefully keeps the head and neck in a neutral position (anteroposteriorly as well as laterally) during the roll.

10. Rescuers 2 and 3 roll the patient up on his side away from them. The patient's arms are kept locked to his side to maintain a splinting effect. The head, shoulders, and pelvis are kept in line during the roll.

11. The backboard is now positioned next to the patient and held at a 30- to 45-degree angle by Rescuer 4. If there are only three rescuers, the board is pulled into place by Rescuer 2 or 3. The board is left flat in this case.

12. When everyone is ready, Rescuer 1 gives the order to roll the patient onto the backboard. This is accomplished by keeping the head, shoulders, and pelvis in line.

13. Now, complete the Rapid Trauma Survey.

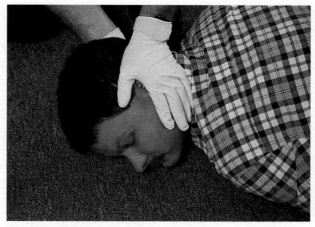

FIGURE 12-3 When stabilizing the neck of the prone (or supine) patient, your thumbs always point toward the face (not the occiput). This prevents having your arms crossed when the patient is rolled over.

Special Considerations: When log-rolling the patient with chest or abdominal injuries, try to roll him onto his uninjured side. The roll should be executed quickly enough to not compromise lung expansion. When log-rolling a patient with injuries to the lower extremities, position Rescuer 2 at the feet of the patient to provide in-line support to the injured leg(s) during the log roll. Again try to roll onto the uninjured side. The side to which you turn the patient during the log-roll procedure is not critical and can be changed in situations where you can only place the backboard on one side of the patient.

The log-roll technique is useful for most trauma patients, but for those patients with a fractured pelvis it may aggravate the injury to roll their weight onto the pelvis. If the pelvic fracture appears stable, the log roll should be carefully performed, turning the patient onto the uninjured side (if it can be identified). Patients with obviously unstable pelvic fractures should not be log-rolled but lifted carefully onto a board using four or more rescuers.

The scoop stretcher (see Chapter 2, Figure 2-5) is a supplemental device that may help move the patient onto the backboard when specific injuries complicate log-rolling. Some newer scoop stretchers have been found to provide equal or superior stabilization when compared to the long backboard (see reference 3 in Bibliography for Chapter 11). Such scoop stretchers can be used in place of a long backboard.

Securing the Patient to the Backboard

There are several different methods of securing the patient using straps. As with all equipment, you should become familiar with your strapping system before using it in an emergency situation.

Two examples of commercial devices for full body immobilization are the Reeves sleeve and the Miller body splint. The Reeves sleeve is a heavy-duty sleeve into which a standard backboard will slide. Attached to this sleeve are the following:

- A head motion-restriction device
- Heavy vinyl-coated nylon panels that go over the chest and abdomen and are secured with seat-belt-type straps and quick-release connectors
- Two full-length leg panels to secure the lower extremities
- Straps to hold the arms in place
- Six handles for carrying the patient
- Metal rings (2,500-lb strength) for lifting the patient by rope

When the patient is in this device, he remains immobilized when lifted horizontally, vertically, or even carried on his side (like a suitcase). This device is excellent for the confused, combative patient who must be restrained for his safety (Figure 12-4).

The Miller body splint is a combination backboard, head immobilizer, and body immobilizer (see Chapter 11, Figure 11-6b). Like the Reeves sleeve, it does an excellent job of SMR with a minimum of time and effort.

PROCEDURE

❊ Applying and Securing a Long Backboard to a Standing Patient

1. Rescuer 1 stands in front of the patient and stabilizes the head and neck in a neutral position. Rescuer 2 applies a semirigid cervical collar while Rescuer 1 continues to maintain the neck in a neutral position.

2. Rescuer 2 places a long backboard against the patient's back.

3. Rescuer 3 secures the patient to the board using nylon straps. These must include an anchor strap high on the chest as well as ones that cross over the shoulders and the pelvis and legs to prevent movement when the board is tilted down.

4. Rescuer 3 places padding behind the patient's head to maintain a neutral position, and applies and secures a blanket roll or commercial head motion-restriction device using elastic wraps or wide tape.

5. Rescuers 2 and 3 carefully tilt the board back onto a stretcher and secure the legs.

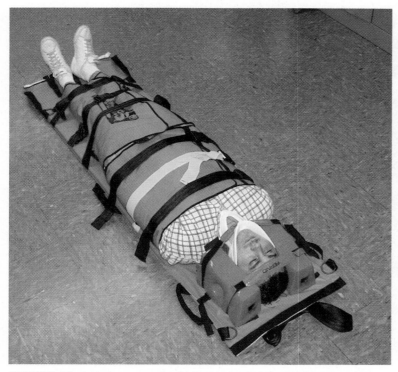

FIGURE 12-4 Patient restrained in a Reeves sleeve. Combative patients can have their arms enclosed within the panels and the straps.

Special Considerations for the Head and Neck: Stabilizing the head and neck in a neutral position sometimes cannot be accomplished safely. If the head or neck is held in an angulated position and the patient complains of pain on any attempt to straighten it, you should stabilize it in the position found. The same is true of the unconscious patient whose neck is held to one side and does not easily straighten with a gentle attempt. You cannot use a cervical collar or commercial head motion-restriction device in this situation. You must use pads or a blanket roll and careful taping to stabilize the head and neck in the position found.

HELMET MANAGEMENT

PROCEDURE

✴ Removing a Motorcycle Helmet from a Trauma Patient

To remove a motorcycle helmet from a patient with a possible cervical-spine injury, take the following steps (Scan 12.5).

1. Position yourself above or behind the patient. Place your hands on each side of the helmet and stabilize the head and neck by holding the helmet and the patient's neck.

2. Your partner positions himself to the side of the patient and removes the chin strap. Chin straps can usually be removed easily without cutting them.

3. Your partner then assumes the stabilization by placing one hand under the neck and the occiput and the other hand on the anterior neck with the thumb pressing on one angle of the mandible and the index and middle fingers pressing on the other angle of the mandible.

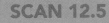

SCAN 12.5

Removing a Motorcycle Helmet

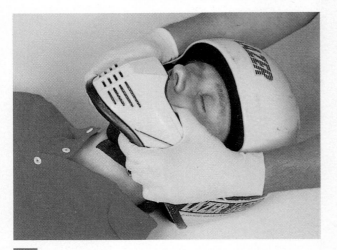

1 One rescuer applies stabilization by placing hands on each side of the helmet with fingers on the patient's mandible. This prevents slippage if the strap is loose.

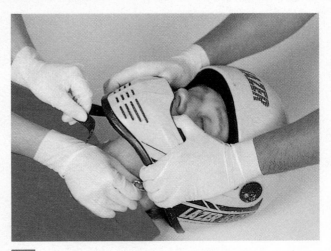

2 A second rescuer loosens the strap at the D-rings while stabilization is maintained.

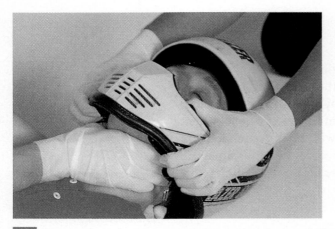

3 The second rescuer places one hand on the mandible at the angle, thumb on one side, long and index fingers on the other.

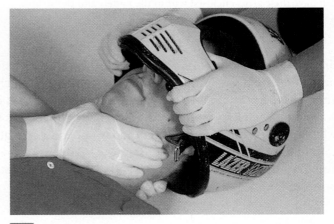

4 With the other hand, the second rescuer holds the occipital region. This maneuver transfers the stabilization responsibility to the second rescuer. The rescuer at the top removes the helmet in two steps, allowing the second rescuer to readjust his hand position under the occipital region. Three factors should be kept in mind: (a) The helmet is egg-shaped and therefore must be expanded laterally to clear the head. (b) If the helmet provides full facial coverage, glasses must be removed first. (c) If the helmet provides full facial coverage, the nose will prevent removal. To clear the nose, the helmet must be tilted backward and raised over it.

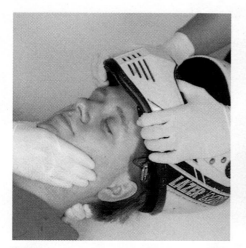

5 Throughout the removal process, the second rescuer maintains in-line stabilization from below in order to prevent head tilt.

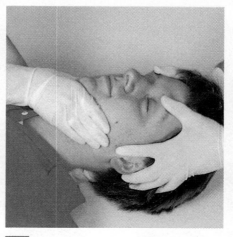

6 After the helmet has been removed, the rescuer at the top replaces his hands on either side of the patient's head with his palms over the ears, taking over stabilization.

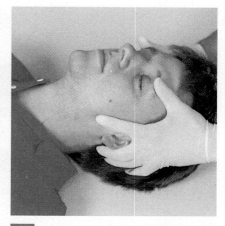

7 Stabilization is maintained from above until SMR is completed.

4. You now remove the helmet by pulling out laterally on each side to clear the ears and then up to remove. Tilt full-face helmets back to clear the nose (tilt the helmet, not the head).

5. If the patient is wearing glasses, remove them through the visual opening before removing the full-face helmet. Your partner maintains stabilization of the neck during this procedure.

6. After removal of the helmet, you again assume stabilization of the neck by grasping the head on either side, with your fingers holding one angle of the jaw and the occiput.

7. Your partner now applies a suitable cervical collar.

PROCEDURE
✴ Alternative Procedure for Removing a Helmet

This alternative has the advantage of one person maintaining stabilization of the neck throughout the whole procedure (Scan 12.6). Note that this procedure does *not* work well with full-face helmets.

1. Position yourself above or behind the patient and place your hands on each side of the neck at the base of the skull. Stabilize the neck in a neutral position. If necessary, you may use your thumbs to perform a modified jaw thrust while doing this.

2. Your partner positions himself over to the side of the patient and removes the chin strap.

3. Your partner now removes the helmet by pulling out laterally on each side to clear the ears and then up to remove. You maintain stabilization of the neck during the procedure.

4. Your partner now applies a suitable cervical collar.

Alternative Procedure for Removing a Helmet

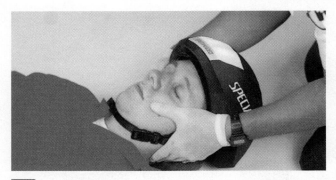

1 Apply steady stabilization in neutral position.

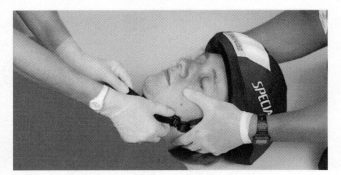

2 Remove the chin strap.

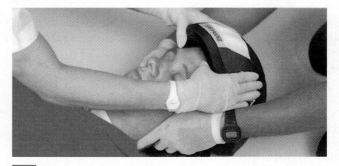

3 Remove the helmet by pulling gently on each side.

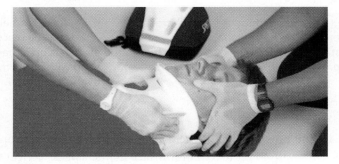

4 Apply a suitable cervical-spine extrication collar and secure the patient to a long backboard.

BIBLIOGRAPHY

1. Johnson, D. R., M. Hauswald, C. Stockhoff. 1996. Comparison of a vacuum splint device to rigid backboard for spinal immobilization. *American Journal of Emergency Medicine* 14: 369–72.

2. Kleiner, D. M., A. Pollak, C. McAdam. 2001. Helmet hazards. Do's and don'ts of football helmet removal. *JEMS* 26: 36–44, 46–48.

3. Krell, J. M., et al. 2006. Comparison of the Ferno scoop stretcher with the long backboard for spinal immobilization. *Prehospital Emergency Care* 10: 46–51.

Abdominal Trauma

Arthur H. Yancey II, MD, MPH, FACEP

Melissa White, MD, MPH

OBJECTIVES

Upon completion of this chapter, you should be able to:

1. Identify the basic anatomy of the abdomen and explain how abdominal and chest injuries may be related.

2. Differentiate between blunt and penetrating injuries and identify complications associated with each.

3. Describe the treatment required for the patient with protruding viscera.

4. Relate how injuries apparent on the exterior of the abdomen can damage underlying structures.

5. Describe possible intra-abdominal injuries based on findings of history, physical examination, and mechanism of injury.

6. Discuss advanced life support interventions for patients with abdominal injuries.

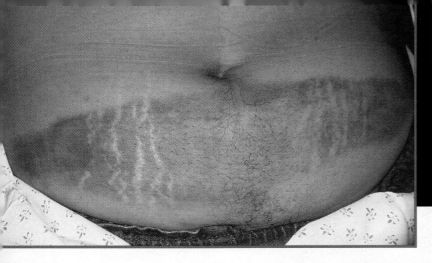

Dan, Joyce, and Buddy of the Emergency Transport System (ETS) have been called to the scene of a single motor-vehicle collision in which the auto ran into a tree. The male victim is still in the auto. He is restrained and currently awake. *What other information about the scene and the patient would be valuable? What injuries would you expect from a mechanism of this type?* Keep these questions in mind as you read the chapter. Then, at the end of the chapter, find out how the rescuers completed this call.

INTRODUCTION

Injury to the abdomen can be a difficult condition to evaluate in the hospital. In the field it is usually even more so. Nevertheless, because intra-abdominal injury is one of the major causes of preventable traumatic death, the possibility of intra-abdominal injury must be recognized, documented, and addressed immediately. Penetrating abdominal injuries obviously need immediate surgical attention; blunt injuries may be more subtle, but potentially are just as deadly. Whether the result of blunt or penetrating trauma, abdominal injury presents two life-threatening dangers: hemorrhage and infection. Hemorrhage has immediate consequences, and thus you must be alert to the danger of early shock in all abdominal-injury patients. Infection, which presents late, may be just as deadly, but does not require field intervention beyond prevention of gross contamination.

The role of prehospital providers in the management of abdominal trauma has been the subject of some controversy. Studies in the mid-1980s demonstrated that appropriate and timely intervention by well-trained paramedics could improve the hemodynamic status of critically injured patients with wounds to the abdomen. More recent studies have suggested that pneumatic antishock garment (PASG) application and/or vigorous IV fluid resuscitation in the prehospital setting may do more harm than good for patients with penetrating abdominal trauma (see Chapter 8 and the Bibliography for this chapter). The effects of fluid resuscitation in blunt trauma are less well studied.

In the field, rapid patient assessment and early treatment of shock is critical in the management of the patient with abdominal trauma.

ANATOMY OF THE ABDOMEN

The abdomen is traditionally divided into three regions: the thoracic abdomen, the true abdomen, and the retroperitoneal abdomen. The thoracic portion of the abdomen is located underneath a thin sheet of muscle, the diaphragm, and is enclosed by the lower ribs (Figure 13-1). It contains the liver, gallbladder, spleen, stomach, and transverse colon. In-

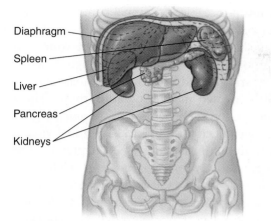

FIGURE 13-1 Intrathoracic abdomen.

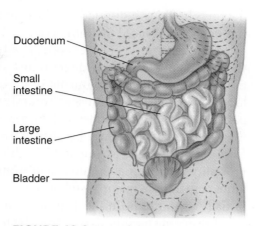

FIGURE 13-2 True abdomen.

jury to the liver and spleen is most common in blunt trauma and can result in life-threatening hemorrhage.

The true abdomen contains the small intestines and the bladder (Figure 13-2). Damage to the intestines can result in infection, peritonitis, and shock. In a female patient, the uterus, fallopian tubes, and ovaries are considered to be part of the pelvic portion of the true abdomen.

The retroperitoneal abdomen lies behind the thoracic and true portions of the abdomen (Figure 13-3). This area includes the kidneys, ureters, pancreas, posterior duodenum, ascending and descending colon, abdominal aorta, and the inferior vena cava. Because of its location away from the body surface, injuries here are difficult to evaluate. While hemorrhage in the true abdomen may cause the anterior abdominal wall to become distended, hemorrhage severe enough to cause shock may occur in the retroperitoneal space without this dramatic sign. In the pelvic part of the retroperitoneal abdomen are the iliac vessels. These vessels and their branches may be damaged by abdominal trauma or pelvic fracture. Injury to them can cause exsanguinating hemorrhage with no early symptoms.

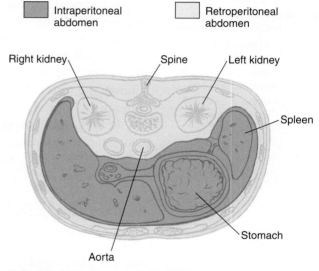

FIGURE 13-3 Retroperitoneal abdomen.

TYPES OF INJURIES

Injuries to the abdomen are usually categorized as blunt or penetrating trauma, but a combination of the two also occurs. Blunt trauma is the most common mechanism of abdominal injury and has relatively high mortality rates of 10 to 30 percent. The reason for this is likely related to the frequency of accompanying injuries to the head, chest, or an extremity(s) in as many as 70 percent of MVC victims. Blunt abdominal injury may be from direct compression of the abdomen, with fracture of solid organs (spleen/liver) and/or blowout of hollow organs (intestines). Injury may also arise from deceleration forces, with tearing of organs and their blood vessels. The patient who has suffered blunt trauma may have no pain and little external evidence of injury, which may give you a false sense of security. Patients with multiple lower rib fractures are notorious for having severe intra-abdominal injuries without significant abdominal pain. The severe pain from the rib

PEARLS
Abdominal Injury

- When mechanisms of trauma or associated injuries like lower rib fractures or gluteal penetrating wounds suggest possible intra-abdominal injury, do not be fooled by the patient's lack of abdominal pain or tenderness. Be prepared to treat hypovolemic shock from occult intra-abdominal bleeding.

- The patient who has had blunt trauma to the abdomen and has abdominal pain and/or tenderness on ITLS Secondary Survey probably has serious abdominal trauma and is likely to develop shock quickly (even if vital signs are initially normal). Load and go, preparing to treat the development of hemorrhagic shock en route to the hospital.

fractures becomes a distracting injury for the less noticeable abdominal pain. As a result, this patient may bleed to death because abdominal injuries are not recognized.

Most penetrating injuries are caused by gunshot or stab wounds. Gunshot wounds to the abdomen may include direct trauma to an organ and vasculature through penetration from the bullet, its fragments, or the energy transmitted from the bullet mass and velocity. As a rule, most gunshot wounds will be treated in the operating room. These patients have mortality rates of between 5 and 15 percent. These rates are much higher than those of stab wounds because of greater incidence of injury to abdominal viscera from the higher energy imparted to the intra-abdominal organs (see Chapter 1). The mortality rate from abdominal stab wounds is relatively low (1–2 percent). Unless the knife penetrates a major vessel or organ, such as the liver or spleen, the patient may not initially appear to be in shock at the scene. However, some of these patients can develop life-threatening peritonitis over the next few hours to days. These wounds need to be carefully evaluated in the hospital because approximately one-third of these patients require surgery.

You should remember that the path of the penetrating object might not be readily apparent from the wound location. Any penetrating wound of the chest may penetrate the abdomen, and vice versa. The course of a bullet may pass through numerous structures in different body locations. It is important to look at the patient's entire posterior surface because penetrating trauma in the gluteal area (iliac crests to the gluteal folds, including the rectum) is associated with up to a 50 percent incidence of significant intra-abdominal injuries.

In the prehospital phase, with both blunt and penetrating trauma, you must be most concerned about intra-abdominal bleeding with hemorrhagic shock.

ASSESSMENT AND STABILIZATION
Scene Size-up

You can glean much important information from the scene by noting the circumstances surrounding the patient's injury. An accurate but rapid assessment of the scene will usually tip you off to the possibility of abdominal trauma. Do circumstances on the scene suggest that the victim has fallen from a height or been hit by a passing vehicle? Has there been an explosion that could have hurled the victim against immobile objects or transmitted blast pressure to organs inside the abdomen? Has the victim of an automobile crash had the shoulder strap under the arm rather than over the shoulder? Or was the lap belt worn too high over the soft true abdomen instead of correctly across the pelvis? Any of these mechanisms can lead to abdominal injury.

If the patient was involved in a motor-vehicle crash, as you do your Scene Size-up, quickly observe the damage to the vehicle, such as passenger compartment intrusion, airbag deployment, broken windows, bent steering wheel/steering column, and location of occupants. If the patient needs to be extricated, note the location of the safety belts; although they certainly save lives, incorrectly worn safety belts can cause blunt abdominal injuries by compressing the intra-abdominal organs against the spine. Remember that lap belts alone, especially in the young adolescent age group may, ironically, predispose an individual to intra-abdominal injuries.

The person who is stabbed or shot may be able to give you some idea as to the size of the instrument or trajectory of the bullet. With gunshot wounds, it is also important to know the caliber, the range from which it was fired, and the number of rounds that were fired. A bystander or the police may be able to provide such information. When you arrive at the hospital (optimally a trauma center), be sure to report any mechanism that suggests abdominal injury. However, while at the scene, it is important not to spend a great deal of time attempting to obtain a history. The major cause of preventable mortality in abdominal trauma is delayed diagnosis and treatment.

Patient Assessment

As in treating any other traumatic condition, the patient should first undergo the ITLS Primary Survey. If the mechanism for abdominal injury is present and the patient has signs of shock, you should assume that abdominal injury is present and possibly the cause of the shock. The essence of the prehospital abdominal examination in the ITLS Primary Survey is rapid visual evaluation and palpation. Observe the torso for deformities, contusions, abrasions, and punctures (DCAP), evisceration, and distention. Note any tenderness or tenseness. The chest is only one thin muscle sheet (the diaphragm) away from the abdominal cavity, so injury to both is not uncommon. The presence of a seat-belt sign, or large abrasion over the abdomen (see the Case Study photo at the beginning of this chapter) and/or upper neck, is indicative of intra-abdominal injury in approximately 25 percent of cases. Be mindful that splenic injury may present with referred left posterior shoulder pain, and liver injury may present with referred right posterior shoulder pain.

Distention of the abdomen should be interpreted as a sign of severe hemorrhage as should tenderness or tenseness over the abdominal wall. Gentle palpation of the iliac crests (pelvic wings) and pubis of the pelvis may reveal the tenderness or bony crepitation associated with fractures. Pelvic fractures frequently result in hemorrhagic shock. Signs of intra-abdominal injury usually do not appear early, so if signs of intra-abdominal injury are present in the prehospital phase, there is usually significant injury. Shock may be imminent (see Chapter 8). Abdominal tenderness or distention is an indication for immediate transport to the hospital. But remember that lack of tenderness does not rule out injury in a patient with an altered mental status and/or spinal injury at or above the level of the abdomen.

Auscultation or percussion in the field loses critical time and little useful information is gained. Abdominal wounds should never be probed with your finger or with an instrument. If clothing must be removed to visualize injury, try to preserve important potential legal evidence by cutting around (rather than through) areas that have signs of possible penetration.

Stabilization

Significant abdominal trauma cannot be stabilized in the field. Interventions should follow the ITLS Primary Survey outlined in Chapter 2. They should proceed in the same order in which assessment occurred: airway (A), breathing (B), and circulation (C). This means that even if a patient has only an abdominal injury, supplemental oxygen by mask or endotracheal tube should be delivered through a confirmed open airway. Breathing should be verified to be adequate or the patient treated to ensure adequate ventilation. Then, and only then, should the consequences of hypovolemic shock from abdominal injury be addressed as part of the circulation assessment.

Apply oxygen at 12 to 15 liters per minute by mask or at 5 liters per minute by nasal cannula (see Chapter 4). Start two large-bore IV lines in the uninjured upper extremities infusing normal saline begun at a KVO (keep vein open) rate. Do this en route to the hospital unless it can be done on scene without delaying transport (during extrication or waiting for arrival of the ambulance). The patient should be readied for rapid transport. If the patient's blood pressure drops below 90 mmHg systolic with signs of impending shock, then the IV fluids should be given at a rate to maintain the systolic blood pressure at 90 to 100 mmHg (see Chapter 8). It is thought that aggressive fluid resuscitation might dislodge protective clots and dilute clotting factors, which would lead to worsening hemorrhage.

SCAN 13.1

Caring for an Evisceration

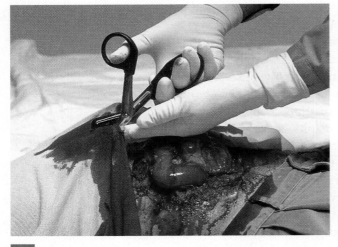

1 Remove clothing from around the abdominal wound.

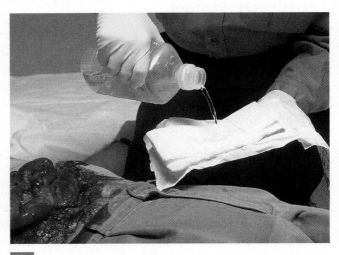

2 Cover the wound with a sterile dressing soaked with normal saline.

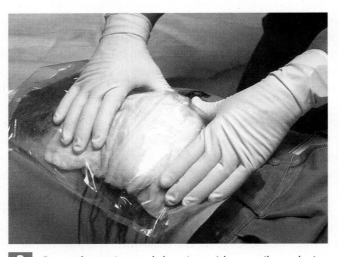

3 Cover the moistened dressing with a sterile occlusive dressing to prevent evaporative drying.

Gently cover any organ or viscera protruding from a wound with gauze moistened with saline or water. If you have a long transport time, you can apply a nonadherent material, such as plastic wrap or aluminum foil, to prevent drying of the gauze and intestines (Scan 13.1). If the intestines are allowed to dry, they may become irreversibly damaged. Do not ever push any abdominal contents protruding from a wound back into the abdomen. Similarly, if a foreign body (such as a knife or glass shard) is impaled in the abdomen, do not attempt removal or manipulation as this may precipitate uncontrollable hemorrhage. Carefully stabilize the object in place without moving it. Pregnant patients deserve the special considerations addressed in Chapter 19.

Case Study continued

Dan, Joyce, and Buddy of the Emergency Transport System (ETS) have been called to the scene of auto versus tree. As they respond they decide that Joyce will act as team leader and prepare for a patient with chest, abdomen, extremity, and/or spinal injuries. Upon their arrival, they find the police and a rescue squad already on scene. The scene is safe. There is only one victim.

The victim was driving an old truck without shoulder straps or airbags. But he did have his lap belt on when he lost control on a curve and ran off of the road, striking a large tree. There was significant impact, with the truck engine being pushed back almost to the passenger compartment. The ETS team helps the rescue squad extricate the patient from the vehicle.

Initial Assessment reveals an obese young male who is awake but confused with the smell of an alcoholic beverage on his breath. He is talking and has an open airway. His breathing is somewhat labored and he complains of pain with each inspiration. He has strong but rapid radial pulses. He was able to move his hands and feet before and after extrication. They use a short backboard device and they extricate him onto a long backboard, where he is secured. As they are extricating him, they note that there are no obvious injuries to the back. Joyce identifies him as a load-and-go patient because of the mechanism along with altered mental status and tachycardia. She performs a Rapid Trauma Survey while Buddy applies a nonrebreather oxygen mask and has suction ready in case the patient vomits. The airway is clear with no obvious trauma to the head or neck. Breath sounds are present but decreased on the left side. There is no obvious chest trauma. The abdomen has a large bruise from the seat belt and is diffusely tender. There are no obvious extremity injuries.

After transferring the patient to the ambulance, Joyce performs a brief neurological exam (patient awake but confused, eyes open spontaneously, and he obeys commands = GCS score 14). She also takes vital signs, while Buddy starts two large-bore IVs. The patient's blood pressure is 140/90, pulse 130, respiration 30, and pulse oximeter 93 percent on 100 percent oxygen. The patient complains of abdominal and chest pain and states he thinks a deer ran in front of his truck and he lost control trying to miss it. He has no allergies, takes no medications, has no past history of serious illness. He ate two hamburgers and drank "three" beers just before the collision.

Joyce reports to medical direction and is instructed to keep IVs at minimum rate unless his blood pressure falls below 90 systolic. The Detailed Exam reveals no other injuries but Joyce thinks she can hear bowel sounds in the left chest. Before arrival (20-minute transport time), the patient becomes pale and diaphoretic and his blood pressure drops to 70/40. IV normal saline is given to raise the blood pressure to 90/50. Upon arrival at the trauma center, he is taken directly to surgery where he is found to have a diaphragmatic hernia on the left as well as a ruptured spleen and a contusion of the liver. After a stormy course complicated by delirium tremens, he eventually survives.

A deceleration motor-vehicle collision can cause injuries to almost any system, but patients wearing only a lap belt are prone to compression fractures of the lumber spine (clasp-knife effect). The lap belt is prone to cause intra-abdominal injuries if it is worn across the abdomen rather than across the pelvis. Sudden compression of the abdomen can cause rupture of the diaphragm and herniation of abdominal contents into the chest. This usually occurs on the left because the large mass of the liver protects the right side. Anyone with significant abdominal trauma is subject to develop hemorrhagic shock, so always be prepared.

SUMMARY

Effective prehospital management of the patient with abdominal trauma entails the following:

- Scene Size-up for mechanisms and pertinent history from the patient and/or witnesses
- Rapid patient assessment
- Rapid transport to the appropriate hospital (optimally, a trauma center)
- IV lines and other interventions as needed (usually performed en route)

The enemies of the abdominal trauma patient are bleeding and time elapsed from injury until optimal care. If you can minimize on-scene delays, you will help to maximize the patient's chance for survival.

BIBLIOGRAPHY

1. Aprahamian, C., B. M. Thompson, J. B. Towne. 1983. The effect of a paramedic system on mortality of major open intra-abdominal vascular trauma. *Journal of Trauma* 23: 687–90.
2. Bickell, W. H., M. J. Wall, et al. 1994. Immediate versus delayed fluid resuscitation for hypotensive patients with penetrating torso injuries. *New England Journal of Medicine* 331 (October): 1105–9.
3. Mattox, K. L., P. E. Bickell, et al. 1989. Prospective MAST study in 911 patients. *Journal of Trauma* 29: 1104–12.
4. Newgard, C. D., et al. 2005. Steering wheel deformity and serious thoracic or abdominal injury among drivers and passengers involved in motor vehicle crashes. *Annals of Emergency Medicine* 45 (January): 43–50.
5. Pepe, P. E., et al. 2002. Prehospital fluid resuscitation of the patient with major trauma. *Prehospital Emergency Care* 6: 81.
6. Pons, P. T., B. Honigman, C. Moore, et al. 1985. Prehospital advanced trauma life support for critical penetrating wounds to the thorax and abdomen. *Journal of Trauma* 25: 828–32.
7. Scalea, T. M., et al. 2004. Trauma of the abdomen. *In Tintinalli's emergency medicine, A comprehensive study guide.* Sec. 22, chap. 260, 6th ed. New York: McGraw-Hill Companies, Inc.
8. Stone, C. K., L. E. Rodriguiz, et al. 2004. Immediate management of life-threatening injuries. In *Current emergency diagnosis and treatment.* 5th ed. New York: McGraw-Hill Companies, Inc.
9. Todd, S. R. 2004. Critical concepts in abdominal injury. *Critical Care Clinics* 20 (January): 119–34.

Extremity Trauma

John E. Campbell, MD, FACEP
S. Robert Seitz, M Ed, RN, NREMT-P

OBJECTIVES

Upon completion of this chapter, you should be able to:

1. Prioritize extremity trauma in the assessment and management of life-threatening injuries.

2. Discuss the major complications and treatment of the following extremity injuries:
   a. Fractures
   b. Dislocations
   c. Amputations
   d. Open wounds
   e. Neurovascular injuries
   f. Sprains and strains
   g. Impaled objects
   h. Compartment syndrome

3. Estimate blood loss from pelvic and extremity fractures.

4. Discuss major mechanisms of injury, associated trauma, potential complications, and management of injury to the following areas:
   a. Pelvis
   b. Femur
   c. Hip
   d. Knee
   e. Tibia/fibula
   f. Clavicle and shoulder
   g. Elbow
   h. Forearm and wrist
   i. Hand or foot

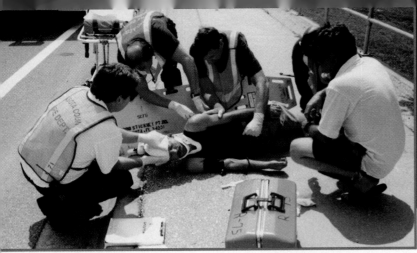

(© Craig Jackson/
In the Dark Photography)

Dan, Joyce, and Buddy of the Emergency Transport System (ETS) have been called to the scene of an auto–pedestrian collision. They are told that the pedestrian is unconscious. *What injuries should they expect with a mechanism of this type? Are head and spinal injuries likely?* Keep these questions in mind as you read the chapter. Then, at the end of the chapter, find out how the rescuers completed this call.

INTRODUCTION

You must never let distorted or wounded extremities occupy your attention when there may be more life-threatening injuries present. These dramatic injuries are easy to identify when you first encounter the patient and they may be disabling, but are rarely immediately life-threatening. It is important to remember that the movement of air through the airway, the mechanics of breathing, the maintenance of circulating blood volume, and the appropriate treatment of shock always come before the splinting of any fracture.

Hemorrhagic shock is a potential danger of very few musculoskeletal injuries. Only direct lacerations of arteries or fractures of the pelvis or femur are commonly associated with enough bleeding to cause shock. Injuries to the nerves or vessels that serve the hands and feet are the most common complications of fractures and dislocations. Such injuries cause the loss of function that we lump under the term *neurovascular compromise*. Thus, evaluation of pulses, motor function, and sensation (PMS) distal to fractures is very important.

INJURIES TO EXTREMITIES

Fractures

Fractures are generally quite painful, and you should consider the use of analgesic medication if your protocols and the situation allow. Fractures may be open (compound) with the broken end of the bone still protruding or having once protruded through the skin (Figure 14-1a), or they may be closed (simple) with no communication to the outside (Figure 14-1b). Fractured bone ends are extremely sharp and are quite dangerous to all the tissues that surround the bone. Since nerves and arteries frequently travel near the bone, across the flexor side of joints, or very near the skin (hands and feet), they are frequently injured. Such neurovascular injuries may be due to lacerations from bone fragments or from pressure due to swelling or hematoma.

Closed fractures can be just as dangerous as open fractures because injured soft tissues often bleed profusely. It is important to remember that any break in the skin near a fractured bone may be considered an opening for contamination.

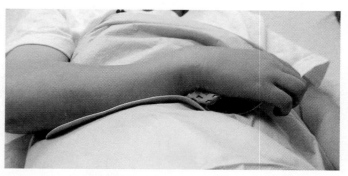

FIGURE 14-1b Closed forearm fracture. *(Photo courtesy of Roy Alson, MD)*

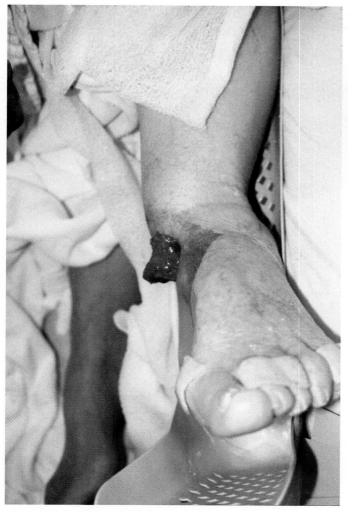

FIGURE 14-1a Open ankle fracture.

A closed fracture of one femur can cause the loss of up to a liter of blood; thus, two fractured femurs can cause life-threatening hemorrhage (Figure 14-2). A fractured pelvis can cause extensive bleeding into the abdomen or the retroperitoneal space. The pelvis usually fractures in several places and may have 500 cc of blood loss for each fracture. Pelvic fractures may lacerate the bladder or the large pelvic blood vessels. Either of these structures can cause fatal hemorrhage into the abdomen. Remember, multiple fractures can cause life-threatening hemorrhage without any external blood loss.

Open fractures add the dangers of contamination as well as loss of blood outside the body. If protruding bone ends are pulled back into the skin when the limb is aligned, bacteria-contaminated debris will be pulled into the wound. Infection from such debris may prevent healing of the bone and may even cause death from septic complications.

Dislocations

Joint dislocations are extremely painful injuries. They are almost always easy to identify because normal anatomy is distorted (Figure 14-3). Major joint dislocations, though not life threatening, are often true emergencies because of the neurovascular compromise that can, if not treated quickly, lead to amputation. It is impossible to know whether or not a fracture exists in combination with a dislocation. It is very important to check for PMS distal to major joint dislocations.

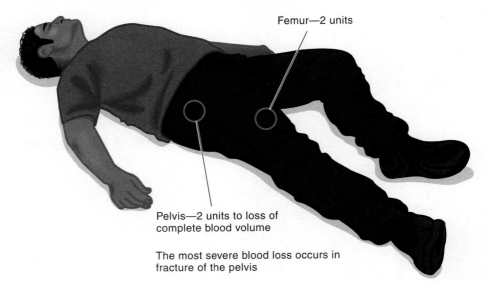

Estimating blood loss by site
and number of fractures

Femur—2 units

Pelvis—2 units to loss of
complete blood volume

The most severe blood loss occurs in
fracture of the pelvis

FIGURE 14-2 Internal blood loss from fractures.

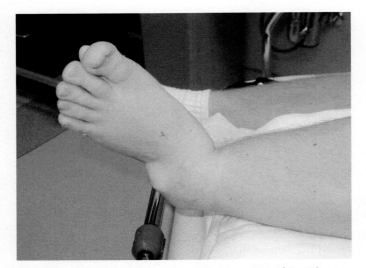

FIGURE 14-3 Ankle dislocation. *(Photo courtesy of Roy Alson, MD)*

Ordinarily, injuries should be splinted in the position in which they are found. However, there are certain exceptions to this rule. It is universally true that one can apply only gentle traction to any distorted extremity in an effort to straighten it. In the few instances that you would use traction to straighten an extremity, use no more than 10 pounds of force. Most often the best treatment for the patient is padding and splinting the extremity in the most comfortable position and rapidly transporting to a facility that has orthopedic care available.

Amputations

Amputations are disabling and sometimes life-threatening injuries. They have the potential for massive hemorrhage, but most often, the bleeding will control itself quite readily with ordinary pressure applied to the stump. The stump should be covered with a damp sterile dressing and an elastic wrap that will apply uniform, reasonable pressure across the entire stump. If bleeding absolutely cannot be controlled with pressure, a tourniquet may be used. Though rarely needed, a tourniquet can be life saving.

You should make an effort to find the amputated part and bring it with you. This sometimes neglected detail can have serious future implications for the patient, since parts can frequently be used for graft material. Reimplantation is attempted only in very limited situations. For this reason, you should not suggest to the patient that reimplantation will be done but rather that the doctor will evaluate whether reimplantation is possible. Small amputated parts should be placed in a plastic bag (Figure 14-4). If ice is available, place the bag in a larger bag or container containing ice and water. Do not use ice alone, and never use dry ice. Cooling the part slows the chemical processes and will increase the viability from 4 hours to up to 18 hours. It is important to bring amputated parts even if reimplantation appears to be impossible.

Open Wounds

Cover wounds with a sterile dressing and bandage carefully. Gross contamination such as leaves or gravel should be removed from the wound, and smaller pieces of contamination can be irrigated from the wound with normal saline in the same manner that you would irrigate a chemically contaminated eye. Bleeding can almost always be stopped with pressure dressings or pneumatic splints. Tourniquets should almost never be needed to stop bleeding from a wound if amputation is not present. If necessary, a blood pressure cuff or pressure on a larger artery proximal to the injury may be appropriate. However, if the patient is having exsanguinating hemorrhage from an extremity injury and you cannot stop the bleeding with pressure, you should not hesitate to use a tourniquet. If you have bleeding that cannot be stopped with pressure or with a tourniquet, such as injuries to the axilla or groin, you should use one of the new hemostatic agents such as QuikClot (Figure 14-5) or Celox. These agents should be packed into the wound (not for use in open abdominal or chest wounds) and pressure applied. Patients with severe hemorrhage should be transported immediately after the ITLS Primary Survey. Obvious exsanguinating hemorrhage is the only time you can change your ABC order of exam to CAB.

Neurovascular Injuries

The nerves and major blood vessels generally run beside each other, usually in the flexor area of the major joints. They may be injured together, and loss of circulation and/or sensation can be due to disruption, swelling, or compression by bone fragments or hematomas. Foreign bodies or broken bone ends may well impinge on delicate structures and cause them to malfunction. Always check for PMS before and after any extremity manipulation, application of splint, or traction.

Impaled Objects

Do not remove impaled objects. Apply a very bulky type of padding to hold the object in place and transport the patient with the object in place. The skin is a pivot point in these cases, and any motion outside the body is translated or magnified within the tissues, where the end of the object may lacerate or harm sensitive structures. Impaled objects in the neck that obstruct the airway or those in the cheek of the face are exceptions to this rule.

Compartment Syndrome

The extremities contain muscle tissue in closed spaces that are surrounded by tough membranes that will not stretch. Trauma (crush injuries, closed or open fracture, or sustained compression) to these areas (forearm and lower leg most commonly) may cause bleeding and swelling within the closed spaces. As the area swells, pressure is transmitted to the

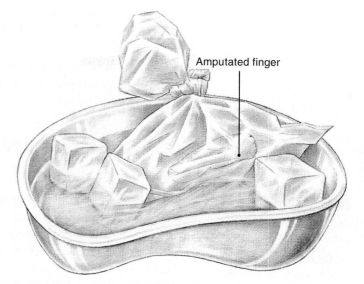

FIGURE 14-4 Amputated parts should be put in a dry bag, sealed, and placed in water that contains a few ice cubes.

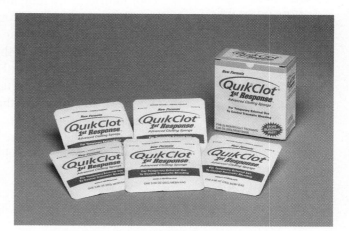

FIGURE 14-5 QuikClot 1st Response is an inexpensive hemostatic agent that can be used to stop bleeding from an exsanguinating extremity injury. *(Photo courtesy of Z-Medica Corp.)*

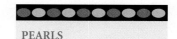

PEARLS
Pulses, Motor Function, Sensation
Always record sensation and circulation initially and after any manipulation, particularly splinting.

blood vessels and nerves. This pressure may compress the blood vessels in such a manner that circulation is impossible. The nerves may also be compromised. These injuries usually develop over a period of hours. Late symptoms are the five Ps: pain, pallor, pulselessness, paresthesia, and paralysis. The early symptoms are usually pain and paresthesia. As with shock, you should think of this diagnosis before the later symptoms develop.

ASSESSMENT AND MANAGEMENT

Scene Size-up and History

When assessing the patient with extremity trauma, it is especially important to get a history because the mechanism of injury may not be apparent in your Scene Size-up. The mechanism of injury and your assessment of the extremity may give you important clues to the potential severity of the injury. If there are rescuers enough, one rescuer can obtain the history while you are performing the ITLS Primary Survey. If not, you should not attempt to elicit a detailed verbal history until you have assessed the status of the airway, breathing, and circulation. In the conscious patient, obtain most of the history at the end of the ITLS Primary Survey.

Foot injuries from long jumps (falls landing on the feet) often have lumbar spine injuries associated with them. Any injury to the knee when the patient is in the sitting position may have associated injuries to the hip. In a like manner, hip injuries may refer pain to the knee, so the knee and the hip are intimately connected and must be evaluated together rather than separately. Falls onto the wrist frequently injure the elbow, and so the wrist and elbow must be evaluated together. The same is true of the ankle and the proximal fibula of the outside of the lower leg. Any injury that appears to be in the shoulder must be carefully examined because it may easily involve either the neck, chest, or shoulder.

Fractures of the pelvis are usually associated with very large amounts of blood loss. Whenever a fracture in the pelvis is identified, shock must be suspected and proper treatment begun.

Assessment

During the ITLS Primary Survey, you are concerned with obvious fractures to the pelvis and large bones of the extremities. You should also find and control major bleeding from the extremities.

During the ITLS Secondary Survey, quickly assess the full length of each extremity, looking for deformity, contusions, abrasions, penetrations, burns, tenderness, lacerations, and swelling (DCAP-BTLS). Feel for instability and crepitation (see Chapters 2 and 3). Check the joints for pain and movement. Check and record distal PMS. Pulses may be marked with pen (ballpoint or felt tip) to identify the area in which the pulse is best felt (Figure 14-6). Crepitation or grating of bone ends is a definite sign of fracture, and once identified, the bone ends should be immediately immobilized to prevent further soft-tissue injury. Checking for crepitation should be done very gently, especially when checking the pelvis. Crepitation means bone ends are grating on one another, and this means you are causing further tissue injury.

Management of Extremity Injuries

Proper management of fractures and dislocations will decrease the incidence of pain, disability, and serious complications. Treatment in the prehospital setting is directed at proper immobilization of the injured part by the use of an appropriate splint. Even with proper immobilization of fractures, the patient may require analgesic medication.

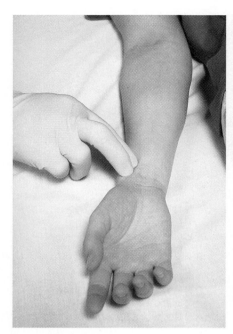

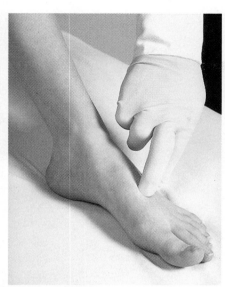

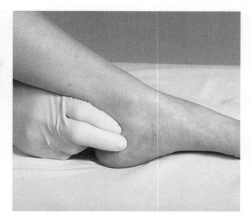

FIGURE 14-6c **Palpate the posterior tibial pulse.** *(Photo courtesy of Michal Heron)*

FIGURE 14-6b **Palpate the dorsalis pedis pulse.** *(Photo courtesy of Michal Heron)*

FIGURE 14-6a **Palpate the radial artery.** *(Photo courtesy of Michal Heron)*

Purpose of Splinting: The objective is to prevent motion in the broken bone ends. The nerves that cause the most pain in a fractured extremity lie in the membrane surrounding the bone. The broken bone ends irritate these nerves, causing a very deep and distressing type of pain. Splinting not only decreases pain, but also eliminates further damage to muscles, nerves, and blood vessels by preventing further motion of the broken bone ends.

When to Splint: There is no simple rule that determines the precise sequence to follow in every trauma patient. In general, the seriously injured patient will be better off if you splint only the spine (long backboard) before transport. The patient who requires a load-and-go approach can have extremity fractures temporarily stabilized by careful packaging on the long backboard. This does not mean that you have no responsibility for identifying and protecting extremity fractures, but implies that it is better to do some splinting in the vehicle en route to the hospital. It is never appropriate to sacrifice time splinting a limb to prevent disability, when that time may be needed to save the patient's life. Conversely, if the patient appears to be stable, extremity fractures should be splinted before moving the patient.

PEARLS
The Golden Hour

- Do not waste the Golden Hour. Be cautious but be rapid, and prioritize life over limb.

- Splint at an appropriate time. The axial skeleton is splinted after the ITLS Primary Survey. Extremities should be splinted en route if a critical situation exists.

PROCEDURE
❈ Rules of Splinting

- You must adequately visualize the injured part. Clothes should be cut off, not pulled off, unless there is only an isolated injury that presents no problem to maintaining immobilization.

- Check and record distal sensation and circulation before and after splinting. Check movement distal to the fracture if possible (for example, ask the conscious patient to wiggle his fingers or observe the motion of the unconscious patient when a painful stimulus is applied). Pulses may be marked with a pen to identify where they were palpated.

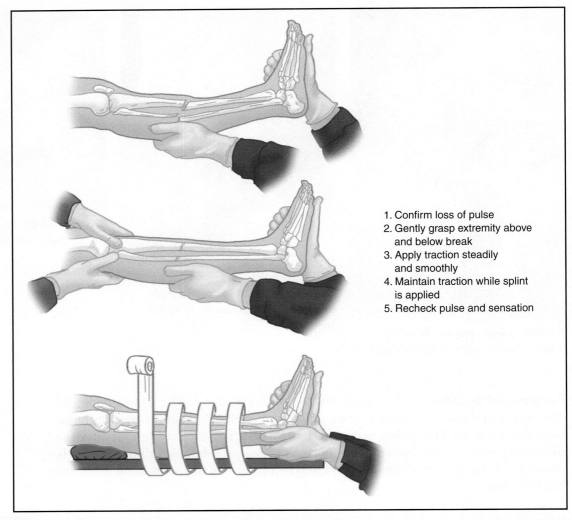

1. Confirm loss of pulse
2. Gently grasp extremity above and below break
3. Apply traction steadily and smoothly
4. Maintain traction while splint is applied
5. Recheck pulse and sensation

FIGURE 14-7 Straightening angulated fractures to restore pulses.

- If the extremity is severely angulated and pulses are absent, apply gentle traction in an attempt to straighten it (Figure 14-7). This traction should never exceed 10 pounds of pressure. If resistance is encountered, splint the extremity in the angulated position. When you are attempting to straighten an extremity, it is very important to be honest with yourself with regard to resistance. It takes very little force to lacerate the wall of a vessel or to interrupt the blood supply to a large nerve. If the trauma center is near, always splint in the position found.

- Open wounds should be covered with a sterile dressing before you apply the splint. Splints should always be applied on the side of the extremity away from open wounds to prevent pressure necrosis.

- Use the splint that will immobilize one joint above and below the injury.

- Pad the splint well. This is particularly true if there is any skin defect or if bony prominences might press against a hard splint.

- Do not attempt to push bone ends back under the skin. If you apply traction and the bone end retracts back into the wound, do not increase the amount of traction. You should not use your hands or any tools to try to pull the bone ends back out, but be sure to notify the receiving physician. Carefully pad bone ends with bandages before applying pneumatic splints to the lower extremities. The healing of bone is improved if the bone ends are kept moist when transport time is prolonged.

■ In a life-threatening situation, injuries may be splinted while the patient is being transported. When the patient appears stable, splint all injuries before moving him.

■ If in doubt, splint a possible injury.

Types of Splints

Rigid Splints. This type of splint can be made from many different materials and includes all cardboard, hard plastic, metal, or wooden types of splints. The type of splint that is made rigid by evacuating air from a moldable splint (vacuum splint) is also classified as a rigid splint. Rigid splints should be padded well and should always extend one joint above and below the fracture.

Soft Splints. This type of splint includes air splints, pillows, and sling- and swathe-type splints. Air splints are good for fractures of the lower arm and lower leg. Air splints have the advantage of compression, which helps to slow bleeding, but they have the disadvantage of increasing pressure as the temperature rises or the altitude increases. They should not be put on angulated fractures since they will automatically apply straightening pressure. Other major disadvantages of air splints include the fact that the extremity pulses cannot be monitored while the splint is in place, and the splints also often stick to the skin and are painful to remove.

Inflating the splints requires you to blow the splints up by mouth or by hand or foot pump (never by compressed air) until they give good support and yet can easily be dented with slight pressure from a fingertip. When using air splints, you must constantly check the pressure to be sure that the splint is not getting too tight or too loose (they often leak).

Remember that if air splints are applied in a cold environment and the patient is moved into the warm environment of the ambulance, the pressure will increase as the splints warm up. Where air ambulances are available, it must be remembered that the pressure in air splints increases if they are applied on the ground and then subsequently the patient is airlifted to the hospital. Continuous monitoring of circulation in the fractured extremity is required. Also remember that if pressure is released during the flight, the pressure will be too low when the patient is returned to the ground.

Pillows make good splints for injuries to the ankle or foot. They are also helpful, along with a sling and a swathe, to stabilize a dislocated shoulder.

Slings and swathes are excellent for injuries to the clavicle, shoulder, upper arm, elbow, and sometimes the forearm. They utilize the chest wall as a solid foundation and splint the arm against the chest wall. Some shoulder injuries cannot be brought close to the chest wall without significant force being applied. In these instances, pillows are used to bridge the gap between the chest wall and the upper arm.

Traction Splint. This device is designed for fractures of the femur. It holds the fracture immobile by the application of a steady pull on the ankle while applying counter traction to the ischium and the groin. This steady traction overcomes the tendency of the very strong thigh muscles to spasm. If traction is not applied, the pain worsens because the bone ends tend to impact or override. Traction also prevents free motion of the ends of the femur, which could lacerate the femoral nerve, artery, or vein. There are many designs and types of splints available to apply traction to the lower extremity (Figure 14-8), but each must be carefully padded and applied with care to prevent excessive pressure on the soft tissues around the pelvis. It is also necessary to use a great deal of care in applying the ankle hitch so as not to interfere with the circulation of the foot. Many of these devices can be used with a buck's boot as an alternative to the ankle hitch.

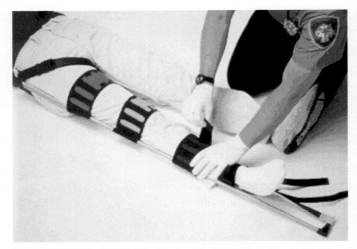

FIGURE 14-8a Kendrick traction device. *(Photo courtesy of Eduardo Romero Hicks, MD)*

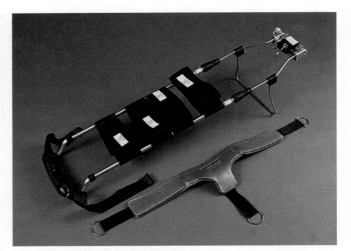

FIGURE 14-8b Hare traction splint.

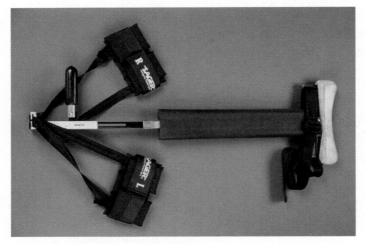

FIGURE 14-8c Sager traction splint.

Management of Specific Injuries

Spine Injuries: Spine injuries are covered elsewhere in the book but included here to remind you that if there is any chance of one, proper SMR (spinal motion restriction) must be done to prevent lifelong paralysis or even death from a spinal-cord injury. In the most urgent cases, careful packaging of the patient on the long backboard may be adequate splinting for a number of different extremity injuries. Remember that certain mechanisms of injury, such as a fall from a height in which the patient lands on both feet, may cause lumbar spine fracture because forces are transmitted all the way up the body.

Pelvis Injuries: It is practical to include injuries to the pelvis with extremities because they are frequently associated. Pelvic injuries are usually caused by motor-vehicle collisions or by severe trauma such as falls from heights. They are identified by gentle pressure being placed on the iliac crests, hips, and pubis during the ITLS Primary Survey. There is always the potential for serious hemorrhage in pelvic fractures, so shock should be expected and the patient rapidly transported (load and go). Internal bleeding from unstable pelvic fractures can be decreased by circumferential stabilization of the pelvis. The PASG or slings made from sheets have been used in the past but there are now commercially available pelvic slings or belts made for this purpose (Figure 14-9).

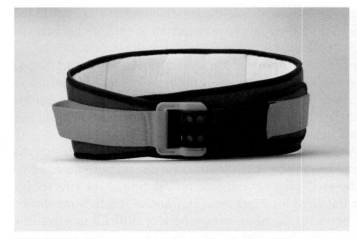

FIGURE 14-9a Commercial pelvic sling device. *(Photo courtesy of Sam Splints)*

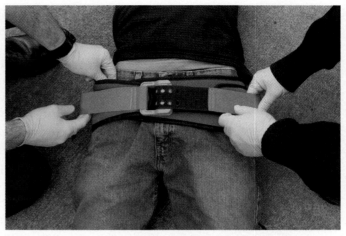

FIGURE 14-9b Pelvic sling applied. *(Photo courtesy of Sam Splints)*

The patient with a pelvic injury should have SMR. The vacuum backboard is especially useful here because it is much more comfortable than the hard backboard. Log-rolling a patient with an unstable pelvic fracture can aggravate the injury. Scoop stretchers or adequate manpower is needed to move these patients to the backboard. As mentioned in Chapter 2, some of the new, more rigid scoop stretchers provide SMR equal to a backboard (Figure 14-10).

Femur Injuries: The femur usually fractures at the midshaft, although hip fractures are quite common. These fractures may have open wounds associated with them and, if so, they must be presumed to be open fractures. There is a lot of muscle tissue surrounding the femur, and when spasm develops after a femur fracture, the bone ends tend to override causing more muscle damage. Because of this, tractions splints are usually used to stabilize the fracture and prevent shortening. Because of the large muscle mass, a great deal of bleeding can occur into the tissue of the thigh. Bilateral femur fractures can be associated with a loss of up to 50 percent of the circulating blood volume.

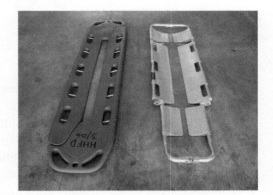

FIGURE 14-10 This scoop stretcher has been found to provide spinal stabilization equal to a backboard. *(Photo courtesy of Leon Charpentier, EMT-P; and Ferno Washington, Inc.)*

Hip Injuries: Hip fractures are most often in the narrow "neck" of the femur, where strong ligaments may occasionally allow this type of fracture to bear weight. The ligaments are very strong, and there is very little movement of the bone ends in the most frequent type of hip fracture. You must consider hip fractures in any elderly person who has fallen and has pain in the knee, hip, or pelvic region. The affected leg will usually (but not always) be externally rotated and shortened. This type of presentation and pain should be considered a fracture until an x-ray proves otherwise. In this age group, pain is frequently well tolerated and sometimes even ignored or denied. In general, the tissues in the elderly patient are more delicate, and less force is required to disrupt a given structure. Always remember that isolated knee pain may well be coming from damage to the hip. Do not use a traction splint for a hip fracture.

Hip dislocation is a different story. Most posterior hip dislocations are a result of the knees being struck by the dashboard, forcing the relatively loose, relaxed hip out of the posterior side of its cup in the pelvis (Figure 14-11). Thus, any patient in a severe automobile crash with a knee injury must have the hip examined very carefully. Posterior hip dislocation is an orthopedic emergency and requires reduction as soon as possible to prevent

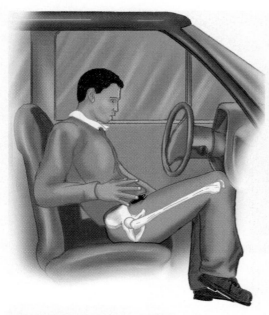

FIGURE 14-11 Mechanism of posterior dislocation of the hip, "down and under."

sciatic nerve injury or necrosis of the femoral head due to interrupted blood supply. This is a very difficult reduction to perform because the amount of force required is very great and the movement must be quite precise. The posterior dislocated hip will usually be flexed, and the patient will not be able to tolerate having the leg straightened. The leg will almost invariably be rotated toward the midline. A posterior hip dislocation should be supported in the most comfortable position by the use of pillows and by splinting to the uninjured leg (Figure 14-12).

The anterior dislocated hip is rare because of the complex mechanism required to produce this injury. The patient with an anterior hip dislocation will present with external rotation of the affected leg much like a fractured hip except you may not be able to bring the leg forward in line with the body. It may be very difficult to place this person in the supine position on a backboard or on the stretcher in the ambulance. While the posterior hip dislocations puts pressure on the sciatic nerve, the anterior hip dislocation puts pressure on the femoral artery and vein. If the vein is collapsed, a clot can form distally producing a large pulmonary embolus as soon as the hip is reduced. Patients with anterior or posterior hip dislocations require rapid transport.

Knee Injuries: Fractures or dislocation of the knee (Figure 14-13) are quite serious because the arteries are bound down above and below the knee joint and are often bruised or lacerated if the joint is in an abnormal position. There is no way to know whether a fracture exists in an abnormally positioned knee and, in either case, the decision must be based on the circulation and neurological function below the knee in the foot. Some authorities state that about 50 percent of knee dislocations have associated injuries to the vessels, and many knee injuries later require amputation. It is important to restore the circulation below the knee whenever possible.

Prompt reduction of knee dislocation is very important. If there is loss of pulse or sensation, apply gentle traction by hand or by way of a traction splint. You must be careful to apply no more than 10 pounds of force. This force must be applied along the long axis of the leg. If there is resistance to straightening the knee, splint it in the most comfortable position and transport the patient rapidly. This may be considered a true orthopedic emergency.

Do not confuse this injury with a patella dislocation. The patella will dislocate to the side and the affected leg will be held slightly flexed at the knee. You can easily see that the patella is out of place. While painful, this is not a serious injury and should simply be splinted with a pillow under the knee and taken to the emergency department. Straightening the leg usually reduces the patella dislocation.

Tibia/Fibula Injuries: Fractures of the lower leg are often open due to thin skin over the front of the tibia and often have significant internal and/or external blood loss. Internal blood loss can interrupt the circulation to the foot if a compartment syn-

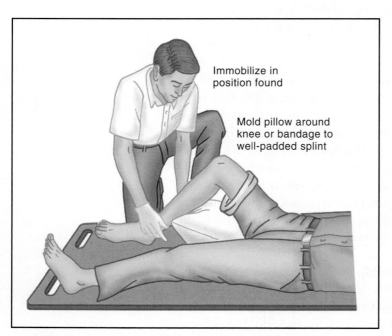

Immobilize in position found

Mold pillow around knee or bandage to well-padded splint

FIGURE 14-12 Splinting posterior dislocation of the hip.

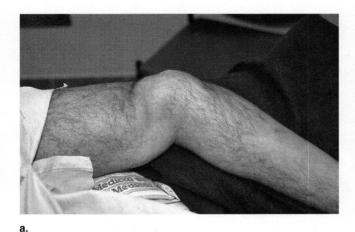
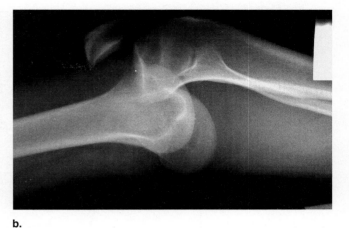

a.   b.

FIGURE 14-13a Knee dislocation: (a) presentation of a knee dislocation; (b) x-ray of the dislocation.

drome develops. It is rarely possible for patients to bear weight on fractures of the tibia, but fractures of the distal fibula are frequently mistaken for sprains. Fractures of the lower tibia/fibula may be splinted with a rigid splint, an air splint, or a pillow (Figure 14-14). Pneumatic splints will adequately splint upper tibia fractures. Here again it is important to dress any wound and pad any bone ends that may be put under an air splint.

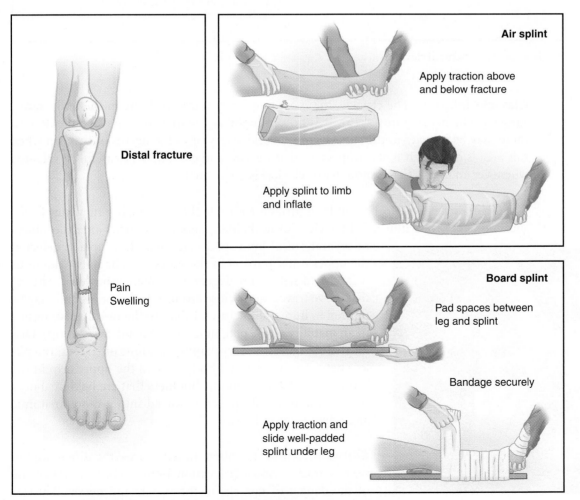

Distal fracture

Pain
Swelling

Air splint

Apply traction above and below fracture

Apply splint to limb and inflate

Board splint

Pad spaces between leg and splint

Bandage securely

Apply traction and slide well-padded splint under leg

FIGURE 14-14 Splinting a lower leg fracture with splint or board splint.

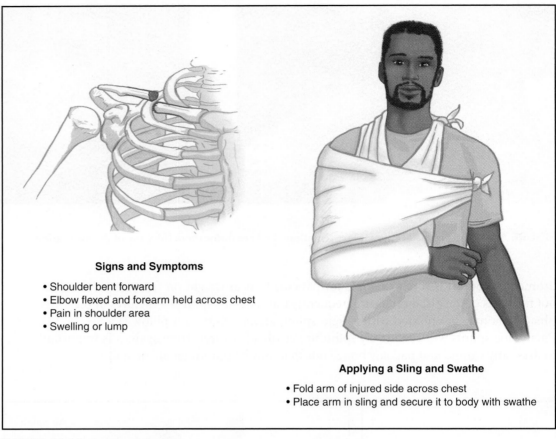

Signs and Symptoms

- Shoulder bent forward
- Elbow flexed and forearm held across chest
- Pain in shoulder area
- Swelling or lump

Applying a Sling and Swathe

- Fold arm of injured side across chest
- Place arm in sling and secure it to body with swathe

FIGURE 14-15 Fractured clavicle.

Clavicle Injuries: The clavicle, the most frequently fractured bone in the body, rarely causes problems (Figure 14-15). It is best immobilized with a sling and swathe. Rarely, there may be injuries to the subclavian vein and artery or to the nerves of the arm when this area is injured. It is also important that the ribs and chest be very carefully evaluated whenever an injury to the shoulder or clavicle is discovered.

Shoulder Injuries: Most shoulder injuries are not life threatening, but they may be associated with severe injuries of the chest or neck. Many shoulder injuries are dislocations or separations of joint spaces and may show up as a defect at the upper outer portion of the shoulder. The upper humerus is fractured with some degree of frequency, however. The radial nerve travels quite close around the humerus and may be injured in humeral fractures. Injury to the radial nerve results in an inability of the patient to lift the hand (wrist drop). Dislocated shoulders are very painful and quite often require a pillow between the arm and body to hold the upper arm in the most comfortable position. Shoulders that are held in abnormal positions should never be forced into a more anatomic alignment (Figure 14-16).

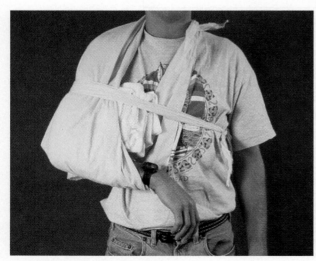

FIGURE 14-16 Dislocated shoulder.

Elbow Injuries: It is often difficult to see the difference between a fracture and a dislocation. Both can be serious because of the danger of damage to the vessels and nerves that run across the flexor surface of the elbow. Elbow injuries should al-

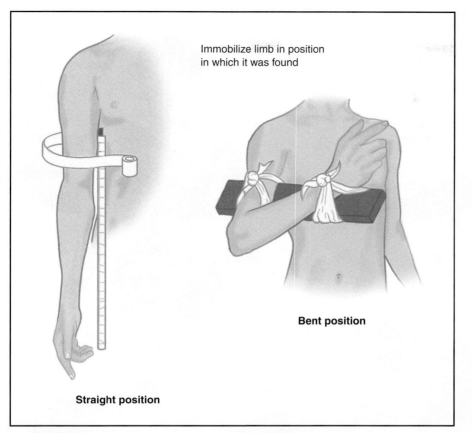

Immobilize limb in position
in which it was found

Bent position

Straight position

FIGURE 14-17 Fractures or dislocations of the elbow.

ways be splinted in the most comfortable position and the distal function clearly evaluated (Figure 14-17). Never attempt to straighten or apply traction to an elbow injury because the tissues are quite delicate and the structure is very complicated.

Forearm and Wrist Injuries: Fractures to the forearm and wrist are very common (Figure 14-18), usually as a result of a fall onto the outstretched arm. Usually, such a fracture is best immobilized with a rigid splint or an air splint (Figure 14-19). If a rigid splint is used, a roll of gauze in the hand will hold the arm in the most comfortable position of

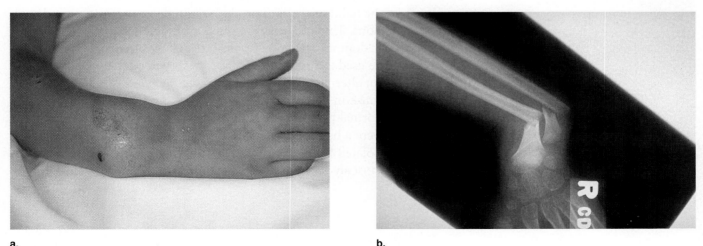

a.   b.

FIGURE 14-18a Presentation of a forearm fracture: (a) a fracture will often present with deformity; (b) an x-ray of the fracture.

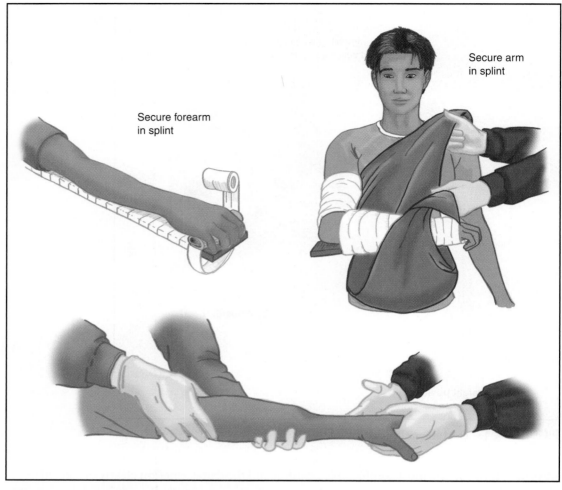

Secure forearm
in splint

Secure arm
in splint

FIGURE 14-19 Fractures of the forearm and wrist.

function. The forearm is also subject to internal bleeding, which can interrupt the blood supply to the fingers and the hand (compartment syndrome).

Hand or Foot Injuries: Many industrial accidents involving the hand or the foot produce multiple open fractures and avulsions. These injuries are often gruesome in appearance but are seldom associated with life-threatening bleeding. A pillow may be used to support these injuries very effectively (Figure 14-20). An alternative method of dressing the hand is to insert a roll of gauze in the palm, then arrange the fingers and thumb in their normal position. The entire hand is then wrapped as though it were a ball inside a very large and bulky dressing. Elevating the isolated hand or foot injury above the level of the heart will almost always reduce bleeding dramatically during transport.

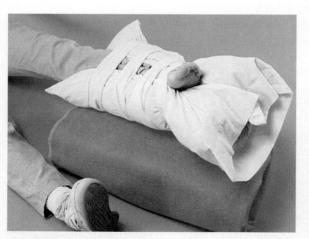

FIGURE 14-20 Pillow splinting an injured foot.

Case Study *continued*

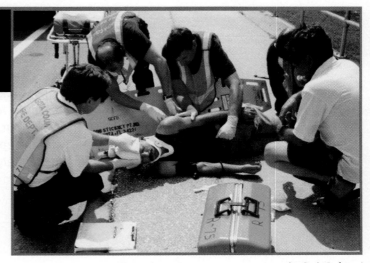

(© Craig Jackson/
In the Dark Photography)

Dan, Joyce, and Buddy of the Emergency Transport System (ETS) are on the way to the scene of an auto–pedestrian collision with an unconscious patient, the pedestrian. During travel to the scene, they decide that Buddy is team leader on this call. As they finish preparing for a patient with serious multisystem injuries, they arrive on the college campus where the male student stepped out in front of a car and was hit. He was thrown about 15 feet, and has been unconscious since the injury. Nothing is known about him, as no bystanders know him. The scene is safe. He is the only victim.

As they approach, their general impression is bad. The patient is lying on his right side with his right leg at an abnormal angle. He is not moving. He does not respond when Buddy speaks to him. Initial Assessment reveals that his airway is open, but his respiration is shallow and slow. He has a weak, rapid pulse at the wrist. The ETS team checks his back (no apparent injuries) as they log-roll him onto a backboard. Joyce begins assisted ventilation with 100 percent oxygen while Buddy performs the Rapid Trauma Survey, which reveals the patient has a hematoma of the right temporal area and only moans when his fingers and toes are pinched. There is no deformity of the neck and the neck veins are flat. The chest has no apparent injuries and breath sounds are present and equal. Heart sounds are easily heard. The abdomen is soft and the patient does not seem to have pain when the abdomen is palpated. The pelvis is stable but seems to be tender, since the patient moans when the pelvis is palpated. There is an obvious deformity of the right thigh but PMS of all extremities is present (the patient withdraws his fingers and toes to pinching).

Buddy immediately gets the team to move the patient to the ambulance and begin transport. A brief neurological exam done en route reveals that the patient opens his eyes to pain (pupils 3 mm and react equally to light), moans to pain, and withdraws to pain. His GCS score is calculated to be 8 (severe brain injury). He has no gag reflex so Joyce intubates him by the oral route with a 7.5 mm endotracheal tube. Vital signs are BP 90/60, pulse 130, and respiration assisted at 10 per minute. His pulse oximeter saturation is 100 percent and his ventilatory rate is adjusted to maintain his CO_2 level at 40 mmHg. While Joyce ventilates the patient, Buddy and Dan start two large-bore IVs and give normal saline to raise the blood pressure to 120/70. They then apply a traction splint to the right leg.

Transport time is only 5 minutes, so by the time they contact medical direction they are almost at the hospital. The patient was found to have an epidural hematoma and this was immediately evacuated with good results. The patient also had a fractured pelvis and right femur, but no other injuries. He responded well to treatment and was back in school by the next semester. He had no residual neurological symptoms.

This patient had multiple-system trauma, which is the usual case with auto–pedestrian collisions. Because he had a GCS score of 8, it was imperative not to let him remain hypotensive, so fluid was given to raise his BP to 120 mmHg systolic. His shock was secondary to the fractured femur and pelvis and not to any other internal injuries. The patient's coma was due to the epidural hematoma, which is one of the few head injuries that usually respond immediately to decompression. The outcome might have been different had he been allowed to remain hypotensive.

SUMMARY

While usually not life threatening, extremity injuries are often disabling. These injuries may be more obvious than more serious internal injuries, but do not let extremity injuries distract you from following the usual steps of the ITLS Primary Survey. Pelvic and femur fractures can be associated with life-threatening internal bleeding, so patients with these injuries are in the load-and-go category. Proper splinting is important to protect the injured extremity from further injury. Dislocations of elbows, hips, and knees require careful splinting and rapid reduction to prevent severe disability to the affected extremity.

BIBLIOGRAPHY

1. Abarbanell, N. R. 2001. Prehospital midthigh trauma and traction splint use: Recommendations for treatment protocols. *American Journal of Emergency Medicine.* 19(2): 137–40.
2. American College of Surgeons Committee on Trauma. 2004. *Advanced trauma life support.* Chicago: American College of Surgeons, 205–30.
3. Bledsoe, B., D. Barnes. 2004. Traction splint. An EMS relic? *JEMS* 29(8): 64–69.
4. Cross, D. A., J. Baskerville. 2001. Comparison of perceived pain with different immobilization techniques. *Prehospital Emergency Care* 5(3): 270–74.
5. Dischinger, P. C., K. Read, J. Kerns, et al. 2004. Consequences and costs of lower extremity injuries. *Annual Proceedings of the Association for the Advancement of Automotive Medicine* 48: 339–53.
6. Friese, G., G. LeMay. 2005. Emergency stabilization of unstable pelvic fractures. *Emergency Medical Services* 34(5): 67–71.
7. Heightman, A. 2006. From the editor: Out of sight, out of mind. *JEMS* 31(7): 2006.
8. Krell, J. M., et al. 2006. Comparison of the Ferno scoop stretcher with the long backboard for spinal immobilization. *Prehospital Emergency Care* 10: 46–51.

Extremity Trauma Skills

Donna Hastings, EMT-P

OBJECTIVES

Upon completion of this chapter, you should be able to:

1. Explain when to use a traction splint.
2. Describe the complications of using a traction splint.
3. Apply the most common traction splints:
   a. Thomas splint
   b. Hare splint
   c. Sager splint
4. Demonstrate pelvic stabilization techniques.

TRACTION SPLINTS

Traction splints are designed to immobilize fractures of the femur. They are not useful for fractures of the hip, knee, or lower leg. Applying firm traction to a fractured or dislocated knee may tear the blood vessels behind the knee. If there appears to be a pelvic fracture, you cannot use a traction splint because it may cause further damage to the pelvis. Fractures below the midthigh that are not angulated or are severely shortened may just as well be immobilized by air splints.

Traction splints work by applying a padded device to the back of the pelvis (ischium) or to the groin. A hitching device is then applied to the ankle, and counter traction is applied until the limb is straight and well immobilized. Apply the splints to the pelvis and groin very carefully to prevent excessive pressure on the genitalia. Also use care when attaching the hitching device to the foot and ankle so as not to interfere with circulation. To prevent any unnecessary movement, do not apply traction splints until the patient is on a long backboard. If the splint extends beyond the end of the backboard, be very careful when moving the patient and when closing the ambulance door so that you do not hit the splint and cause movement in the fracture site. You must check the circulation in the injured leg, so remove the shoe before attaching the hitching device.

In every case at least two people are needed to apply traction. One must hold steady, gentle traction on the foot and leg while the other applies the splint. When dealing with load-and-go situations, do not apply the splint until the patient is in the ambulance (unless the ambulance has not arrived).

PROCEDURE

❋ Applying a Thomas Traction Splint (Half-Ring Splint)

The Thomas splint was used exclusively prior to the advent of modern traction devices. During World War I, its use decreased the mortality rate for battlefield femur fractures from 80 percent to 40 percent. At that time it was considered one of the greatest advancements in medical care. It is still used in some countries and in the absence of other options. To apply a Thomas traction splint, follow these steps (Figure 15-1).

1. Have your partner support the leg and maintain gentle traction while you cut away the clothing and remove the shoe and sock to check the pulse and sensation at the foot.
2. Position the splint under the injured leg. The ring goes down and the short side goes to the inside of the leg. Slide the ring snugly up under the hip, where it will be pressed against the ischial tuberosity.
3. Position two support straps above the knee and two below the knee.
4. Attach the top ring strap.
5. Apply padding to the foot and ankle.
6. Apply the traction hitch around the foot and ankle (Figure 15-2).
7. Maintain gentle traction by hand.
8. Attach the traction hitch to the end of the splint.
9. Increase traction by Spanish windlass action using a stick or tongue depressors.
10. Release manual traction and reassess circulation and sensation.
11. Support the end of the splint so that there is no pressure on the heel.

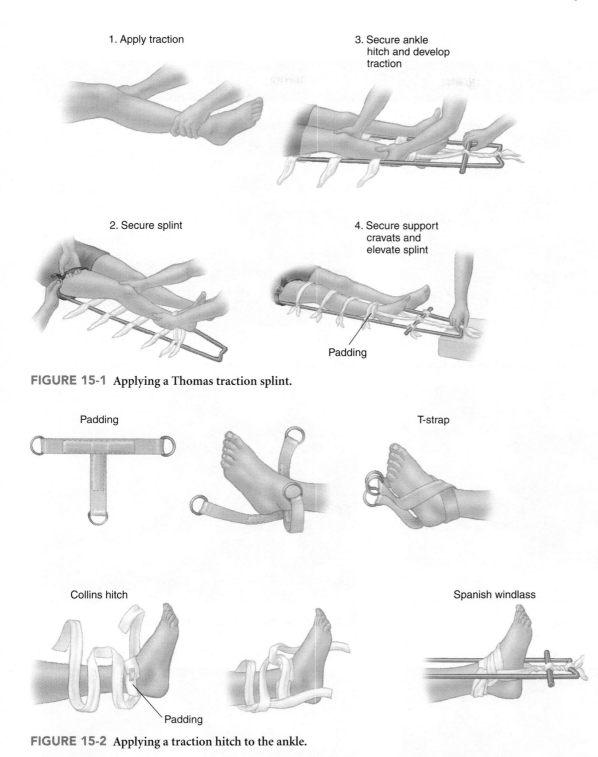

1. Apply traction

2. Secure splint

3. Secure ankle hitch and develop traction

4. Secure support cravats and elevate splint

Padding

FIGURE 15-1 Applying a Thomas traction splint.

Padding

T-strap

Collins hitch

Padding

Spanish windlass

FIGURE 15-2 Applying a traction hitch to the ankle.

PROCEDURE

� Applying a Hare Traction Splint

The Hare traction splint is the modern version of the Thomas splint. To apply the Hare traction splint, follow these steps (Scan 15.1).

1. Position the patient on the backboard or stretcher.

2. Have your partner support the leg and maintain gentle traction, while you cut away the clothing and remove the shoe and sock to check pulse and sensation at the foot.

SCAN 15.1

APPLYING A HARE TRACTION SPLINT

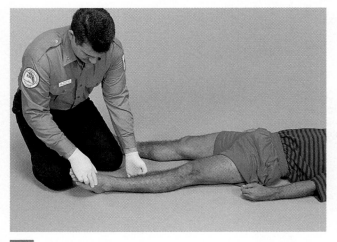

1 Assess distal pulses and motor and sensory function.

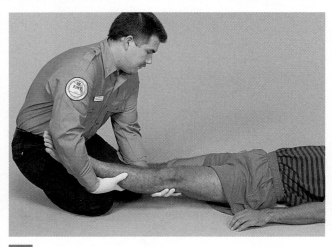

2 Stabilize the injured leg by applying manual traction.

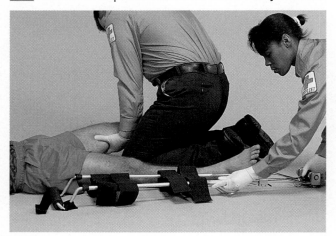

3 Adjust the splint for proper length.

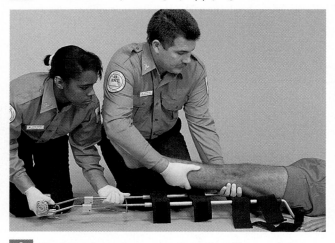

4 Position the splint under the injured leg until the ischial pad rests against the bony prominence of the buttocks. Once the splint is in position, raise the heel stand.

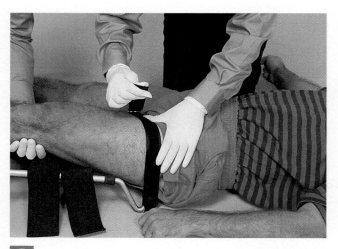

5 Attach the ischial strap over the groin and thigh.

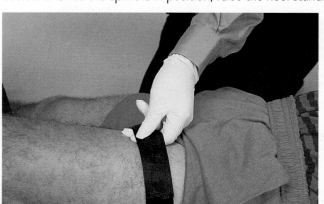

6 Make sure the ischial strap is snug but not tight enough to reduce distal circulation.

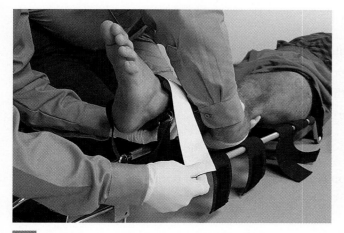

7 With the patient's foot in an upright position, secure the ankle hitch.

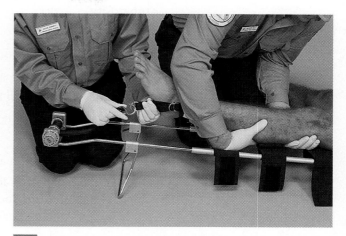

8 Attach the S-hook to the D-ring and apply mechanical traction. Full traction is achieved when the mechanical traction is equal to the manual traction and the pain and muscle spasms are reduced. In an unresponsive patient, adjust the traction until the injured leg is the same length as the uninjured leg.

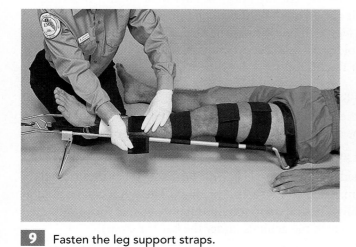

9 Fasten the leg support straps.

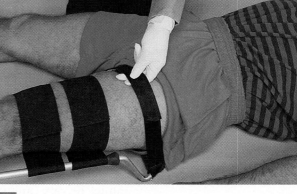

10 Reevaluate the ischial strap and ankle hitch to ensure that both are securely fastened.

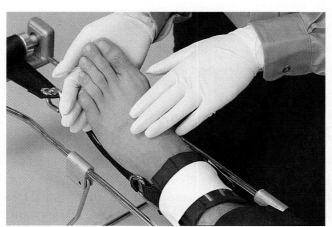

11 Reassess distal pulses and motor and sensory function.

3. Using the uninjured leg as a guide, pull the splint out to the correct length.

4. Position the splint under the injured leg. The ring goes down and the short side goes to the inside of the leg. Slide the ring up snugly under the hip against the ischial tuberosity.

5. Attach the ischial strap.

6. Apply the padded traction hitch to the ankle and foot.

7. Position and attach two support straps above the knee and two below the knee.

8. Attach the traction hitch to the windlass by way of the S-hook.

9. Turn the ratchet until the correct tension is applied.

10. Reassess PMS of leg.

11. Release manual traction and recheck circulation and sensation.

12. To release mechanical traction (when too tight or when removing splint), pull the ratchet knob outward and then slowly turn to loosen.

PROCEDURE

❄ Applying a Sager Traction Splint

The Sager traction splint is different in several ways. It works by providing counter traction against the pubic ramus and the ischial tuberosity medial to the shaft of the femur; thus it does not go under the leg. The hip does not have to be slightly flexed, as with the Hare. The Sager splint is also lighter and more compact than other traction splints. You can also splint both legs with one splint if needed. The current Sager splints are significantly improved over older models and may represent the state of the art in traction splints. To apply a Sager traction splint, follow these steps (Scan 15.2).

1. Position the patient on a long backboard or stretcher.

2. Have your partner support the leg and maintain gentle traction while you cut away the clothing and remove the shoe and sock to check the pulse and sensation at the foot.

3. Using the uninjured leg as a guide, pull the splint out to the correct length.

4. Position the splint to the inside of the injured leg with the padded bar fitted snugly against the pelvis in the groin. Attach the strap to the thigh. The splint can be used on the outside of the leg, using the strap to maintain traction against the pubic ramus. Be very careful not to catch the genitals under the bar (or strap).

5. While your partner maintains gentle manual traction, attach the padded hitch to the foot and ankle.

6. Extend the splint until the correct tension is obtained.

7. Apply the elastic straps to secure the leg to the splint.

8. Release manual traction and recheck circulation and sensation.

PELVIC STABILIZATION TECHNIQUES

Pelvic fractures involve either the iliac crest or the pelvic ring. Fractures to the iliac crest indicate serious trauma; however, they are not life threatening like fractures of the pelvic ring with resulting blood loss. In either case, the actual technique for stabilizing the fracture is the same and may be accomplished by either of two common approaches.

APPLYING A SAGER TRACTION SPLINT

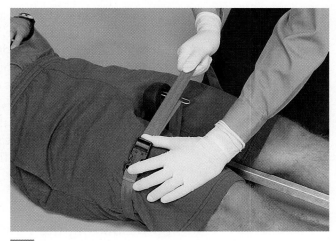

1 Place the splint along the medial aspect of the injured leg. Adjust it so that it extends about 4 inches beyond the heel.

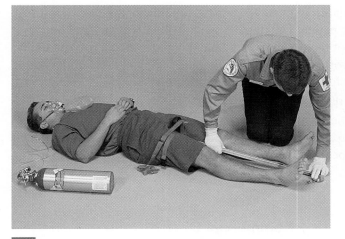

2 Secure the strap to the thigh.

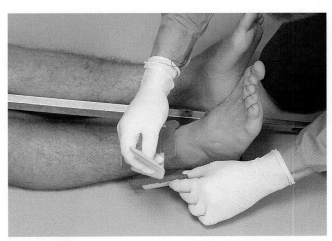

3 Apply the ankle hitch and attach it to the splint.

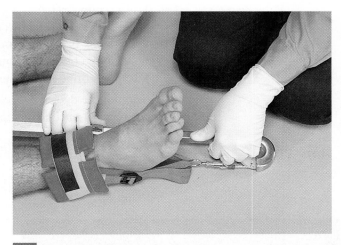

4 Apply traction by extending the splint. Adjust the splint to 10 percent of the patient's body weight.

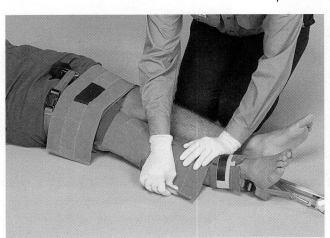

5 Apply the straps to secure leg to splint. Reassess distal pulses and motor and sensory function.

PROCEDURE

❈ Stabilizing the Pelvis with a Sheet or Blanket

1. Place a sheet or blanket horizontally on the lower half of the backboard prior to moving the patient.

2. Use a scoop stretcher, if available, to move the patient onto the backboard. If a scoop stretcher is not available, the patient will need to be log-rolled as gently and quickly as possible. If you have one of the newer more stable scoop stretchers, you can use it instead of a backboard but you will have to slide the sheet or blanket up under the patient after he is on the stretcher.

3. Tie two diagonal corners of the sheet or blanket together with the knot formed at the hip on one side. Repeat the tie with the remaining two corners and the knot formed on the opposite hip. In each case, gently and smoothly increase the tension until firm support is provided for the pelvis (Figure 15-3).

PROCEDURE

❈ Stabilizing the Pelvis with a Commercial Device

1. Open the device and place it horizontally on the lower half of the backboard prior to moving the patient.

2. Use a scoop stretcher, if available, to move the patient onto the backboard. If a scoop stretcher is not available, the patient will need to be log-rolled as gently and quickly as possible. If you have one of the newer more stable scoop stretchers, you can use it instead of a backboard but you will have to slide the device up under the patient after he is on the stretcher.

3. Tighten the device as the manufacturer recommends. Gently and smoothly increase the tension until firm support is provided for the pelvis (Figure 15-4).

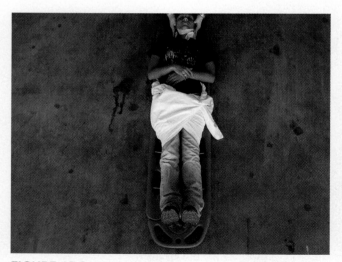

FIGURE 15-3 Manual stabilization of unstable pelvic fracture using a sheet. *(Photo courtesy of Leon Charpentier, EMT-P)*

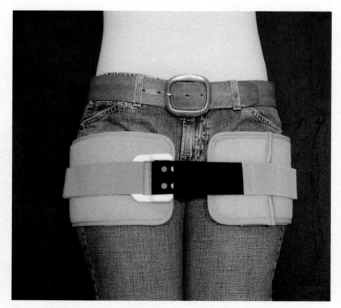

FIGURE 15-4 Stabilization of an unstable pelvic fracture using a commerical device. *(Photo courtesy of Sam Medical Products)*

Burns

Roy L. Alson, PhD, MD, FACEP

OBJECTIVES

Upon completion of this chapter, you should be able to:

1. Identify the basic anatomy of the skin including:
   a. Epidermal and dermal layers
   b. Structures found within
2. List the basic functions of the skin.
3. Describe types of burns as a function of burn depth.
4. Estimate depth of burn based on skin appearance.
5. Estimate extent of burn using the rule of nines.
6. Identify complications and describe the management of:
   a. Thermal burns
   b. Chemical burns
   c. Electrical burns
7. List situations and physical signs that:
   a. Indicate inhalation injury
   b. Suggest carbon monoxide poisoning
8. Discuss how carbon monoxide causes hypoxia.
9. Describe the treatment for carbon monoxide poisoning.
10. Identify which patients may require transport to a burn center.

(© Craig Jackson/
In the Dark Photography)

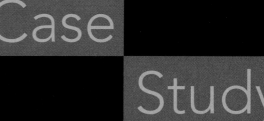

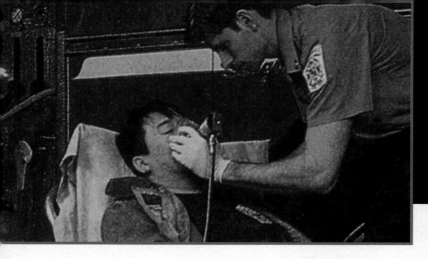

Dan, Joyce, and Buddy of the Emergency Transport System (ETS) have been called to the scene of a warehouse fire. They are told that the watchman has just been rescued after being trapped in an upstairs bathroom. *What injuries should they expect with a mechanism of this type? Is carbon monoxide poisoning possible? Are there medical problems that can be precipitated or aggravated by this mechanism?* Keep these questions in mind as you read the chapter. Then, at the end of the chapter, find out how the rescuers completed this call.

INTRODUCTION

According to the American Burn Association, there are over 1 million burn injuries per year in the United States, resulting in more than 4,500 deaths. Thousands more are injured. Many who survive their burns are left severely disabled and/or disfigured. While the number of those killed or injured has decreased in the last 30 years, particularly with the use of smoke detectors and the improvements in burn care, burn injury is still a major problem for our society. Applying the basic principles taught here can help decrease death, disability, and disfigurement from burn injuries. As the rescue of burn patients can be extremely dangerous, following the rules of scene safety is extremely important. Multiple agents (Table 16-1) can cause burn injuries, but in general, pathologic damage to the skin is similar. Specific differences among the types of burns will be discussed in later sections.

TABLE 16-1 *Types of Burn Injuries*	

1. Thermal
  a. Flame
  b. Scald
  c. Steam
	2. Electrical
	3. Chemical
	4. Radiation

ANATOMY AND PATHOPHYSIOLOGY

The Skin

The largest organ of the body, the skin, is made up of two layers. The outer layer, which we can see on the surface, is called the *epidermis.* It serves as a barrier between the environment and our body. Underneath the thin epidermis is a thick layer of collagen connec-

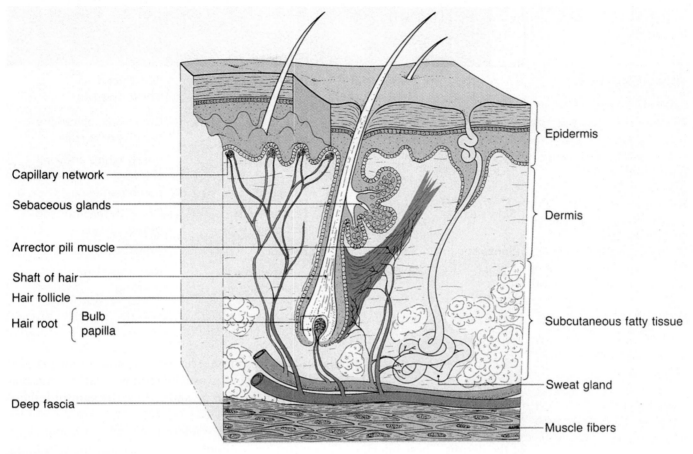

Capillary network

Sebaceous glands

Arrector pili muscle

Shaft of hair

Hair follicle

Hair root { Bulb
            papilla

Deep fascia

Epidermis

Dermis

Subcutaneous fatty tissue

Sweat gland

Muscle fibers

FIGURE 16-1 The skin.

tive tissue called the *dermis.* This layer contains the important sensory nerves and also the support structures such as the hair follicles, sweat glands, and oil glands (Figure 16-1). The skin has many important functions, which include acting as a mechanical and protective barrier between the body and the outside world, sealing fluids inside, and preventing bacteria and other microorganisms from readily entering the body. The skin is also a vital sensory organ that provides input to the brain on general and specific environmental data and serves a primary role in temperature regulation. Damage to the skin renders it unable to carry out these functions and puts the body at risk for serious problems.

Burn damage to the skin occurs when heat or caustic chemicals come in contact with the skin and damage its chemical and cellular components. In addition to actual tissue injury, the body's inflammatory response to the skin damage may also result in additional injury or increase the severity of a burn. The portions of the skin that are necrosed by the thermal insult are referred to as the *Zone of Coagulation* and have suffered irreversible injury. Surrounding this area is a *Zone of Stasis;* blood flow is compromised and tissues will die if blood flow is not restored. This condition is seen in the deeper areas of partial-thickness burns and is helped by good burn care and fluid resuscitation. Surrounding this is the *Zone of Hyperemia,* where there is increased blood flow to the tissues as a result of the actions of inflammatory mediators released by damaged skin.

Classifying Burns by Depth

Burns are characterized, based on the depth of tissue damage and skin response, as superficial (first degree), partial thickness (second degree), or full thickness (third degree). Superficial burns result in minor tissue damage to the outer epidermal layer only, but do

TABLE 16-2 *Characteristics of Various Depths of Burns*

	Superficial (first degree)	Partial Thickness (second degree)	Full Thickness (third degree)
Cause	Sun or minor flash	Hot liquids, flashes, or flame	Chemicals, electricity, flame, hot metals
Skin color	Red	Mottled red	Pearly white and/or charred, translucent and parchmentlike
Skin surface	Dry with no blisters	Blisters with weeping	Dry with thrombosed blood vessels
Sensation	Painful	Painful	Anesthetic
Healing	3–6 days	2–4 weeks, depending on depth	Requires skin grafting

cause an intense and painful inflammatory response. The most common injury of this type is "sunburn." Although no medical treatment is usually required, various medications can be prescribed that significantly speed healing and reduce the painful inflammatory response.

Partial-thickness burns cause damage through the epidermis and into a variable depth of the dermis. These injuries will heal (usually without scarring) because the cells lining the deeper portions of the hair follicles and sweat glands will multiply and grow new skin for healing. Antibiotic creams or various specialized types of dressings are routinely used to treat these burns and, therefore, appropriate medical evaluation and care should be provided for patients with these injuries. Emergency care of partial-thickness burns involves cooling the burn and covering with a clean dry dressing.

Full-thickness burns cause damage to all layers of the epidermis and dermis. No more skin cell layers are left, so healing by regrowth of epidermal cells is impossible. All full-thickness burns leave scars that later may contract and limit motion of the extremity (or restrict movement of the chest wall). Deeper full-thickness burns usually result in skin protein becoming denatured and hard, forming a firm, leatherlike covering that is referred to as *eschar*. Characteristics of these burns are listed in Table 16-2, and the depth levels and examples are shown in Figures 16-2, 16-3, and 16-4.

Determining the Severity of Burns

The body's normal inflammatory response to the burn injury can result in progressive tissue damage for a day or two following burn injury, which may well result in an increase in burn depth. Any condition that either reduces circulation

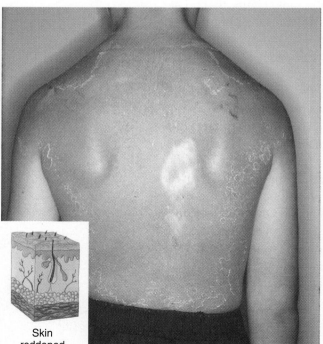

Skin reddened

FIGURE 16-2 Superficial (first-degree) burn.

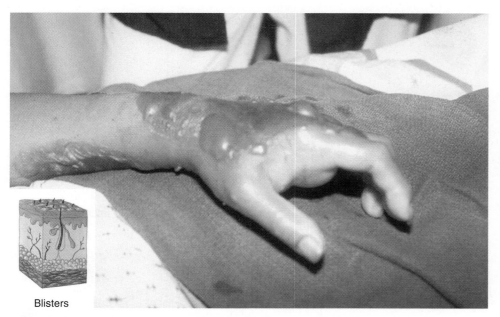

Blisters

FIGURE 16-3 **Partial-thickness (second-degree) burn.** *(Courtesy of Roy Alson, MD)*

(shock) to this damaged tissue or by itself causes further tissue damage will lead to burn progression with increasing burn depth. Because of this process of burn progression, it is not essential to determine exactly the burn depth in the field. You should, however, be able to clearly discern between superficial and deep burns. Because transport to a burn center depends on both depth and extent of the burn, you should be able to estimate the amount of body surface involved in the burn.

The burn size is best estimated in the field using the rule of nines (Figure 16-5). The body is divided into areas that are either 9 percent or 18 percent of the total body

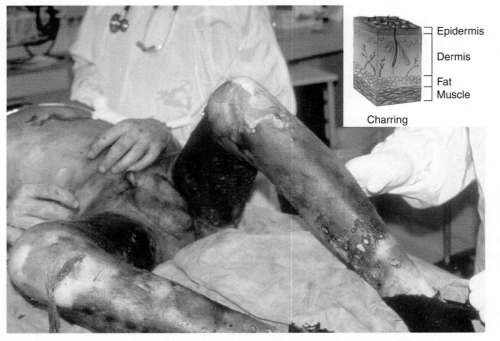

Epidermis

Dermis

Fat
Muscle

Charring

FIGURE 16-4 **Full-thickness (third-degree) burn.** *(Courtesy of Roy Alson, MD)*

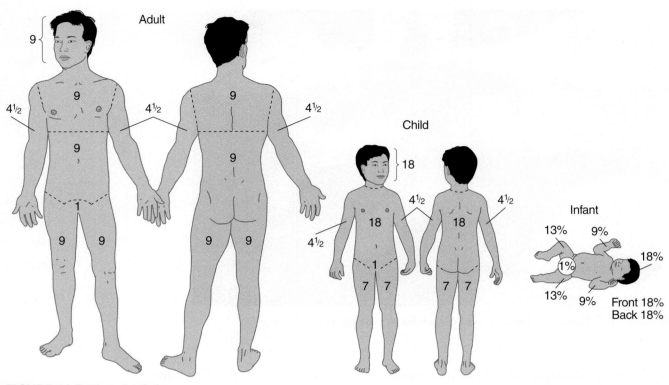

FIGURE 16-5 The rule of nines.

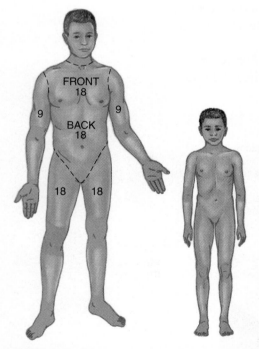

FIGURE 16-6 Areas in which small burns are more serious: Second- or third-degree burns in these areas (shaded portions) should be treated in the hospital.

surface and by roughly drawing in the burned areas, the extent can be estimated. Only partial-thickness and full-thickness burns are used for this calculation. In small children there are some differences in body size proportions and a Lund and Browder chart is helpful (Table 16-3). For smaller or irregular burns, the size can be estimated using the palmar surface (including the fingers) of the patient's hand, which is about 1 percent of the total body surface area. Even small burns can be serious if they involve certain parts of the body that affect function or appearance (Figure 16-6).

Initial care that is directed specifically toward the burn should concentrate on limiting any progression of the burn depth and extent.

PATIENT ASSESSMENT AND MANAGEMENT

Evaluation of the burn patient is often complicated by the dramatic nature of the injuries. You can easily be overwhelmed by the extent of the injury. You must remember that even patients with major burns rarely expire in the initial postburn period from the burn injury. Death in the immediate postburn period is a consequence of associated trauma or conditions such as airway compromise or smoke inhalation. A careful, systematic approach to patient evaluation will allow you to identify and manage critical life-threatening problems and to improve patient outcome.

TABLE 16-3	*Lund and Browder Chart*							

		Age (Years)				%	%	%
Area	0–1	1–4	5–9	10–15	Adults	2°	3°	Total
Head	19	17	13	10	7			
Neck	2	2	2	2	2			
Ant. Trunk	13	17	13	13	13			
Post. Trunk	13	13	13	13	13			
R. Buttock	2½	2½	2½	2½	2½			
L. Buttock	2½	2½	2½	2½	2½			
Genitalia	1	1	1	1	1			
R.U. Arm	4	4	4	4	4			
L.U. Arm	4	4	4	4	4			
R.L. Arm	3	3	3	3	3			
L.L. Arm	3	3	3	3	3			
R. Hand	2½	2½	2½	2½	2½			
L. Hand	2½	2½	2½	2½	2½			
R. Thigh	5½	6½	8½	8½	9½			
L. Thigh	5½	6½	8½	8½	9½			
R. Leg	5	5	5½	6	7			
L. Leg	5	5	5½	6	7			
R. Foot	3½	3½	3½	3½	3½			
L. Foot	3½	3½	3½	3½	3½			
					Total			

Weight _____

Height _____

Patient Assessment

The ITLS Primary and Secondary Surveys should follow the standard format described in Chapter 2.

Scene Size-up: The steps for assessing a major burn patient are the same as for any other major trauma patient. Begin by performing a Scene Size-up as outlined in Chapter 1, with an emphasis on your own safety. After the size-up is completed, your next priority is to remove the patient from the source of the burn. This is the first step in treating a burn patient, and involves both maintaining your safety and the safety of your patient.

There are specific and significant dangers in removing the burn source in all types of burn injuries. As a structure fire progresses, there is a point at which flashover occurs. Flashover is the sudden explosion into flame of everything in the room, with the temperature rising instantaneously to over 2,000 degrees centigrade. There is often little warning before this happens; thus removal of patients from burning buildings takes priority over all other treatment. Remember also that fire consumes oxygen and produces large quantities of toxic products and smoke. Thus, personnel making entry to carry out rescue should wear breathing apparatus or risk becoming victims themselves.

PEARLS
Assessment

Treat burn patients as trauma patients: ITLS Primary Survey, critical interventions, and transport decision, ITLS Secondary Survey, and ITLS Ongoing Exam.

Chemicals are not always easy to detect, either on patients or on objects in the environment. Rescuers have suffered severe chemical burns because of the failure to note sources of toxic and caustic chemicals and use appropriate personal protective equipment. Special training in hazardous materials management is recommended for all rescuers.

Electricity is exceptionally dangerous, and handling of high-voltage wires is extremely hazardous. Specialized training and knowledge are required to appropriately deal with these situations, and you should not attempt to remove wires unless specifically trained and equipped to do so. Even objects commonly felt to be safe, such as wooden sticks, manila rope, and firefighter's gloves, may not be protective and may result in electrocution. If at all possible, the source of electricity should be turned off before any attempt at rescue is made.

Initial Assessment: People do not actually die rapidly from burn injuries. Early burn deaths are usually the result of airway or trauma. Death from shock due to fluid loss from the burn will not be seen for many hours (or days) and sepsis takes days to develop. Burn victims may sustain multiple trauma from falls or other mechanisms. Hemorrhagic shock will develop rapidly compared to burn shock, so that management of the patient's trauma using ITLS guidelines is very important. Even though the burn is highly visible and makes an intense impression at the scene, care of the burn itself has a lower priority than airway management. You should manage burn patients the same as any other trauma patients and perform an Initial Assessment as soon as the burn victim is in a safe area.

Begin by assessing and, if necessary, securing the airway, while simultaneously checking the initial level of consciousness and protecting the cervical spine. Assessment of breathing, circulation, and control of major hemorrhage is then carried out.

Rapid Trauma Survey: Based upon the findings from the Scene Size-up and the Initial Assessment, a Rapid Trauma Survey is then performed, a baseline set of vital signs is obtained, and if possible, a SAMPLE history obtained. At this point a determination is made on the need for immediate transport and critical interventions. Critical problems in the burn patient that require immediate intervention include airway compromise, altered level of consciousness, or the presence of major injuries in addition to the burn. Clues from the mechanism of injury that point to critical problems include a history of being confined in a closed space with the fire or smoke, electrical burns, chemical exposure, falls from a height, or other major blunt force trauma. Supplemental oxygen should be initiated as soon as possible for all major burn patients.

The Rapid Trauma Survey of the burn patient is directed toward identification of airway and circulatory compromise. Besides clues from the mechanism of injury, other findings that should alert the responder to potential airway problems are the presence of facial and scalp burns, sooty sputum, and singed nasal hair and eyebrows. Examine the oral cavity and look for soot, swelling, or erythema (redness). Ask the patient to speak. A hoarse voice or persistent cough suggests involvement of deeper airway structures. Auscultate the chest. Wheezing or rales should alert you to the presence of lower airway injury from inhalation. Examine burned areas and check for distal pulses.

In your assessment of the burn patient, note and record the type of burn mechanism and the particular circumstances such as entrapment, explosion, mechanisms for other possible injuries, smoke exposure, chemical/electrical details, and so forth. An appropriate past medical history should also be documented in writing. If the patient is unable to speak, ask other witnesses and/or fire personnel about the circumstances of the injury.

ITLS Secondary Survey: Perform a standard Detailed Exam on stable patients. This survey should include an evaluation of the burn, estimating the depth based on appearance, and also estimating the burn size. These findings are important in determining the level of medical care that is appropriate for the burn victim.

Patient Management

Once the immediate life-threats have been addressed, you should attend to the burn wound itself. Try to limit burn wound progression as much as possible. Rapid cooling early in the course of a surface burn injury can help limit this progression. Following removal from the source of the burn, the skin and clothing are still hot and this heat continues to injure the tissues, causing an increase in burn depth and seriousness of the injury. Cooling halts this process and, if done appropriately, is beneficial. Cooling should be done with any source of clean water, but this should be undertaken for no more than a minute or two. Cooling for longer periods of time can induce hypothermia and subsequent shock.

Following the brief period of cooling, manage the burn by covering the patient with clean, dry sheets and blankets to keep the patient warm and to prevent hypothermia. It is not necessary to have sterile sheets. The patient should be covered even when the environment is not cold because damaged skin loses temperature regulation capacity. Patients should never be transported on wet sheets, wet towels, or wet clothing and ice is absolutely contraindicated. Ice will worsen the injury as it causes vasoconstriction and thus reduces the blood supply to already damaged tissue. Cooling the burn wound improperly can cause hypothermia and additional tissue damage and could be worse than not cooling the burn at all. Initial management of chemical and electrical burn injuries will be described later in this chapter in the sections on those injuries.

During the evaluation of the extent of the burn injury, you should remove the patient's loose clothing and jewelry. Cut around burned clothing that is adherent, but do not try to pull the clothing off of the skin. IV line insertion is rarely needed on scene during initial care unless delay in transport to a hospital is unavoidable. It takes hours for burn shock to develop; therefore, the only reason to initiate IV therapy is if other factors indicate a need for fluid volume or medication administration. Attempting to start IV therapy on scene in major burn patients is often difficult and routinely delays initial transport and arrival at the hospital. IV access may be established during transport.

Pain medication administration in the multiple-trauma patient remains controversial. A risk of masking associated trauma and also both central nervous system and cardiovascular depression are associated with the use of pain medication. In isolated burns without coexisting trauma and long transport times, administration of analgesics in appropriate dosages will improve patient comfort. Therefore, prior to administration of pain medication, consultation with medical direction is recommended.

It is appropriate that a physician see burn injuries. There are now available specialized forms of therapy that offer specific advantages to the treatment of superficial, partial-thickness, and full-thickness burns. We have all seen partial-thickness burns become infected and progress to full-thickness burns because of poor care. The sooner specialized burn therapy can be initiated, the more rapid and satisfactory the results will be. Table 16-4 lists conditions that would benefit from care at a burn center. Based upon available local resources and protocols, it may be appropriate to bypass a local facility and transport these patients directly to the burn center.

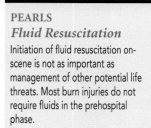

PEARLS
Cooling
Early after the burn event, properly cool the surface thermal injury, but do not cause hypothermia.

PEARLS
Fluid Resuscitation
Initiation of fluid resuscitation on-scene is not as important as management of other potential life threats. Most burn injuries do not require fluids in the prehospital phase.

Special Problems in Burn Management

The following sections review management of specific types of burns, based upon the injury mechanism. Be aware that more than one type of burn can be present in a patient. For example, a high-voltage electrical burn injury may also produce flame burns due to ignition of the patient's clothing.

Flash Burns: Flash burns are virtually always superficial or partial-thickness burns. A flash burn occurs when there is some type of explosion, but no sustained fire. The single

TABLE 16-4 *Injuries That Benefit from Care at a Burn Center*

- Partial-thickness burns greater than 10% total body surface area (TBSA)
- Burns that involve the face, hands, feet, genitalia, perineum, or major joints
- Third-degree burns in any age group
- Electrical burns, including lightning injury
- Chemical burns
- Inhalation injury
- Burn injury in patients with preexisting medical disorders that could complicate management, prolong recovery, or affect mortality
- Any patients with burns and concomitant trauma (such as fractures) in which the burn injury poses the greatest risk of morbidity or mortality. In such cases, if the trauma poses the greater immediate risk, the patient may be initially stabilized in a trauma center before being transferred to a burn unit. Physician judgment will be necessary in such situations and should be in concert with the regional medical control plan and triage protocols.
- Burned children in hospitals without qualified personnel or equipment for the care of children
- Burn injury in patients who will require special social, emotional, or long-term rehabilitative intervention

Source: American College of Surgeons, Committee on Trauma. 1999. *Guidelines for the operations of burn units* (55–62); *Resources for optimal care of the injured patient.*

heat wave traveling out from these explosions results in such short patient–heat contact that full-thickness burns almost never occur. Only areas directly exposed to the true heat wave will be injured. Typically, face and hands are involved. An example of this type of burn is seen when someone pours gasoline on a charcoal fire in order to get it to heat up faster. In situations of possible flash explosion risk, you should *always* wear proper protective clothing and avoid entry into explosive environments. Other injuries (fractures, internal injuries, blast chest injuries, and so on) may occur as a result of explosion.

Inhalation Injuries: Inhalation injuries account for more than half of the 4,500 plus burn-related deaths in the United States each year. Inhalation injuries are classified as carbon monoxide poisoning, heat-inhalation injuries, or smoke (toxic) inhalation injuries. Most frequently, inhalation injuries occur when a patient is injured in a confined space or is trapped; however, even victims of fires in open spaces may have inhalation injuries. Flash explosions (no fire) practically never cause inhalation injuries.

Carbon Monoxide Poisoning. Carbon monoxide poisoning and asphyxiation are by far the most common causes of early death associated with burn injury. Carbon monoxide is a by-product of combustion and is one of the numerous chemicals in common smoke. It is present in high concentrations in auto exhaust fumes and fumes from some types of home space heaters. Since it is colorless, odorless, and tasteless, its presence is virtually impossible to detect. Carbon monoxide binds to hemoglobin (257 times stronger than oxygen), resulting in the hemoglobin being unable to transport oxygen. Patients quickly become hypoxic even in the presence of low concentrations of carbon monoxide. An alteration in level of consciousness is the predominant sign of this hypoxia (Table 16-5). A cherry-red skin color or cyanosis is rarely present as a result of carbon monoxide poison-

TABLE 16-5 *Symptoms Associated with Increasing Levels of Carboxyhemoglobin Binding*

Carboxyhemoglobin Level (%)	Symptoms
20	Headache common, throbbing in nature; shortness of breath on exertion
30	Headache present; altered central nervous system function with disturbed judgment; irritability, dizziness; decreased vision
40–50	Marked central nervous system alteration with confusion, collapse; also fainting with exertion
60–70	Convulsions; unconsciousness; apnea with prolonged exposure
80	Rapidly fatal

ing and, therefore, cannot be used in the assessment of patients for carbon monoxide poisoning. Pulse oximetry will remain normal to high in the presence of carbon monoxide and cannot be used to assess these patients. Some newer model pulse oximeters can now specifically measure carboxyhemoglobin levels and, if available, should be used on all persons who have the possibility of exposure to carbon monoxide. Death usually occurs because of either cerebral or myocardial ischemia or myocardial infarction due to progressive cardiac hypoxia.

Treat patients suspected of having carbon monoxide poisoning with high-flow oxygen by mask. If such a patient loses consciousness, begin Advanced Life Support with intubation and ventilation using 100 percent oxygen. If a patient is simply removed from the source of the carbon monoxide and allowed to breathe fresh air, it takes up to 7 hours to reduce the carbon monoxide–hemoglobin complex to a safe level. Having the patient breathe 100 percent oxygen decreases this time to about 90 to 120 minutes, and use of hyperbaric oxygen (100 percent oxygen at 2.5 atmospheres) will decrease this time to about 30 minutes (Figure 16-7). All suspected cases of carbon monoxide poisoning or toxic inhalation should be transported to an appropriate hospital. The decision to transport the patient to a hyperbaric chamber should be made by medical direction.

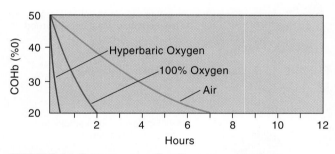

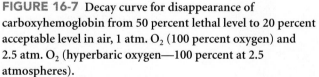

FIGURE 16-7 Decay curve for disappearance of carboxyhemoglobin from 50 percent lethal level to 20 percent acceptable level in air, 1 atm. O_2 (100 percent oxygen) and 2.5 atm. O_2 (hyperbaric oxygen—100 percent at 2.5 atmospheres).

Heat-Inhalation Injuries. Heat-inhalation injuries are confined to the upper airway, because breathing in flame and hot gases does not result in heat transport down to the lung tissue itself. The water vapor in the air in the tracheal-bronchial tree effectively absorbs this heat. Steam inhalation is the exception to this rule, as steam is superheated water vapor. A second exception to this rule is if the patient has inhaled a flammable gas that then ignites and causes thermal injury to the level of the alveoli (example: a painter in a closed space where the paint fumes are ignited by a spark).

As a result of the heat injury, tissue swelling occurs just as it does with surface burns. The vocal cords themselves do not swell because they are dense fibrous bands of connective tissue. However, the loose mucosa in the supraglottic area (the hypopharynx) is where the swelling occurs, and can easily progress to complete airway obstruction and

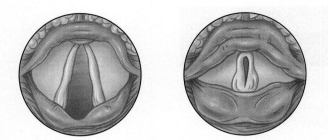

FIGURE 16-8 Heat inhalation can cause complete airway obstruction by swelling of the hypopharynx: left side—normal anatomy; right side—swelling proximal to cords.

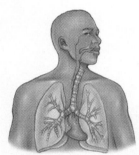

- Burns of the face
- Singed eyebrows or nasal hair
- Burns in the mouth
- Carbonaceous (sooty) sputum
- History of being confined in a closed space while being burned
- Exposure to steam

FIGURE 16-9 Danger signs of upper airway burns.

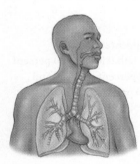

- Victims exposed to smoke in an enclosed place
- Victims who were unconscious while exposed to smoke or fire
- Victims with a cough after being exposed to smoke or fire
- Victims short of breath after being exposed to smoke or fire
- Victims with chest pain after being exposed to smoke or fire

FIGURE 16-10 Patients in whom you should suspect smoke inhalation.

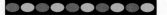

PEARLS
Chemical Burns
Chemical injuries, in general, require prolonged and copious irrigation.

death (Figure 16-8). There is usually some time between the injury and the development of airway edema, so loss of airway due to direct thermal injury is rare in the initial prehospital phase. Be aware that once the swelling begins, the airway can obstruct rapidly. Aggressive fluid resuscitation can hasten this swelling. During secondary transport to a burn center, the risk of airway swelling can become significant and can cause airway obstruction as volume-resuscitation IV fluids are being administered. For this reason, if there is any potential for airway burns, the patient should be sedated and intubated before a transfer. It is much easier to electively intubate a patient in the emergency department than do a crash intubation in the back of an ambulance.

Figure 16-9 lists signs that should alert you to the danger of your patient having upper airway burns. Swollen lips indicate the presence of thermal injury at the airway entrance, and hoarseness (indicating altered airflow through the larynx area) is a warning of early airway swelling. Stridor (high-pitched inspiratory breathing and/or a seal-bark cough) indicates severe airway swelling with pending airway obstruction and represents an immediate emergency. The only appropriate treatment is airway stabilization, preferably via nasotracheal intubation or by paralysis and rapid sequence intubation. This procedure may be far more difficult than under other routine circumstances because of significant anatomic alterations due to swelling. Additionally, because of irritation of inflamed damaged tissue, lethal laryngospasm may occur when the endotracheal tube first touches the laryngeal area. Therefore, this procedure is best undertaken in a hospital emergency department and should be done in the field only when absolutely necessary following communication and orders from medical direction. You should be prepared to perform a surgical airway in these patients if unable to intubate.

Smoke-Inhalation Injuries. Smoke-inhalation injuries (Figure 16-10) are the result of inhaled toxic chemicals that cause structural damage to lung cells. Smoke may contain hundreds of toxic chemicals that damage the delicate alveolar cells. Smoke from plastic and synthetic products is the most damaging. Tissue destruction in the bronchi and alveoli may take hours to days. However, as these toxic products in the smoke are very irritating, they may precipitate bronchospasm or coronary artery spasm in susceptible individuals. Treat bronchospasm with inhaled beta agonists (albuterol) and oxygen.

Chemical Burns: Thousands of different types of chemicals can cause burn injuries. Chemicals may not only injure the skin, but also be absorbed into the body and cause internal organ failure (especially liver and kidney damage). Volatile forms of chemicals may be inhaled and cause lung tissue damage with subsequent severe life-threatening respiratory failure. The effects of the chemical agents on the other organ systems, such as the lung or liver, may not be immediately apparent after exposure. Chemical injuries are frequently deceiving in that initial skin changes may be minimal even when a severe injury is present. This may lead to secondary contamination of rescuers. Minimal burns on the patient may not be obvious. As a result, you can get these chemicals on your own skin unless appropriate precautions are taken. Factors that lead to tissue damage include chemical concentration, amount, manner and duration of skin contact, and the mechanism of action of the chemical agent. The pathologic process causing the tissue damage continues until the chemical is either consumed in the damage process, detoxified by the body, or is physically removed. Attempts at inactivation with specific neutralizing chemicals are dangerous because the process of neutralization may generate other chemical reactions (heat) that may worsen the injury. Therefore, you should aim treatment at chemical removal by following these four steps.

PROCEDURE
✴ Removing the Source of Chemical Burns

1. Wear appropriate protective gloves, eyewear, and respiratory protection if needed. In some situations you will need to wear a chemical protective suit as well.

2. Remove all the patient's clothing. Place in plastic bags to limit further contact.

3. Flush chemicals off the body by irrigating copiously with any source of available water or other irrigant. If dry chemicals are on the skin, they should first be thoroughly brushed off before performing copious irrigation. Remember: *The solution to pollution is dilution.*

4. Remove any retained agent adhering to the skin by any appropriate physical means such as wiping or gentle scraping. Follow this by further irrigation (Figures 16-11 and 16-12).

Ideally, all contaminated patients should be decontaminated prior to transport, so as to limit skin damage and prevent contamination of the ambulance or hospital. Critical interventions including airway management can be initiated prior to and during the decontamination process. If the patient has not been fully decontaminated prior to transport, notify the receiving hospital as soon as possible, so that they can be prepared to manage the patient.

Irrigation of caustic chemicals in the eye is exceptionally important because irreversible damage will occur in a very short period of time (less than the transport time to get to the hospital). Irrigation of injured eyes may be difficult because of the pain associated with eye opening. However, you must begin irrigation to prevent severe and permanent damage to the corneas (Figure 16-13a, b). Check for contact lenses or foreign bodies

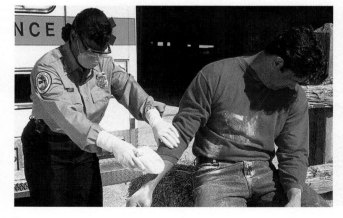
a.
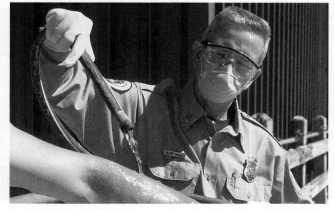
b.

FIGURE 16-11 For a chemical burn, (a) brush away dry powders, and then (b) flood the area with water. (*Photos courtesy of Michal Heron*)

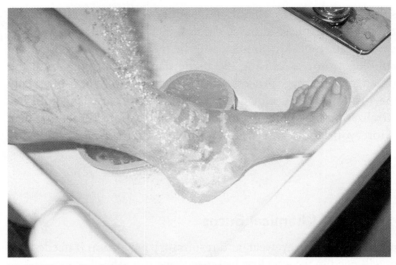

FIGURE 16-12 Acid burn of the ankle being irrigated. *(Courtesy of Roy Alson, MD)*

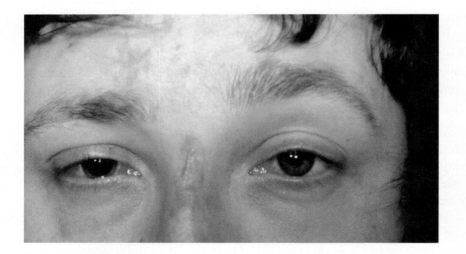

a.

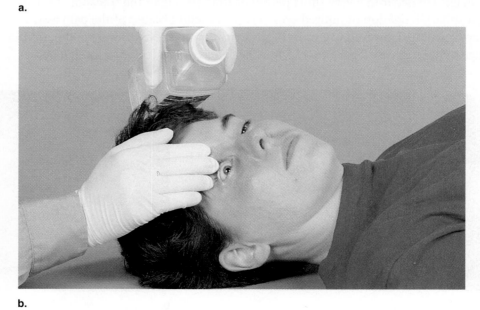

b.

FIGURE 16-13 (a) Chemical burns to the eyes; (b) emergency care of chemical burns to the eye.

and, if present, remove them early during irrigation. A nasal cannula hooked to an IV bag of normal saline and placed over the bridge of the nose makes an excellent bilateral eye wash system during transport.

Electrical Burns: In cases of electrical burns, damage is caused by electricity entering the body and traveling through the tissues. Injury results from the effects of the electricity on the function of the body organs and from the heat generated by the passage of the current. Extremities are at risk for more significant tissue damage, versus the torso, because their small size results in higher local current density (Figure 16-14). The factors that determine severity of electrical injury include the following:

- Type and amount of current (alternating versus direct current and also the voltage)
- Path of the current through the body
- Duration of contact with the current source

The most serious and immediate injury that results from electrical contact is cardiac arrhythmia. Any patient who receives an electric current injury, regardless of how stable he looks, should have a careful immediate evaluation of his cardiac status and continuous monitoring of cardiac activity. The most common life-threatening arrhythmias are premature ventricular contractions, ventricular tachycardia, and ventricular fibrillation. Aggressive Advanced Life Support management of these arrhythmias should be undertaken, since these patients usually have normal healthy hearts and the chances for resuscitation are excellent. For a patient in ventricular fibrillation with only basic life support available, start cardiopulmonary resuscitation (CPR) and transport immediately to a hospital facility. Most of these victims do not have preexisting cardiovascular disease, and their heart muscle tissue is usually not damaged as a result of the electricity. Even under circumstances of prolonged CPR, resuscitation is often possible. Once those efforts at managing cardiac status are complete, provide field care as previously described for thermal burns.

Electrical injuries cause skin burns at the entrance and exit sites because of high temperatures generated by the electric arc (2,500 degrees centigrade) at the skin surface. Additional surface flame burns may result if the patient's clothing is ignited. Fractures

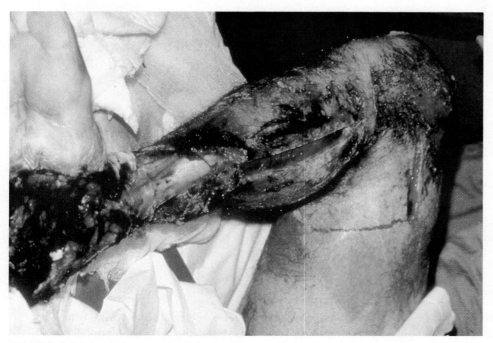

FIGURE 16-14 Electrical burn of the lower leg and foot. *(Courtesy of Roy Alson, MD)*

and/or dislocations may be present due to the violent muscle contractions that electrical injuries cause. Often victims are involved in construction and may sustain fractures or other injuries due to falls after an electric shock. Internal injuries usually involve muscle damage, nerve damage, and possible intravascular blood coagulation due to electrical current passage. Internal chest or abdominal organ damage due to electrical current is exceedingly rare.

At the scene of an electrical injury, your first priority is scene safety. Determine if the patient is still in contact with the electrical current. If so, you must remove the patient from contact without becoming a victim yourself (Figure 16-15). Handling high-voltage electrical wires is extremely hazardous. Special training and special equipment are needed to deal with downed wires; never attempt to move wires with makeshift equipment. Tree limbs, pieces of wood, and even manila rope may conduct high-voltage electricity. Even firefighter gloves and boots do not offer adequate protection in this situation. If possible, leave the handling of downed wires to power company personnel or develop a special training program with your local power company to learn how to use the special equipment designed to handle high-voltage lines.

In the field setting, it is impossible to tell the total extent of the damage in electrical burns. So, all electrical burn patients should be transported for hospital evaluation. Due to the potential for arrhythmia development, routine IV access should be initiated in the ambulance, along with continuous cardiac monitoring. IV fluid resuscitation should be started during transport in this situation. Because of extensive tissue destruction, the fluid needs during interfacility transport of an electrical burn patient are often higher than those with thermal burns. Electrical burn patients are at risk for developing rhabdomyolysis and renal failure.

Lightning Injury: Lightning kills more persons in North America each year than any other weather-related phenomenon. Injuries from lightning are very different from other electrical injuries in that lightning produces extremely high voltages (>10,000,000 volts) and currents (>2,000 amps), but has a very short duration (<100 msec) of contact.

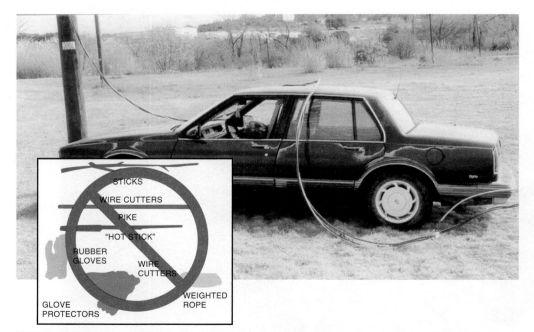

FIGURE 16-15 Removal of high-voltage electrical wires. Do not try to remove wires with safety equipment (or sticks) unless specially trained. Turn off the electricity at the source or call the power company to remove the wires. *(Courtesy of Leon Charpentier, EMT-P)*

Lightning produces a "flashover" phenomenon, in which the current flows around the outside of the victim's body. Consequently, the internal damage from current flow seen with generated electricity is not seen in a lightning strike. Most of the effects from a lightning strike are the result of the massive DC (direct current) shock that is received. Classic lightning strike burns produce a fernlike or splatter pattern across the skin (Figure 16-16). The victim does not need to be struck directly to sustain an injury. Lightning may strike an adjacent object or nearby ground and still produce an injury to a victim. Often the victim's skin is wet, from either sweat or rain. This water, when heated by the lightning current, is quickly vaporized, producing superficial and partial-thickness burns, and may literally explode the clothing off the victim. As these burns are superficial, aggressive fluid resuscitation is not required.

The most serious effect of a lightning strike is cardiorespiratory arrest, with the massive current acting like a defibrillator to briefly stop the heart. Cardiac activity often spontaneously resumes within minutes. However, the respiratory drive centers of the brain are also depressed by the current discharge, and these areas take longer to recover and resume the normal respiratory drive. Consequently, the victim remains in respiratory arrest, which is followed by a second cardiac arrest from hypoxia.

The essential component of the management of the lightning strike victim is restoration of cardiorespiratory function, while protecting the cervical spine. Follow standard guidelines for CPR and Advanced Cardiac Life Support (ACLS). Since lightning strikes can occur at sporting events and other outdoor gatherings, strikes often become multiple-casualty events. It must be stressed that in a multiple-casualty lightning strike, the conventional triage approach of a pulseless or nonbreathing patient equaling a dead patient should not be followed. If a patient is awake or breathing after a lightning strike, he will most likely survive without further intervention. Resuscitative efforts should concentrate on those victims who are in respiratory or cardiac arrest, since prompt CPR and ACLS represent the only chance that these victims have for survival.

Long-term problems have been seen in lightning strike patients, such as the development of cataracts, or neurological and/or psychological difficulties. Perforation of the eardrum is quite common, and rarely long bone or scapular fractures, as seen in the

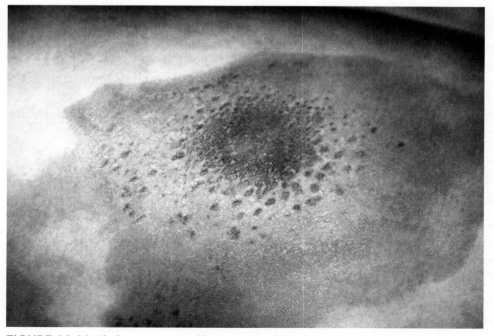

FIGURE 16-16 Flashover pattern of burns on the skin of a victim of a lightning strike.

victims of generated high-voltage electrical injuries, may be seen. These fractures are managed as described in Chapter 14.

There are over 200 reported deaths in North America each year due to lightning strike. This represents only 30 percent of lightning strike victims; thus it is possible that you will have to care for such a victim. These events often involve multiple victims, with varying degrees of severity. Prompt CPR greatly improves the chances of survival. When confronted with a naked (or partially unclothed) unconscious or confused patient, with perforated eardrums and a fernlike or splatter burn pattern on his body, think lightning strike.

Radiation Burns: Ionizing radiation damages cells by breaking molecular bonds. Skin burns from radiation look exactly like thermal burns and cannot be differentiated by their appearance alone. However, radiation burns develop slowly over days and so generally do not present as an emergency. Because of the damage to the skin cells, radiation burns heal very slowly. They can cause fluid loss like thermal burns and are even more prone to infection. Patients with radiation burns are not radioactive unless they are contaminated with radioactive material. If there is any danger that they might be contaminated, you should call for the hazardous materials team to scan them for radiation and perform decontamination if needed. Noncontaminated radiation-burn patients are treated the same as any burn patient. Decontamination of patients contaminated by radioactive material is beyond the scope of this course.

Circumferential Burns: Circumferential full-thickness burns may lead to neurovascular compromise. While this is rarely a problem on the fire scene, this may become significant during an interfacility transfer. Full-thickness burns that are circumferential around an extremity can act as a tourniquet as edema progresses. Early on, the patient may complain of loss of sensation, tingling and eventually develop ischemic pain with loss of pulses. Circumferential full-thickness burns on the extremities will require an escharotomy by the physician, especially if long transport times are involved. Circumferential burns of the chest can interfere with chest expansion and thus compromise respirations. Again, escharotomy in this setting can improve ventilatory status.

Be sure to alert the receiving facility if you are transporting a patient with full-thickness circumferential burns.

Secondary Transport: Major burns often do not occur in locations where immediate transport to a burn center is possible. As a result, transport from a primary hospital to a burn center is commonly necessary. After the initial stabilization, prompt transfer to a burn center can improve patient outcome. During this transport, it is important for the ambulance crew to continue resuscitation initiated at the referring facility.

Prior to secondary transport, the transferring physician should have completed the following:

- Stabilization of respiratory and hemodynamic function. This may include intubation and IV access for fluid administration.
- Assessment and management of associated injuries
- Review of appropriate lab data (specifically, blood gas analysis)
- Insertion of nasogastric tube in patients having burns covering more than 20 percent of the body surface area
- Placement of a Foley (urinary) catheter to allow measurement of urine output, which can assist in determining the adequacy of ongoing fluid resuscitation
- Assessment of peripheral circulation and appropriate wound management
- Proper arrangements with the receiving hospital and physician

PEARLS
Secondary Transport

- Plan all secondary transports to burn centers and effectively continue resuscitation during such transports.
- Do not begin a secondary transport of a patient with a possible airway burn without the patient being intubated before transport.

You should specifically discuss the transport with either the referring or the receiving physician to determine what special functions may need monitoring and to determine the appropriate range for fluid administration, since burns often require extremely large hourly IV rates for appropriate cardiovascular support. Initial resuscitative fluid needs in a burn patient are calculated using the Parkland formula:

$$4 \text{ cc/kg of Ringer's lactate or normal saline} \times \% \text{ burn area} \times \text{body weight (kg)}$$
$$= \text{fluid needs in first 24 hours}$$

Half of this fluid is given in the first 8 hours and the remainder over the next 16 hours.

It is important for you to maintain careful records indicating patient condition and treatment during transport. You should also make an in-depth report to the receiving facility.

Pediatric Burns: Children represent nearly one-half of all patients who seek treatment for burns. Because of their thinner skin, they are at greater risk for severe injury following a burn. Postburn problems, such as hypothermia, are more likely to occur in children because of their larger surface area to body mass ratio. Because of differences in anatomy, the rule of nines must be modified, as in small children the head represents a larger portion of the body surface (see Figure 16-5). The Lund and Browder chart is better for estimating burn size in children (see Table 16-2). The palmar surface (1 percent) rule applies to children as well as adults.

Sadly, burns in children may be the result of intentional abuse and, in fact, 10 percent of abuse cases in the United States involve burns. You should be alert for signs of abuse. These include burns that match shapes of objects such as curling irons, irons, or cigarette burns. Also suspicious for abuse are multiple stories of how the injury occurred or stories of the burn being caused by activities by the child that are inconsistent with the child's development. Burns to the genitalia, perineum, or in a stocking or glove distribution (Figure 16-17) should also raise suspicion. If there is a suspicion of abuse, this must be reported to child protective services or law enforcement.

Fire and EMS personnel can help reduce burns in children through community education. Programs to teach parents about limiting the temperature on household water heaters to 120 degrees Fahrenheit and programs to teach children about fire safety can make a significant impact on the incidence of pediatric burns in your community. You should also be aware that the elderly may also be victims of abuse by burns (see Chapter 18).

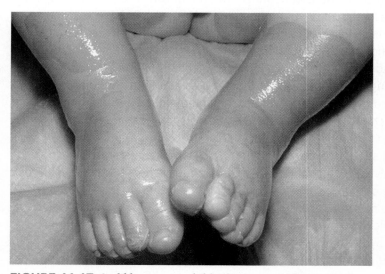

FIGURE 16-17 Scald burns on a child. This is a typical pattern of child abuse burns. (*Courtesy of Roy Alson, MD*)

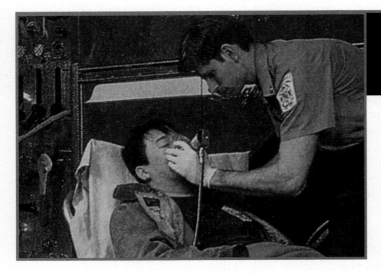

Dan, Joyce, and Buddy of the Emergency Transport System (ETS) have been called to the scene of a warehouse fire where the watchman has just been rescued from an upstairs bathroom. They prepare to care for a patient with burns and/or inhalation injuries. During travel to the scene, they decide that Buddy will be team leader on this call.

They arrive in the industrial district to find a large warehouse engulfed in flames. The victim has been removed from the area of the fire to a local staging area. As they approach, their general impression is bad, as the patient appears to be having difficulty breathing. He is alert but can only speak in one- and two-word sentences because of dyspnea. His voice is hoarse and there is audible wheezing. Initial assessment reveals that his airway is open but he is having wheezing and rapid, stridorous respiration. There are obvious burns of the face. He has a strong but rapid pulse at the wrist.

Dan applies an oxygen mask attached to a demand valve (a flow-restricted oxygen-powered ventilation device, or FROPVD) while Buddy continues a Rapid Trauma Survey. There is erythema and some blistering of the face. The nose hairs are singed. There is soot in the mouth and nose. There is no deformity of the neck and the neck veins are flat. The chest has no apparent injuries but there are inspiratory and expiratory wheezes bilaterally. Heart sounds are rapid and faint. The abdomen is soft and the patient denies pain with palpation. The pelvis is stable and nontender. There is some erythema of the hands but no blistering. There is normal PMS of the extremities.

Buddy gets the team to immediately move the patient to the ambulance and they begin transport. Vital signs are BP 160/100, pulse 140, and respiration 40 per minute. His pulse oximeter saturation is 100 percent, but Buddy realizes that the pulse oximeter is worthless in carbon monoxide inhalation victims so he attaches no significance to the reading. While Dan initiates an albuterol nebulizer treatment with 100 percent oxygen, Buddy starts a large-bore IV at a keep-vein-open rate and gets the SAMPLE history.

The patent states he is 45 years old and has a history of asthma. He denies any allergies and his medication is an albuterol inhaler that he uses as needed. He was upstairs making his rounds when he heard a loud explosion. When he opened the door to the stairs, they were engulfed in flames. He went to the back of the building, where he was eventually rescued by the fire department. He complains of burning of his face and hands and also has chest pain and severe dyspnea. He had just finished eating his evening meal when the explosion occurred. Because of the stridor, Dan decides to intubate. Using the rapid sequence intubation protocol, Dan administers a sedative agent followed by a paralytic. He easily passes a 7-mm endotracheal tube and confirms position. (In the absence of permission for RSI, Dan would attempt to insert a 9-mm endotracheal tube by the nasotracheal route.)

Buddy contacts medical direction and is instructed to give a bolus of IV steroids. Given the injuries found by the crew, medical direction instructs them to transport the patient to the regional burn center in the next county. When doing the Secondary Survey, Buddy attaches a cardiac monitor and does a 12-lead EKG, which reveals an acute injury pattern. He immediately notifies medical direction and fills out the thrombolytic information sheet. The burn team and the acute cardiac care team meet them at the emergency department of the burn center. Because of the rapid treatment the patient eventually makes a complete recovery.

A blast of flame can cause upper airway burns, leading to loss of the airway from swelling. The patient with facial burns and burns in the mouth or nose and who has stridor is in danger of immediate loss of the airway. Not only does smoke inhalation cause hypoxia and poisoning by multiple toxic gases, it can also precipitate bronchospasm in susceptible individuals. The hypoxia can precipitate a myocardial infarction in individuals who already have borderline coronary arteries. The toxic gases can precipitate coronary spasm, leading to myocardial infarction or arrhythmias. Giving 100 percent oxygen is the best prehospital treatment of carbon monoxide poisoning. The pulse oximeter is unable to tell the difference between oxyhemoglobin and carboxyhemoglobin, so will give false results and is not to be trusted in this case.

SUMMARY

Burn injuries are potentially deadly for both you and your patient. You must never forget the rules of scene safety. Half of all burn deaths are from inhalation injuries; do not forget the airway. Give 100 percent oxygen if there is any chance of inhalation injury. Cool the burn to halt the burning process, but do not cause hypothermia. You must begin irrigating chemical burns in the field, or the burn damage will continue during transport. This is one of the few instances in trauma care when extra time spent in the field may be beneficial to the patient. Electrical burns are commonly associated with cardiac arrest, but rapid evaluation and management are usually life-saving. High-voltage electricity is extremely dangerous; get trained personnel to turn it off. Do not begin secondary transfer of a burn patient until the patient has been properly stabilized and the airway protected.

BIBLIOGRAPHY

1. American Burn Association. 2003. Inhalation injury: Diagnosis. *Journal of the American College of Surgeons* 196(2): 307–12.
2. Committee on Trauma, American College of Surgeons. 2004. Injuries due to burns and cold. *Advanced Trauma Life Support*. Chicago: The College, 231–42.
3. Criss, E., and others. 1998. Not just blowing smoke. *Emergency Medical Services* (March 2003): 27–39.
4. Danks, R. R. 2003. Burn management: A comprehensive review of the epidemiology & treatment of burn victims. *JEMS* 28(5): 118–41.
5. Miller, K. 2003. Acute inahaltion injury. *Emergency Medical Clinics of North America*, 21, (2): 533–57.
6. Naradzay, J. F., R. Alson. 2005. Thermal burns. *Emedicine: On-line Emergency Medicine Text*. Boston: Boston Medical Publishers.
7. Shehan, H., R. Papini. 2004. Initial management of a major burn: Overview. *British Medical Journal*. 328: 1555–57.
8. Singer, A. J. 2000. Thermal burns rapid assessment and treatment. *EM Practice* 2(9).
9. Wald, D. A. 1998. Burn management: Systematic patient evaluation, fluid resuscitation, and wound management. *Emergency Medicine Reports*. 19: 45–52.

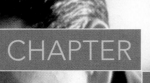

17

Trauma in Children

Ann Marie Dietrich, MD, FACEP, FAAP
Jonathan I. Groner, MD, FACS, FAAP

OBJECTIVES

Upon completion of this chapter, you should be able to:

1. Describe effective techniques for gaining the confidence of children and their parents.

2. Predict pediatric injuries based on common mechanisms of injury.

3. Describe the ITLS Primary and Secondary Surveys in the pediatric patient.

4. Demonstrate understanding of the need for immediate transport in potentially life-threatening circumstances, regardless of the lack of immediate parental consent.

5. Differentiate the equipment needs of pediatric patients from those of adults.

6. Describe the various ways to perform SMR on a child and how this differs for an adult.

7. Discuss the need for involvement of EMS personnel in prevention programs for parents and children.

Note: Because of increasing demand for further training in management of the injured child, ITLS has developed a one-day course (Pediatric ITLS) that covers this subject in detail. You may get more information about this course by calling ITLS International at 888-495-4875 (outside the United States call 630-495-6442).

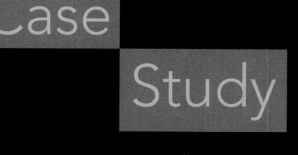

Case Study

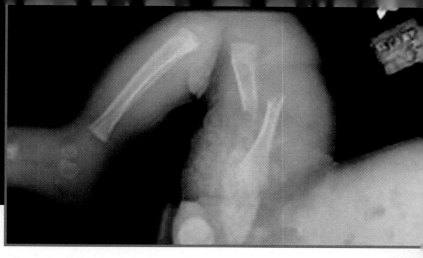

Joyce, Dan, and Buddy have received a call to a home for an 18-month-old child who fell from a couch. They are told that the infant appears to be unconscious. As they respond to the scene, they decide that Joyce will be team leader. *What sort of injuries should they expect from this mechanism? How does evaluation and treatment of a 1-year-old differ from an adult?* Keep these questions in mind as you read the chapter. Then, at the end of the chapter, find out how the rescuers completed this call.

INTRODUCTION

Children are not just little adults. They differ from adults in that they have different patterns of injuries, frequently have different responses to those injuries, require special equipment for assessment and treatment, are difficult to assess and communicate with, and come with parents and other family members. Doctors as well as EMTs are uncomfortable treating children because of these differences and the fact that we treat them less frequently and thus do not develop as much expertise as we would like. Those of us with children of our own are further hampered by the intense emotions we feel when treating a seriously injured child. For all these reasons you should study this chapter carefully.

COMMUNICATING WITH THE CHILD AND FAMILY

A child is part of a family unit. To a child, the one constant factor in life is family. So family-centered care for an injured child is critical. (Remember that the caregiver of a child will not always be a parent, but for simplicity the generic term "parent" is used in this chapter when referring to the guardian of a child.) Following an injury to a child, parents should be involved as much as possible in emergency care. They should be supported and encouraged to provide love and concern to their child. Parents who receive careful instructions and guidance in how they may do so are assets in the field. Explain to them what you are doing and why you are doing it, and then use their trust relationship with the child to enhance your history, physical examination, and care of the patient. Inclusion and respect of the family will improve the performance of all aspects of stabilization of an injured child.

The best way to get parent confidence is to demonstrate your competence and compassion in managing the child. Parents are more likely to be cooperative if they see that you are confident, organized, and using equipment that is designed for children. Show the parents you know how important they are by involving them in the care of their child.

Whenever possible, keep parents in physical and verbal contact with the child. They can perform simple tasks such as holding a pressure dressing or holding the child's hand. Parents can explain to the child what is going on or sing their favorite songs.

Show your concern for the child, but do not freeze. One technique is to pretend that the parent is one of your examiners. You can then talk your way through the examination, using language that is understandable to both the child and parents. You will also be able to better assess mental status. A child who can be consoled or distracted by a person or a toy has a normal mental status (most sensitive indicator of adequate perfusion). On the other hand, a child who cannot be consoled or distracted may have a head injury, may be in shock, or may be experiencing hypoxia or severe pain. Changes in distractibility and ability to be consoled are important observations about the level of consciousness of a child. Record and report them just as you would report changes in level of consciousness of an adult. Since they are familiar with a child's baseline mental status, parents are your best resource for detecting subtle changes in the child's level of consciousness. They will notice when the child is "not acting right" before you will.

A child less than 9 months old likes to hear "cooing" sounds, the jingle and sight of keys, and often feels more comfortable when swaddled. For the child under 2 years, the flashlight is a good distraction. Use appropriate language for the developmental level of the child. Children less than 1 year of age know many "ah" sounds, like "mama" and "papa." Try to use those. Older children, especially 2-year-olds, are typically negative and often difficult to distract or comfort. Expect all questions to be answered by "no." Therefore, tell the child and the parents what you are going to do and do it. For example, "We are going to hold your head still. Mom, this is important in case he has hurt his neck." Speak simply, slowly, and clearly. Be gentle and firm. The toddler and young child can benefit from a toy or doll being with them. Ask the parent to get one favorite belonging, if easily available, for the ride to the hospital. It will make the trip to and through the hospital easier. If time allows and the patient is stable, you can make an airplane out of two tongue blades or a doll out of a rubber glove (if child is over 3 years old and will not choke on the rubber).

Do not get caught in the trap of asking the child if he wants to take a trip in the ambulance or to be placed in a cervical collar. The child will answer "no" most of the time. Tell the child what you are doing with a smile on your face. Show it does not hurt, perhaps by doing it to a parent or yourself. Size is intimidating. When approaching a child, try to make yourself small by getting on the child's level. In the care of a child, it is appropriate that EMTs spend much field time on their knees.

Frightened children, especially around the ages of 2 to 4 years, may try to defend themselves by biting, spitting, or hitting. They are acting out of fear. Stay calm, recognize that the behavior is normal, reassure the child, and use firm, not painful, physical control of the patient as needed. Parents and children do not understand packaging, which makes them more likely to resist it. Explain why packaging is necessary. Most parents will understand if you explain that even though the chances are low that there is anything seriously wrong with the spine, the stakes are high if there is. Make a game of packaging with the child. If the parent refuses to let you package the child, write it down on your run report and get the parent to sign it.

Whenever possible, allow parents to accompany their child in the vehicle. It is very frightening for a child and a family to be separated, especially if the injuries are severe. Give the parents specific instructions and position them to provide comfort and support to their child without interfering with the care that must be given.

Before you leave the scene with the child, be sure to ask the parent about other children. Sometimes they are so concerned about one that they forget other small children who may be in a high-risk situation, such as alone in the house.

PARENTAL CONSENT

Many states have consent laws that exist to protect children. Although consent is necessary for children who are stable, and desirable in children who are injured, any critically injured child should *not* have care delayed while attempting to obtain consent. EMTs have to make a decision on whether or not it will take too long to find a parent to obtain consent. In a situation in which a child needs emergency care (such as a child in a bicycle/motor-vehicle collision and no parent present), you must treat that child appropriately. Transport before you receive permission, document why you are transporting without permission, and notify medical direction of this action.

If the parents or legal guardians do not want you to transport or treat, try to persuade them. If you cannot, document your actions on the written report and try to get them to sign it. If the child has a critical injury and the parents refuse transport, notify law enforcement and the appropriate social authorities immediately and try to continue your care of the child until they arrive. If you suspect abuse, notify authorities at the appropriate time. You do not have to confront the possible abuser.

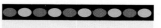

PEARLS
Abuse

You are the only one to see the scene of the injury. Be alert to signs of child abuse.

ASSESSMENT AND CARE

Pediatric Equipment

Table 17-1 contains a list of suggested pediatric equipment for the prehospital provider. You would not want to approach a 170-pound man who is having a heart attack with a 3.5-mm endotracheal tube, nor should you approach a child with adult equipment. Keep pediatric equipment in a separate trauma box. Equipment for each size child could be kept in different trauma boxes, so that everything for that size child would be at your fingertips. However, lack of storage space makes multiple boxes impractical for most rescue vehicles and ambulances. In addition, it is impractical to make multiple trips back to the vehicle if the dispatch information was inaccurate. The solution is a length-based tape (Broselow or Standard Pediatric Aid to Resuscitation Card system [SPARC]) that, when used to measure the length of a child, gives you the estimated weight of the child, precalculated doses of fluid and medications, and estimated sizes of common equipment needed. You could have equipment and supplies sorted into boxes or bags coded to the color panels on the length-based tape (compact color-coded bags are commercially available).

PEARLS
Equipment

Children require special equipment. Without this equipment, you cannot provide the pediatric patient with adequate care.

Using a length-based drug dose chart or tape (such as the Broselow tape or SPARC system) has become an essential component for determining the appropriate equipment and medication doses for a child (Figures 17-1 and 17-2). These devices allow you to focus on the patient instead of remembering the correct equipment size and drug dose. These tape systems estimate weight better than emergency medicine professionals, and endotracheal tube size as well as anesthesiologists (see Chapter 9).

Common Mechanisms of Injury

Children are most commonly injured from falls, MVCs, auto–pedestrian crashes, burns, airway obstruction from a foreign body, and child abuse. Children who fall usually land on their heads because the head is the largest and heaviest part of a small child's body. Serious head injury is unusual in a fall from under 27 inches. The use of motorcycles and dirt bikes, especially if a helmet is not worn, may result in serious injury. Motor-vehicle collisions, especially if lap belt restraints are improperly used, may result in the seat-belt syndrome, and injury may occur to the liver, spleen, intestines, or lumbar spine. Any situation

TABLE 17-1 *Prehospital Pediatric Equipment and Supplies*

BLS Equipment and Supplies

Essential	Desirable
• Oropharyngeal airways: infant, child, and adult sizes (sizes 00–5) with tongue blades for insertion • Self-inflating resuscitation bag, child and adult sizes • Masks for bag-valve mask device: neonatal, infant, child, and adult sizes • Oxygen masks; infant, child and adult sizes • Nonrebreathing mask: pediatric and adult sizes • Stethoscope • Pediatric femur traction splint • Pediatric backboard with head immobilizer • Pediatric cervical collars (rigid) • Blood pressure cuff, infant and child • Portable suction unit with a regulator • Suction catheter: tonsil-tip and 6F–14F • Extremity splints: pediatric size • Bulb syringe • Obstetric pack • Thermal blanket • Water-soluble lubricant	• Infant car seat • Nasopharyngeal airways: sizes 18F–34F, or 4.5–8.5 mm • Glasgow Coma Score reference • Small stuffed toy • Finger-stick blood glucose device • Pulse oximeter

ALS Equipment and Supplies

ALS units should carry everything on the BLS list, plus the following items.

Essential	Desirable
• Transport monitor • Defibrillator with adult and pediatric paddles • Monitoring electrodes: pediatric sizes • Endotracheal tubes, uncuffed sizes 2.5–6 mm, cuffed sizes 6–8 mm, • Endotracheal tube stylets: pediatric and adult sizes • Infant and child laryngoscope straight blades sizes 0–3 and curved blades sizes 2–4 • Nasogastric tubes, sizes 8F–16F • KID (immobilization device) • Magill forceps: pediatric and adult • Intraosseous needles, sizes 16, 18, 20 • Butterfly cannulae, 23 and 25 gauge • Over-the-needle catheters, 16–24 gauge • Pediatric armboards • Broselow tape • Nebulizer	• Disposable CO_2 detection device • End-tidal CO_2 monitors • Blood glucose analysis system

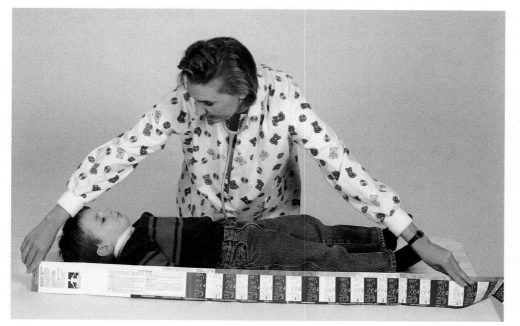

a.

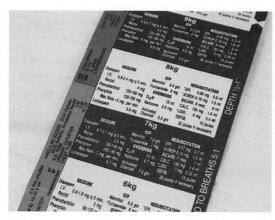

b.

FIGURE 17-1 Use of Broselow tape.

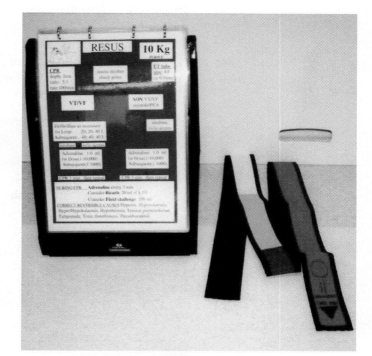

FIGURE 17-2 Standard Pediatric Aid to Resuscitation Card system has color-coded tape and booklet of precalculated doses of fluids, medications, and equipment. *(Photo Courtesy of Kyee Han, MD)*

in which the injury pattern and mechanism differ may be child abuse. Suspect abuse if the history does not match the injury, if there is a delay in seeking health care, or if the story keeps changing.

Assessment of the Airway

As you begin the assessment be sure to stabilize the neck in a neutral position with your hands. Do not take time to apply a cervical collar until you have finished the ITLS Primary Survey. Recognize the signs of airway obstruction in children: apnea, stridor, or "gurgling" respiration. So that the neck does not have to be moved, the jaw thrust should be the first airway maneuver in the unconscious child who has sustained trauma. In small children, the occiput is so big that it will flex the neck and may occlude the airway when the child is lying flat. It is often necessary to place a pad underneath the torso to keep the neck in a neutral position (see Figure 17-3 and Chapter 11). Hyperextension of the neck also may cause airway occlusion.

Inspecting the airway is easier in the child than in the adult (Figure 17-4). It is true that the child's tongue is large, the tissue is soft, and the airway is easy to obstruct, but other characteristics make it easier to manage the child's airway. For example, neonates are obligatory nose breathers, so just opening the mouth or clearing the nose with a bulb syringe can be life-saving. To use the bulb syringe, collapse the bulb end of the syringe, put the point end in the nose of the child, and release the bulb. Remove the syringe from the nose, squeeze the bulb to empty the mucus, blood, or vomit, and repeat. The bulb syringe can be used to remove secretions from the posterior pharynx of infants as well.

For the unconscious child with no gag reflex, an oral airway is very helpful to get the tongue out of the way and keep the airway open (see Chapter 5). If a tooth is loose, be sure to remove it from the mouth so that the child does not choke on it while you are inserting the airway adjunct. The oral airway can stimulate a gag reflex, which is very sensitive in the conscious child, thus limiting the use of this airway adjunct to unconscious children with no gag reflex. Nasopharyngeal airways are too small to work predictably in children; do not use them. Give ventilation instructions to your partner as soon as you complete your evaluation of breathing.

Check the neck for signs of injury (bruises, marks, and lacerations), carotid pulse, and distended neck veins, and feel for a deviated trachea. What appears to be minor blunt trauma

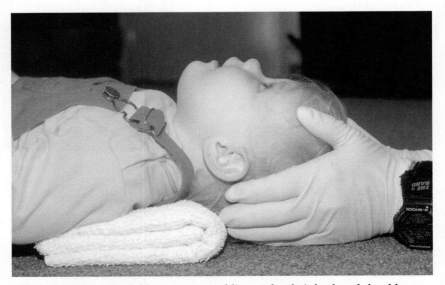

FIGURE 17-3 Most children require padding under their back and shoulders to keep the C-spine in a neutral position. *(Courtesy of Bob Page, NREMT-P)*

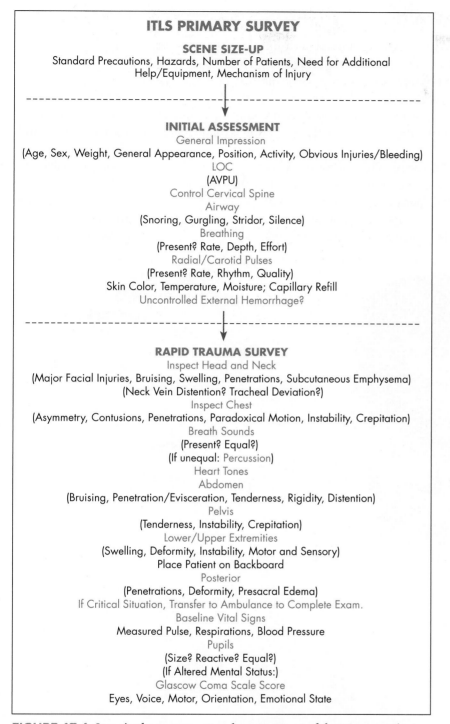

ITLS PRIMARY SURVEY

SCENE SIZE-UP
Standard Precautions, Hazards, Number of Patients, Need for Additional
Help/Equipment, Mechanism of Injury

INITIAL ASSESSMENT
General Impression
(Age, Sex, Weight, General Appearance, Position, Activity, Obvious Injuries/Bleeding)
LOC
(AVPU)
Control Cervical Spine
Airway
(Snoring, Gurgling, Stridor, Silence)
Breathing
(Present? Rate, Depth, Effort)
Radial/Carotid Pulses
(Present? Rate, Rhythm, Quality)
Skin Color, Temperature, Moisture; Capillary Refill
Uncontrolled External Hemorrhage?

RAPID TRAUMA SURVEY
Inspect Head and Neck
(Major Facial Injuries, Bruising, Swelling, Penetrations, Subcutaneous Emphysema)
(Neck Vein Distention? Tracheal Deviation?)
Inspect Chest
(Asymmetry, Contusions, Penetrations, Paradoxical Motion, Instability, Crepitation)
Breath Sounds
(Present? Equal?)
(If unequal: Percussion)
Heart Tones
Abdomen
(Bruising, Penetration/Evisceration, Tenderness, Rigidity, Distention)
Pelvis
(Tenderness, Instability, Crepitation)
Lower/Upper Extremities
(Swelling, Deformity, Instability, Motor and Sensory)
Place Patient on Backboard
Posterior
(Penetrations, Deformity, Presacral Edema)
If Critical Situation, Transfer to Ambulance to Complete Exam.
Baseline Vital Signs
Measured Pulse, Respirations, Blood Pressure
Pupils
(Size? Reactive? Equal?)
(If Altered Mental Status:)
Glascow Coma Scale Score
Eyes, Voice, Motor, Orientation, Emotional State

FIGURE 17-4 Steps in the assessment and management of the trauma patient
are the same for both children and adults.

to the neck can be life threatening. A deviated trachea is difficult to detect in a small child, but has the same significance as in adults. Make a mental note of the child's initial level of consciousness as you begin your survey. Although a preschool child may appear to be sleeping rather than unconscious from an injury, remember that most children will not sleep through the arrival of emergency vehicles. Ask the parents to wake the child so you can get an initial assessment of the airway and level of consciousness. Following a traumatic event, a decreased level of consciousness may suggest hypoxia, shock, head trauma, or seizure.

Assessment of Breathing

Assess the child for breathing difficulty. Count the child's respiratory rate. Most children breathe fast when they are having trouble and then, when they can no longer compensate, they have periods of apnea or a very slow respiratory rate. Note whether the child is "work-ing" to breathe, demonstrated by retractions, flaring, or grunting. Look at the chest rise, listen for air going in and out, and feel the air coming out of the nose. If there is no move-ment, you must breathe for the child. If ventilation is inadequate, you must assist the child.

Artificial Ventilation: When performing mouth-to-mouth ventilation for a small child, you may cover both the child's nose and mouth with your mouth. If a BVM face mask does not fit well when performing bag-valve mask ventilation, try turning the mask upside down for a better seal. Pay attention to your hand placement, too (Figure 17-5). Your large hands can easily obstruct the airway or injure the child's eyes. Give the breaths slowly at

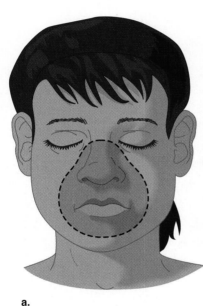

a.

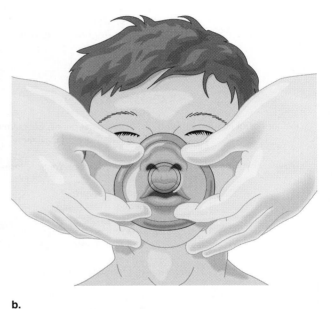

b.

c.

FIGURE 17–5 (a) The mask should fit on the nose and the cleft above the chin; (b) two-handed face mask seal; (c) one-handed face mask seal.

low pressure, less than 20 cm H_2O, to keep from inflating the stomach or causing a pneumothorax. The rates are 20 per minute for a child less than a year of age, 15 per minute for greater than 1 year of age, and 10 per minute for an adolescent. When using a bag-valve mask, it is best to monitor your ventilation with capnography. Studies have found that we tend to hyperventilate even when consciously trying not to.

Most importantly, watch for chest rise when you ventilate. If the chest is rising, air is getting into the lungs. Check air entry on both sides of the chest with your stethoscope. Gentle cricoid pressure (Sellick maneuver; see Chapter 4) is useful and recommended in a child. Some self-inflatable bag-valve masks have a pop-off valve at about 40 cm H_2O pressure. The pressure generated by these devices is more than adequate most of the time. However, lungs are sometimes stiff from a near-drowning, bronchospasm, or aspiration, and more pressure is needed. Be familiar with your equipment. Make sure that your bag-valve mask does not have a pop-off valve.

Endotracheal Intubation: If bag-valve mask ventilation of the child is effective, then intubation is an elective procedure. ***It is usually better not to intubate the child in the field.*** Intubation is extremely difficult to perform even in a dry, well-lighted emergency department. If you must intubate in the field, get ready by preoxygenating (not hyperventilating) the child and preparing your equipment. The oral route should be used on all children. Blind nasotracheal intubation is not recommended in the child less than 8 years old because the nares are too small and the larynx is too far anterior. For oral endotracheal intubation, choose an endotracheal tube size suggested by the length-based tape system, or about the same diameter as the tip of the child's little finger. Another guide is as follows:

$$4 + \frac{\text{age in years}}{4} = \text{size of tube (mm)}$$

In small children the smallest part of the airway is just below the cords, so you can get a good seal using an uncuffed tube until the tube size is at least 6 mm. There is a significant risk of neck movement with any tracheal intubation, so have someone stabilize the neck with his hands during intubation. Using a straight blade, gently move the tongue to the left by entering on the right side of the mouth; place the blade in the vallecula, and lift. Compared to adults, the small child's larynx is closer to the mouth, and this technique is often effective. If you cannot see the cords, advance the laryngoscope blade to the epiglottis and lift again. The cords should be easily seen.

Remember to hold your breath when no one is breathing for the child. As soon as you get an urge to breathe, but after no more than 15 seconds, stop trying to intubate, bag the child to reoxygenate, and try again in a few minutes. Another effective method for reminding you when to ventilate is to have the team member who is stabilizing the neck to count aloud to 15 slowly.

Check to see if the tube is in place by following the confirmation protocol (Chapter 5). Be sure to keep the tube in place. A simple flexion of the neck can push the tube into the right mainstem bronchus, and extension of the neck can pull the tube out of the trachea. Hold the tube firmly in place with your thumb and forefinger on the lip and gum margin so if the child's head moves, the endotracheal tube will stay in place. Capnography is the best way to monitor the position of the endotracheal tube. Apply benzoin to the cheek and lip, being careful not to let any drop in the eye. Firmly tape (or tie with linen tape) the tube to the corner of the mouth and stabilize the head with a head motion-restriction device. Ideally a commercial endotracheal tube holder should be used if available.

Supplemental Oxygen: As you package a child, you will often have to improvise. Tape and straps can restrict the child's chest movement, so assess ventilation frequently en route. Any child with a significant injury should receive supplemental oxygen (as close to

PEARLS
Endotracheal Intubation
The uncuffed endotracheal tube in a child may become dislodged easily, especially during movement of the child. Frequent reassessment is very important. Constant expired CO_2 monitoring (capnography) is very helpful.

100 percent oxygen as possible), even if there seems to be no difficulty breathing. Injury, fear, and crying all increase oxygen demands on tissues. Children with any type of injury are likely to vomit; be prepared. Remember to give ventilation instructions to your teammate before moving to assessment of circulation.

Assessment of Circulation

Signs of Shock: Early shock is far more difficult to diagnose in a child than an adult. Persistent tachycardia is the most reliable indicator of shock in a child. Since pulses may be difficult to find and assess in a child, practice feeling them on most of your pediatric runs and on your own children. In a child, the brachial pulse is usually easy to feel, whereas the carotid is not. Feeling a dorsalis pedis pulse causes less anxiety and may be easier to find than a femoral pulse. A weak rapid pulse with a rate over 130 is usually a sign of shock in children of all ages except neonates (Table 17-2). Prolonged capillary refill and cool extremities may indicate decreased tissue perfusion. Capillary refill may be used along with other methods to assess the circulation, but do not depend on it alone to diagnose shock. Although currently controversial, capillary refill should still be included as part of the Initial Assessment for shock in a child. To test capillary refill, compress the nail bed, the entire foot, or the skin over the sternum for 2 seconds and release to see how quickly the blood returns. Skin color should return to the precompressed state within 2 seconds. If it does not, the child has vasoconstriction, which can be a sign of shock.

Individual variances may make some of the signs of shock normal for a particular child. Tachycardia may occur because of fear or fever. Mottling may be normal in an infant less than 6 months of age, but it also may be a sign of poor circulation, so note it. Extremities may be cold because of nervousness, cold weather, or poor perfusion. Capillary refill may be prolonged in a child who is cold. In general, a child should be carefully evaluated and assumed to have signs of shock if there is persistent tachycardia or signs of poor peripheral perfusion (prolonged capillary refill or cool extremities).

The child's level of consciousness is also a useful indicator of circulatory status, yet note that circulation can be poor even though the child appears to be awake. As mentioned earlier, if the child is able to focus on his parent, or is consolable by the parent or a member of the EMS team, there is enough circulation to allow the child's brain to be working.

Low blood pressure is a sign of late shock, but measuring blood pressure in a frightened child can be time consuming, especially for the inexperienced. To make it easier and more reliable to obtain blood pressure in an emergency, practice taking it at every opportunity. The rule of thumb for cuff size is to use the largest one that will fit snugly on the patient's upper arm. If there is too much noise, you can perform a blood pressure by palpation. Find the radial pulse, pump up the blood pressure cuff until you no

---

●●●●●●●●●●

PEARLS
Shock

Because of strong compensatory mechanisms, children can look surprisingly good in early shock. When they deteriorate, they often "crash." If you have a long transport time and the mechanism of injury or the assessment suggests the possibility of hemorrhagic shock, be prepared. When you give fluid resuscitation to a child, give 20 mL/kg in each bolus, then reassess. Make sure the total amount of fluid you give is reported to the hospital.

TABLE 17-2 *Ranges for Vital Signs*

Age	Weight (kg)	Respiration (per minute)	Pulse (per minute)	Systolic Blood Pressure (mmHg)
Newborn	3–4	30–50	120–160	>60
6 mo.–1 yr	8–10	30–40	120–140	70–80
2–4 yr	12–16	20–30	100–110	80–95
5–8 yr	18–26	14–20	90–100	90–100
8–12 yr	26–50	12–20	80–100	100–110
>12 yr	>50	12–16	80–100	100–120

longer feel the pulse, and allow air to leak slowly while observing the dial on the blood pressure cuff. Record the pressure at which you first feel the pulse and label it "p," for palpation. This will be a systolic blood pressure only and will be slightly lower than a blood pressure that can be auscultated. A systolic blood pressure less than 80 in children, and less than 70 in young infants, is a sign of shock.

Shock may be secondary to occult bleeding in the abdomen, chest, or in a femur fracture. Also, although we teach that patients do not go into shock from intracranial blood loss, in rare circumstances, this can happen in the very young infant.

NOTE: The antishock garment (MAST or PASG) is no longer recommended for treatment of shock except in special circumstances.

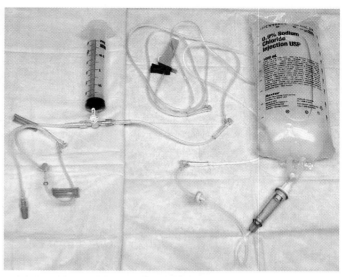

FIGURE 17-6 Equipment for giving bolus treatment for shock. *(Photo Courtesy of Roy Alson, MD)*

Fluid Resuscitation: If hypovolemic shock is present, the child requires fluid resuscitation. You should establish vascular access and give a fluid bolus. The initial bolus should be 20 mL/kg of normal saline, given as rapidly as possible. See the appropriate equipment set up to do this in Figure 17-6. If there is no response, another 20 mL/kg can be given. If the child is in late shock and you cannot see or feel a vein, or cannot start an IV in two attempts or 90 seconds, you may need to perform intraosseous infusion (see Figure 17-7; and Chapter 9). There is *no* scientific data available at this time to suggest that any child in hemorrhagic shock should not be given IV fluids.

Control of Bleeding

Obvious bleeding sources must be controlled to maintain circulation. Remember, the child's blood volume is about 80–90 mL/kg, so a 10-kg child has less than 1 liter of blood. Three or four lacerations can cause a 200-mL blood loss, which is about 20 percent of the child's total volume. Therefore, pay closer attention to blood loss in a child than you do in an adult. Use pressure firm enough to control arterial bleeding if necessary. If you ask the parent or a bystander to help hold pressure, monitor them to be sure they are applying enough pressure to stop the bleeding. Use a bandage tight enough to control venous bleeding, not one that will just soak up the blood so that you do not see it. Elevating an injured extremity also can help to control bleeding. Hemostatic agents can be used to control exsanguinating hemorrhage in children.

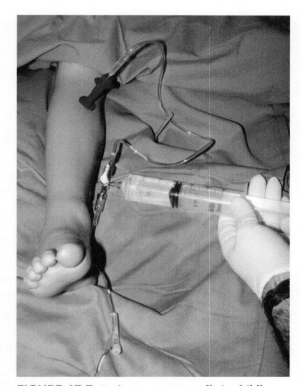

FIGURE 17-7 An intraosseous needle in child's proximal tibia being used for venous access. *(Photo Courtesy of Bob Page, NREMT-P)*

The Critical Trauma Situation

If you have found a critical trauma situation, the child needs rapid transport. Log-roll the child onto a pediatric backboard and leave the scene as quickly as possible. Remember to use a pad under the torso to align the neck in a neutral position. Appropriately sized rigid cervical collars are useful, especially in children over 1 year of age, and can help remind the patient and providers not to move the head. Do not depend on the cervical collar alone;

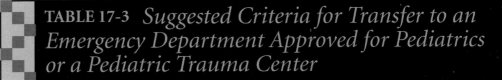

TABLE 17-3 *Suggested Criteria for Transfer to an Emergency Department Approved for Pediatrics or a Pediatric Trauma Center*

Criteria

- Obstructed airway
- Need for an airway intervention
- Respiratory distress
- Shock
- Altered mental status
- Dilated pupil
- Glasgow Coma Scale score <13
- Pediatric Trauma Score <8
- Mechanism of injury (less reliable indicators) associated with severe injuries:
  — Fall from a height of 10 feet or more
  — Motor-vehicle collision with fatalities
  — Ejection from an automobile in a MVC
  — In a MVC, significant intrusion into the passenger compartment
  — Hit by a car as a pedestrian or bicyclist
  — Fractures in more than one extremity
  — Significant injury to more than one organ system

restrict motion of the head with tape and a head motion-restriction device. Children are portable and they can (and should) be transported rapidly. There are very few procedures that should be done in the field. Minutes count, especially in children. On-scene times of less than 5 minutes are desirable.

Administer 100 percent oxygen to all critical pediatric patients. Bag-valve mask ventilation of the critical child is preferable to placing an endotracheal tube if the transport time to an appropriate emergency department is short. Not all emergency departments have the equipment or personnel to handle pediatric emergencies. Transfer arrangements for more severe problems should be worked out in advance so that when the injury occurs, confusion will be minimized and time will be saved. See Table 17-3 for a partial list of mechanisms of injury that are criteria for transport to an emergency department approved for pediatrics or a pediatric trauma center. These, plus pediatric burns, near-drowning, and head injuries with loss of consciousness should go to facilities qualified to handle major pediatric trauma.

If the child needs a procedure, you must decide whether it is worth the time. You should consider how long it will take to perform, how urgent the procedure is, how difficult it will be at the scene versus at the hospital, and how much it will delay reaching definitive care. If you have a 3-minute procedure (an IV) and a 30-minute transport, the IV probably should be started. If you are awaiting the arrival of a helicopter, you also may attempt the procedure, but be sure to have the child packaged and ready when transportation arrives. Your life-saving procedures can be performed in an ambulance while en route to the hospital. Call ahead so that the emergency department can have the necessary equipment and personnel ready. Perform the ITLS Secondary Survey and Ongoing Exams en route if there is time.

If, after completing the ITLS Primary Survey, you find no critical trauma situation, place the child on a backboard and do a methodical ITLS Secondary Survey.

		>1 year	**<1 year**	
Eyes Opening	4	Spontaneously	Spontaneously	
	3	To verbal command	To shout	
	2	To pain	To pain	
	1	No response	No response	
		>1 year	**<1 year**	
Best Motor Response	6	Obeys		
	5	Localizes pain	Localizes pain	
	4	Flexion—withdrawal	Flexion—normal	
	3	Flexion—abnormal (decorticate rigidity)	Flexion—abnormal (decorticate rigidity)	
	2	Extension (decerebrate rigidity)	Extension (decerebrate rigidity)	
	1	No response	No response	
		>5 years	**2–5 years**	**0–23 months**
Best Verbal Response	5	Oriented and converses	Appropriate words and phrases	Smiles, coos, cries appropriately
	4	Disoriented and converses	Inappropriate words	Cries
	3	Inappropriate words	Cries and/or screams	Inappropriate crying and/or screaming
	2	Incomprehensible sounds	Grunts	Grunts
	1	No response	No response	No response

TABLE 17-4 *Glasgow Coma Scale*

ITLS Secondary Survey

As in adults, record accurate vital signs, take a SAMPLE history, and perform a complete head-to-toe exam, including a more detailed neurological exam. During your neurological exam make a notation of whether the child is consolable or distractible. Finish bandaging and splinting, and transport the child while continuously monitoring. Notify medical direction. Calculate the Glasgow Coma Scale (GCS) score or Pediatric Glasgow Coma Scale score (Table 17-4).

POTENTIALLY LIFE-THREATENING INJURIES

Head Injury

Head injuries are the most common cause of death in pediatric patients. The head is the primary focus of injury in the child because the child's head is proportionately larger than the adult's. The force of impact does some damage to the brain, but much of the brain damage from head injuries comes after impact, from preventable causes. To avoid this, you must do three things:

1. *Give oxygen.* Head injury increases brain cell metabolic rate and decreases blood flow in at least part of the brain.

2. *Keep blood pressure up.* Blood must get to the brain to carry oxygen, so systolic pressure must be at least 80 mmHg in the preschool child and 90 mmHg in older children. It is therefore critical to recognize early signs of shock (tachycardia and poor perfusion) and aggressively correct hypovolemia. Early hypotension has been shown to be a predictor of poor outcome.

3. *Be prepared to prevent aspiration.* Head-injury patients frequently vomit. The Sellick maneuver should be used during bag-valve mask ventilation and any intubation attempts. Suction should be readily assessable for any child with a head injury.

Changing level of consciousness is the best indicator of head trauma. A child entering the emergency department with a GCS score of 10 that has come down from 13 will be approached very differently from the child who has a GCS score of 10 that has come up from 7. Assessments using vague words like "semiconscious" are not helpful. Instead, note specific points such as whether the child is distractible, consolable, reaches for the parent, or reacts to pain or voice.

Assessment of pupils is as important in the child as in the adult. Note also whether the eyes are moving both left and right or whether they remain in one position. Do not move the head to determine this!

Children with head injury often fare much better than adults with the same degree of injury. Children with head trauma and low GCS scores may do well if they receive aggressive medical management that focuses on maintenance of oxygenation, ventilation, and perfusion of the brain. Pediatric patients, similar to adults, should not be hyperventilated unless they have evidence of the cerebral herniation syndrome (see Chapter 10). The best way to prevent inadvertent hyperventilation is to monitor ventilation with capnography. Children with certain types of head injuries, such as epidural hematoma, may need immediate surgical intervention to give the brain the maximum chance of complete healing. Transport children with serious head injuries to a trauma center equipped to provide definitive care.

Chest Injury

Children with chest injuries generally give visible signs of respiratory distress, such as tachypnea, grunting, nasal flaring, and retractions. Be aware that children's normal respiratory rates are higher than adults' (Table 17-2). A child breathing faster than 40, or an infant faster than 60, usually has respiratory distress and would benefit from supplemental oxygen. A few grunts are not significant, but persistent grunting indicates a need for ventilatory assistance. A child in respiratory distress often breathes with the nose like a rabbit, which is called *flaring*. Retractions relate to caving in of the suprasternal, intercostal, or subcostal areas with inspiration. Retractions suggest the child is straining to breathe. If any of these signs are persistent, they should alert you to something wrong with the respiratory system (pneumo/hemothorax, foreign body, pulmonary contusion).

Children with blunt chest injury are at risk for pneumothorax. Because the chest is small, a difference in breath sounds from side to side may be more subtle than in the adult. You may not be able to tell a difference, even by listening carefully. It is also difficult to diagnose tension pneumothorax in young children, who usually have short, fat necks that mask both neck vein distension and tracheal deviation. If a tension pneumothorax develops, the heart and trachea should eventually shift away from the side of the pneumothorax. To help detect a shift of a child's heart, place an "X" over the point of maximum impulse (PMI) of the heart. Repeatedly check the location of the PMI. This will help confirm the stethoscope findings and guide chest decompression. Needle thoracostomy (see Chapter 7) can be life-saving.

Children in the preadolescent age group have highly elastic chest walls. Rib fractures, flail chest, pericardial tamponade, and aortic rupture are, therefore, seldom seen in this group. However, pulmonary contusion is common. If a child does have rib fractures or a flail chest, he has sustained a significant force to his chest and should be assumed to have significant internal injuries.

Abdominal Injury

The second leading cause of traumatic death in most pediatric centers is internal bleeding secondary to rupture of the liver and/or spleen. In children, the liver and spleen both protrude below the ribs, exposing the organs to blunt trauma. This poor protection and the relatively large size of the liver and spleen in children allow these organs to be easily torn. Abdominal injuries are difficult to diagnose in the field. A child may have a severe abdominal injury with minimal signs of trauma. Any child with seat-belt marks, bicycle handlebar marks, or bruises to the abdomen should be assumed to have internal injuries. If a child has blunt injury to the chest or abdomen, be prepared to treat for shock. The capsule of a child's liver and spleen are thicker than an adult's; therefore, bleeding is often contained within the organ. If a child with blunt trauma is in shock with no obvious source of bleeding, your decision should be to load and go.

Life-saving interventions should be made en route to the hospital. If you have a short (5–10 minute) transport time to a trauma center, it is not necessary to attempt an IV line. If the child is critical and the transport time is long, you should make no more than two attempts at IV lines before going to an intraosseous infusion. Any child who has been crying or suffered an abdominal injury will develop gastric distention and a tendency to vomit; be prepared.

Spinal Injury

Although children have short necks, big heads, and loose ligaments, cervical spine injuries are uncommon before adolescence. Children less than 9 years of age usually have upper cervical-spine injuries in contrast to older children and adults who usually have lower cervical-spine injuries. There is also a higher incidence of spinal-cord injury without radiographic abnormality (SCIWORA) than in the adult population. Therefore, you should perform appropriate SMR on all children with a potential spinal injury. A cervical collar is not necessary if the head is properly restricted in a padded device. Again, try to make a game of packaging the child. You can promise you will give him a ride in the ambulance as a reward after you get him all wrapped up and ready. Have a parent or other familiar person assist, if possible. Be sure your packaging does not restrict chest movement. As mentioned before, children up to about 8 years of age will need a pad under the torso to keep the neck in a neutral position.

CHILD RESTRAINT SEATS

A child in a motor-vehicle collision while properly restrained is much less likely to have a serious injury than an unrestrained passenger. If in a car seat, the child can usually be transported without being removed from the device. Assess the child as you would other trauma patients. If no injury is found, place padding around the child's head, and tape the head directly to the car seat (Scan 17.1). This method of transportation should be used only after a complete assessment that has revealed *no* injury to the child. If the child has evidence of any serious injuries, then remove the child from the car seat and package. Some cars have built-in infant restraint seats. These seats cannot be removed, so the child who is restrained in one of these will have to be extricated and placed on a pediatric spinal motion-restriction device.

SCAN 17.1

STABILIZING AN APPARENTLY UNINJURED CHILD IN A CAR SEAT

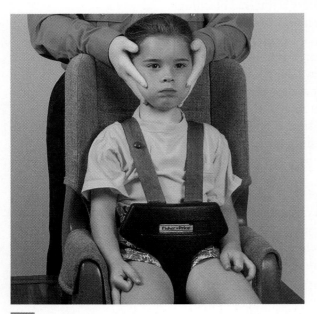

1 One EMT stabilizes the car seat in an upright position and applies and maintains manual in-line stabilization throughout the SMR processs

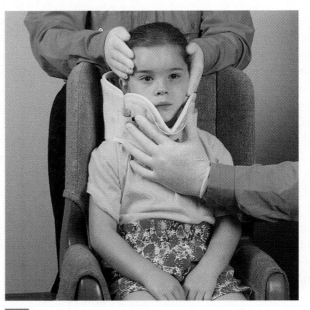

2 A second EMT applies an appropriately sized cervical collar. If one is not available, improvise using a rolled hand towel.

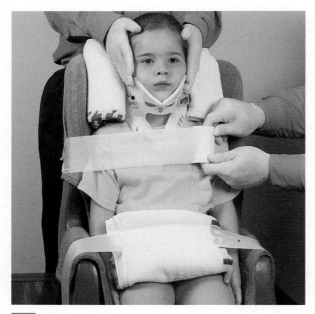

3 The second EMT places a small blanket or towel on the child's lap, then uses straps or wide tape to secure the chest and pelvic areas to the seat.

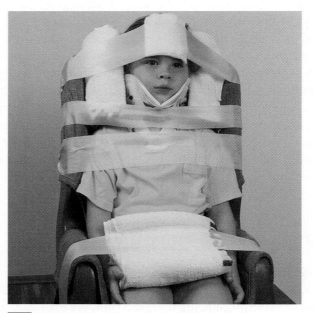

4 The second EMT places towel rolls on both sides of the child's head to fill the voids between the head and seat. The medic tapes the head into place, taping across the forehead and the collar, but avoiding taping over the chin, which would put pressure on the neck. The patient and seat can be carried to the ambulance and strapped to the stretcher, with the stretcher head raised.

Case Study
continued

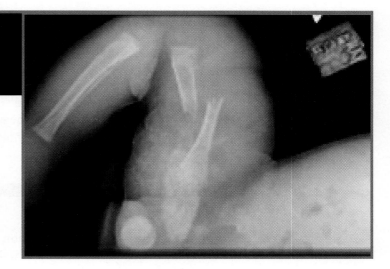

Joyce, the team leader on this call, Dan, and Buddy receive a call to a home for an injured child. They are told that the child had a fall from a couch and is unconscious. When they arrive at an apartment, they see the couch is only 12 inches high and the child is limp on the couch. A man who identifies himself as the stepfather says, "Donnie fell off the couch and wouldn't move. I picked him up and called 9-1-1." They see an 18-month-old child lying on the couch. The general impression is not good, as the child is neither awake nor moving. He is not clothed and there are obvious old full-thickness burns of his buttocks and multiple bruises of varying ages on his body. These are not injuries that would have come from a fall off a couch.

Donnie does not respond to Joyce when she speaks to him. She immediately checks the airway and finds it open but respiration is slow and shallow. Donnie has a slow but strong pulse at the wrist. Dan immediately places a clean sheet on the backboard and they carefully log-roll Donnie onto it. Buddy stabilizes the neck with his knees and begins ventilation with a bag-valve mask. He makes sure that Joyce sees the right pupil is slightly larger than the left.

Joyce performs a Rapid Trauma Survey, which reveals the child has an obvious hematoma of the right temporal area, with bruising of the face. The neck has no obvious deformities; the neck veins are flat and trachea is in the midline. The chest has multiple bruises and abrasions and there is crepitation of the ribs on the left side. Donnie moans in pain when his ribs are palpated and localizes with his hands. Buddy notes that he opens his eyes to pain. Breath sounds are present and equal. The heart can be heard and the rate is about 60 beats per minute. Donnie does not respond when Joyce palpates his abdomen. She notes that the abdomen is not distended but has several bruises in a loop pattern such as an electrical cord would make. The pelvis feels stable. Examination of the extremities reveals normal PMS, but the right thigh is very swollen and the child moans when it is palpated. There are also multiple bruises in linear and loop patterns and some small burns that look like they might have been made with a cigarette. Buddy reports that Donnie has a gag reflex, so he continues bag-valve mask ventilation.

Joyce decides to transport immediately due to the critical nature of the child's injuries. As they are going out the front door, they meet a woman with a bruise on her cheek. She appears to be coming home from work. She sees the child and cries, "My God! Lester, what have you done to Donnie now?" He glares at her and she begins crying. Neither asks to ride in the ambulance, but she asks where they are taking him and says she will be there soon. Dan drives. Joyce takes vital signs: BP 110/70, respiration 8 per minute when Buddy is not ventilating, and pulse 60 per minute. She calculates the GCS score as 9 (eyes, 2; motor, 5; and verbal, 2) and then starts a large-bore IV at a keep-vein-open rate. She also attaches the cardiac monitor (sinus bradycardia) and pulse oximeter (95 on 100 percent oxygen). She performs an ITLS Secondary Survey, which reveals no new information except that both eyes react to light.

Joyce notifies medical direction that they have an unconscious 18-month-old child with multiple injuries including blunt head trauma, burns, bruises, broken ribs, and probably a broken femur. When they arrive, she immediately notifies the doctor and nurse of what they saw and heard at the scene.

The police and social services were notified; the mother and live-in boyfriend were both arrested. The boyfriend was convicted of child abuse and sent to jail but the mother, because she was also an abuse victim, was placed on probation with loss of child custody. The child required surgery for his subdural hematoma and skin grafting for his burns but eventually recovered and went to live with his grandparents. Joyce suffered nightmares, and the whole team went though critical incident stress debriefing.

Case Study

Wrap-up

Child abuse is alarmingly common in our society and is a leading cause of pediatric traumatic death. The common thread among EMS providers is care for others. When confronted with child abuse, our initial reaction can be rage. We must be alert to the signs of child neglect or abuse but never let our emotions prevent us from focusing on treatment of the child. (Always transport the child to the hospital if you have suspicions of abuse.) The investigation is better left to specially trained professionals. Most countries have laws requiring the reporting of suspected child abuse and providing legal protection for those who do so. It is extremely important that you report suspicions, as you may be the only chance that child has for survival. If you report your suspicions to the emergency physician or nurse and they ignore them, you must make your report directly to the appropriate organization. When making a report, always include local law enforcement. Most social service organizations do an excellent job, but many carry heavy workloads and some do not include local law enforcement in their investigation. Child abuse is a crime.

SUMMARY

To provide good trauma care for children, you must have the proper equipment, know how to interact with frightened parents, know the normal vital signs for various ages (or have them posted in your trauma box), and be familiar with the injuries that are more common in children. Fortunately, the assessment sequence is the same for children as for adults. If you perform your assessment well, you will obtain the information needed to make the right decisions in management. Focusing on assessment and management of the child's airway (with cervical-spine control), breathing, and circulation will result in the best possible outcome.

While assessment and management of the injured child are life-saving skills, all responders involved in the care of the seriously injured child should be concerned also about prevention (see Appendix H). Car seats, bicycle helmets, seat belts, all-terrain vehicle injuries, water safety, scald burn injuries, firearm safety, and fire drills are within our area of concern. We should donate our time to teaching safety (Figure 17-8), and we should speak out for laws (infant seat restraints, seat belts, drunk driving) that save lives.

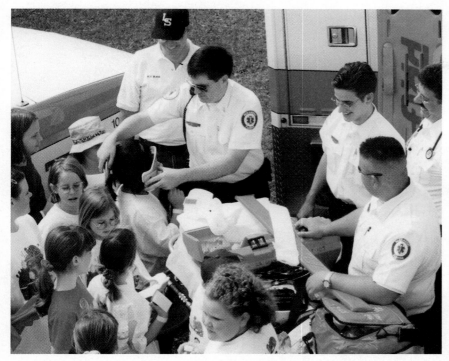

FIGURE 17-8 It is important to organize or participate in programs that educate children about injury prevention and health care. *(© Craig Jackson/In the Dark Photography)*

BIBLIOGRAPHY

1. Dietrich, A., S. Shaner, J. Campbell. 2002. *Pediatric basic trauma life support.* 2nd ed. Oakbrook Terrace, IL: Basic Trauma Life Support International.
2. DiRusso, S. M., et al. 2005. Intubation of pediatric trauma patients in the field: Prediction of negative outcome despite risk stratification. *Journal of Trauma* 59 (July): 84–91.
3. Gausche M., R. J. Lewis, et al. 2000. Effect of out-of-hospital pediatric endotracheal intubation on survival and neurological outcome: A controlled clinical trial. *JAMA* 283(6): 783.

Trauma in the Elderly

Leah J. Heimbach, JD, RN, EMT-P

Jere F. Baldwin, MD, FACEP, FAAFP

OBJECTIVES

Upon completion of this chapter, you should be able to:

1. Describe the changes that occur with aging, and explain how these changes can affect your assessment of the geriatric trauma patient.

2. Describe the assessment of the geriatric trauma patient.

3. Describe the management of the geriatric trauma patient.

(Photo courtesy of Eddie M. Sperling/
Eddie Sperling Photography)

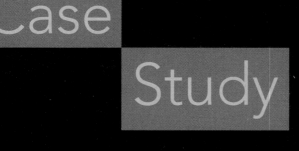

Case Study

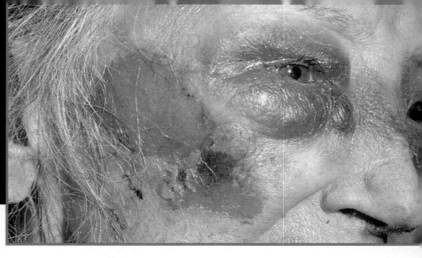

Dan, Joyce, and Buddy are dispatched to the home of an elderly woman whose neighbor called 9-1-1 and said she was hurt. The dispatcher asked the neighbor to remain with the patient until they arrived. As they respond, they decide that Dan will be team leader and they discuss common home injuries in the elderly. *What should you expect if you answered this call? How does evaluation of the elderly differ from that of younger adult patients?* Keep these questions in mind as you read the chapter. Then, at the end of the chapter, find out how the rescuers completed this call.

INTRODUCTION

Citizens over the age of 65 comprise about 12 percent of the U.S. population, but that number is expected to double in the next 25 to 30 years. The age group 85 and older is now the fastest growing segment of the U.S. population. The geriatric population already comprises a significant number of the patients being transported by ambulance. In the United States, over 30 percent of all patients transported by ambulance are over the age of 65.

"Elderly" is often understood as being 65 years or older because retirement benefits are usually initiated at about this point in life. However, chronological age is not the most reliable definition of "elderly." It is more appropriate to consider the biological processes that change with time, such as fewer number of neurons, decreased functioning of the kidneys, and decreased elasticity of the skin and tissues.

As a group, geriatric patients tend to respond to injury less favorably than the younger adult population. Geriatric patients who are injured are more likely to experience fatal outcomes, even if the injury is of a relatively low severity. According to the U.S. National Safety Council, falls, thermal injury, and MVCs have been identified as common causes of traumatic death in the geriatric population. This is an even greater concern given that as a whole the elderly population continues to assume more active lifestyles, making them more prone to injury.

Falls account for the majority of injuries in the geriatric population, the most common pathology being fractures of the hip, femur, and wrist, and head injuries. MVCs account for approximately 25 percent of geriatric deaths, although the elderly drive fewer miles. The geriatric population has a higher incidence of collision than other age groups, second only to that group under the age of 25. Eight percent of deaths are attributable to thermal injuries. These injuries include inhalation, contact with the heat source resulting in scalding and flame burns, and electrical injury.

Little has been written on the response of the geriatric patient to trauma. The existing literature is retrospective in nature and offers little explanation for the more adverse outcomes experienced by the elderly. By gaining an understanding of the normal physiological changes involved in the aging process, you will be better prepared to provide optimum care to the geriatric trauma victim.

This chapter addresses aging processes, highlights illnesses to which the geriatric patient is susceptible, and shows how those processes and illnesses make it difficult to predict the physiological response to trauma in the geriatric patient.

PATHOPHYSIOLOGY OF AGING

Aging is a gradual process whereby changes in bodily functions may occur. These changes are in part responsible for the greater risk of injury in the geriatric population.

The Aging Body

Airway: Changes in airway structures of the geriatric patient may include tooth decay, gum disease, and use of a dental prosthesis. Caps, bridges, dentures, and fillings all present potential airway obstructions in the geriatric trauma patient.

Respiratory System: Changes in the respiratory system begin to appear in the early adult years and increase markedly after the age of 60. Circulation to the pulmonary system decreases 30 percent, reducing the amount of carbon dioxide and oxygen exchanged at the alveolar level. There is a decrease in chest wall movement and in the flexibility of the muscles of the chest wall. These changes cause a decreased inhalation time, resulting in rapid breathing. There is a decreased vital capacity (or decrease in the amount of air exchanged per breath) because of an increased residual volume (volume of air in the lungs after deep exhalation). Overall breathing capacity and maximal work rate may also decrease. If there is a history of cigarette smoking, or a history of working in an area with pollutants, these changes in breathing are even more significant.

Cardiovascular System: Circulation is reduced due to changes in the heart and the blood vessels. Cardiac output and stroke volume may decrease, and the conduction system may degenerate. The ability of the valves of the heart to operate efficiently may decline. These changes may predispose the patient to congestive heart failure and pulmonary edema. Arteriosclerosis occurs with increasing frequency in the course of the aging process, resulting in an increased peripheral vascular resistance (and perhaps systolic hypertension). There may be a normally higher blood pressure in the elderly. Thus a significant change may occur in a patient when the normal blood pressure of 160 drops to 120 as a result of trauma.

Neurological and Sensory Function: Several changes occur in the brain with age. The brain shrinks, and the outermost meningeal layer, the dura mater, remains tightly adherent to the skull. This creates a space or an increased distance between the brain and the skull. Instead of protecting the brain during impact, this space allows an increased incidence of subdural hematoma following trauma. There is also a hardening, narrowing, and loss of elasticity of some arteries in the brain. A deceleration injury may cause blood vessel rupture and potential bleeding inside the skull.

There is decreased blood flow to the brain. The patient may experience a slowing of sensory responses such as pain perception and decreases in hearing, eyesight, or in other sensory perceptions. Many older patients may have a higher pain tolerance from living with conditions such as arthritis, or from being on analgesic medications chronically. This can result in their failure to identify areas in which they have been injured. Other signs of decreased cerebral circulation due to the aging process may include confusion, irritability, forgetfulness, altered sleep patterns, and mental dysfunctions such as loss of memory and regressive behavior. There may be a decrease in the ability, or even an absence of the ability, to compensate for shock.

Thermoregulation: Mechanisms to maintain normal body temperature may not function properly. The geriatric patient may not be able to respond to an infection with a fever, or the patient may not be able to maintain a normal temperature in the face of injury. The geriatric patient with a broken hip who has been lying on the floor in a room where the temperature is 64 degrees Fahrenheit can experience hypothermia.

Renal System: A decrease in the number of functioning nephrons in the kidneys of the geriatric patient can result in a decrease in filtration and a reduced ability to excrete urine and drugs.

Musculoskeletal System: The geriatric patient may exhibit signs of changes in posture. There may be a decrease in total height due to the narrowing of the vertebral discs, slight flexion of the knees and hips, and decreased muscle strength. This may result in a kyphotic deformity of the spine, resulting in the "S" curvature of the spine often seen in the stooped elderly. The geriatric patient may also have advanced osteoporosis—a thinning of the bone resulting in a decrease in bone density. This renders the bone more susceptible to fractures.

There is frequently diminished subcutaneous tissue that decreases protection from falls and blunt trauma. This lack of subcutaneous tissue can also decrease the person's ability to respond to temperature changes. Finally, there may be a weakening in the strength of the muscle and bone from the decrease in physical activity; this will also render the geriatric patient more susceptible to fractures with only a slight fall.

Gastrointestinal System: Saliva production, esophageal motility, and gastric secretion may decrease. This may result in decreased ability to absorb nutrients. Constipation and fecal impactions are common. The liver may be enlarged because of disease processes or may be failing due to disease or malnutrition. This may result in a decreased ability to metabolize medications.

Immune System: As the aging process continues, the geriatric patient may be less able to fight off infection. The patient in a poor nutritional state will thus be more susceptible to infection from open wounds, IV access sites, and lung and kidney infections. The geriatric trauma patient who is not otherwise severely injured may die from sepsis from an impaired immune system.

Other Changes: The total body water and total number of body cells may be decreased, and there is an increase in the proportion of the body weight as fat. There may be a loss in the capacity of the systems to adjust to illness or injury.

Medications

Many geriatric patients take several medications that can interfere with their ability to compensate after sustaining trauma. Anticoagulants may increase bleeding time. Antihypertensives and peripheral vasodilators can interfere with the body's ability to constrict blood vessels in response to hypovolemia. Beta-blockers can inhibit the heart's ability to increase the rate of contraction even in hypovolemic shock.

A number of the aging processes contribute to the increased risk of injury to the geriatric patient. The changes that may increase susceptibility to injury include the following:

- Slower reflexes
- Failing eyesight

- Hearing loss
- Arthritis
- Fragile skin and blood vessels
- Fragile bones

Causative factors related to the aging process have been linked with specific injuries such as tripping over furniture and falling down stairs. Further investigation reveals that these falls are often related as much to a decrease in the function of special senses, such as loss in peripheral vision, as they are to syncope, postural instability, transient impairment of cerebrovascular perfusion, alcohol ingestion, or medication usage. Alterations in perception and delayed response to stressors may also contribute to injury in the geriatric patient. When treating the geriatric trauma patient, remember that the priorities are the same as for all trauma patients. However, you must give consideration to three important issues.

- General organ systems may not function as effectively as those in the younger adult, especially the cardiovascular, pulmonary, and renal systems.
- The geriatric patient also may have a chronic illness that may complicate the effectiveness of trauma care.
- Bones may fracture more easily with less force. Fractures of major bones such as hips or femurs can be life-threatening even with proper care.

ASSESSMENT AND MANAGEMENT

Geriatric patient assessment, as any assessment, must take into account priorities, interventions, and life-threatening conditions. However, you must be acutely aware that geriatric patients can die from less severe injuries than younger patients. In addition, it is often difficult to separate the effects of the aging process or of a chronic illness from the consequences of the injury. The chief complaint may seem trivial because the patient may not report truly important symptoms. You must search for important signs or symptoms. In the geriatric patient, it is not uncommon for the patient to suffer from more than one illness or injury at the same time. Remember that the elderly patient may not have the same response to pain, hypoxia, or hypovolemia as a young person. Do not underestimate the severity of the patient's condition.

You may have difficulty communicating with the patient. This could result from the patient's diminished senses, hearing or sight impairment, or depression. The geriatric patient nonetheless should not be approached in a condescending manner. Do not allow others to take over the reporting of events from the patient who is able and willing to communicate reliable information. Unfortunately, the patient may minimize or even deny symptoms out of fear of becoming dependent, bedridden, institutionalized, or even of losing a sense of self-sufficiency. It is important that you explain any actions, including removing any clothing, before initiating the physical assessment.

There are other considerations in assessing the geriatric trauma patient. Peripheral pulses may be difficult to evaluate. Older patients often wear many layers of clothing, which can impede physical assessment. You must also distinguish between signs and symptoms of a chronic disease and an acute problem, for instance:

- The geriatric patient may have nonpathologic rales.
- The loss of skin elasticity and the presence of mouth breathing may not necessarily represent dehydration.
- Dependent edema may be secondary to venous insufficiency with varicose veins or inactivity rather than congestive heart failure.

Pay attention to deviation from expected ranges in vital signs and other physical assessment findings in the geriatric patient. An injury that is isolated and uncomplicated in the young adult may be debilitating in the older adult. This may be due to the patient's overall condition, lowered defenses, or inability to keep the effects of an injury localized.

When obtaining the past medical history, it is important to note what medications the patient may be taking. Medications may not only account for an abnormal pulse, but may also mask normal circulatory responses that would indicate deterioration in the circulatory system. The result can be a rapid decompensation without warning. Knowledge of the medications that the patient is taking can alert you to the fact that the patient's condition may be more unstable than that presented by current signs and symptoms. Antihypertensives, anticoagulants, beta-blockers, sedatives, and hypoglycemic agents may profoundly influence the response of the geriatric patient to traumatic injury.

ITLS Primary Survey

Scene Size-up: Size up the scene to decide if it is safe, to determine the number of patients, and to identify the mechanism of injury. After the ITLS Primary Survey, it may be helpful to obtain further information and to verify the patient's history from reliable family members or neighbors. This is best done in an area where the patient is unable to overhear the conversation; otherwise it may suggest that the geriatric patient is less than a competent adult. Observe the surrounding area for indications that the patient is able to provide his own care, for signs of alcohol abuse or ingestion of multiple medications, and for signs of violence, abuse, or neglect. Abuse and neglect of the elderly are common. When your assessment of the patient and surroundings is suspicious for abuse or neglect, do not fail to notify the proper authorities. Be sure to gather the patient's medications and bring them to the hospital.

Initial Assessment: As with any trauma patient, you must evaluate and provide an adequate airway and maintain motion restriction of the cervical spine while assessing the initial level of consciousness. The initial level of consciousness has more significance with elderly patients than with younger patients, because subsequent health-care providers may attribute a decreased level of consciousness to a preexisting condition rather than to the trauma. This is more likely to occur if you have not clearly indicated that the patient was clear, lucid, and cooperative at the scene.

> **PEARLS**
> *Altered Mental Status*
> Elderly patients with altered mental status should always be checked for hypoglycemia, shock, and head trauma, rather than assuming they are senile.

If patients respond appropriately to the initial verbal statements, they have an open airway and are conscious. If they do not respond, gently open the airway with a modified jaw thrust while maintaining the neck in a neutral position. This position may be difficult to determine with certainty because of arthritis and kyphosis of the spine. It is important to recognize this and not to forcibly place the occiput flat on the backboard or ground. You should add padding to the backboard to maintain the patient's usual spinal position.

The airway is likely to be partially obstructed. Clear the airway, being alert to possible teeth fragments due to decay and gum disease and dental devices such as caps, bridges, dentures, and fillings. Look, listen, and feel for movement of air. Ensure that the rate and volume of air exchange is adequate. The geriatric patient with unresolved airway difficulty or a decreased level of consciousness should be transported immediately. In such a case, frequently monitor the respiratory effort and level of consciousness (remember to check blood glucose). Consider in-line endotracheal intubation.

Place your face over the patient's mouth to look at the chest rise, to listen to the quality of the breath sounds from the mouth, and to feel the patient's breath against your ear. If the breathing is so fast that there is inadequate air exchange (more than 20 breaths per minute), or if it is too slow (fewer than 10 breaths per minute), or if the volume of air being exchanged is inadequate, provide assisted ventilation with 100 percent supplemental oxygen. Capnography is the best way to objectively monitor the patient's ventilation. Check the rate and quality of the pulse at the wrist (check at the neck if there is no pulse at the wrist). Evaluate skin color and condition. Scan the patient for bleeding, and control any bleeding with pressure.

Rapid Trauma Survey or Focused Exam: The choice between the Rapid Trauma Survey and the Focused Exam depends on the mechanism of injury and/or the results of the Initial Assessment. If there is a dangerous generalized mechanism of injury (auto crash, fall from a height, for instance) or if the patient is unconscious, you should perform a Rapid Trauma Survey. If there is a dangerous focused mechanism of injury suggesting an isolated injury (bullet wound of thigh, stab wound to the chest, and so on), you may perform the Focused Exam that is limited to the area of injury. If there is no significant mechanism of injury (dropped rock on toe) and the Initial Assessment was normal (alert with no history of loss of consciousness, breathing normally, radial pulse less than 120, not complaining of dyspnea or chest, abdominal, or pelvic pain), you may move directly to the Focused Exam based on the patient's chief complaint.

To perform a Rapid Trauma Survey, examine the head, neck, chest, abdomen, pelvis, and extremities. That is, briefly assess the head and neck for injuries and to see if the neck veins are flat or distended and the trachea is in the midline. You may apply a rigid extrication collar at this time. Now look, feel, and listen to the chest. Look for both asymmetrical and paradoxical movement. Note if the ribs rise with respiration or if there is only diaphragmatic breathing. Look for signs of blunt trauma or open wounds. Feel for tenderness, instability, or crepitation (TIC). Now listen to see if breath sounds are present and equal bilaterally.

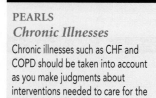

PEARLS
Chronic Illnesses
Chronic illnesses such as CHF and COPD should be taken into account as you make judgments about interventions needed to care for the elderly trauma patient.

Make appropriate interventions for chest injuries. Remember that chest injuries are more likely to cause serious problems in older people with poor pulmonary reserve. Be especially alert to problems in patients with chronic lung disease. Those patients usually have borderline hypoxia even when not injured. Briefly notice the heart sounds so you will have a baseline for changes such as development of muffled heart sounds. Rapidly expose and look at the abdomen (distention, contusions, penetrating wounds), and gently palpate the abdomen for tenderness, guarding, and rigidity. Check the pelvis and extremities for wounds, deformity, and TIC. Note whether the patient can move fingers and toes before transferring to a backboard.

Critical Transport Decisions

There are a few procedures that may be initiated on scene, but do not delay transport. Examples of critical interventions that may be initiated at the scene are the following:

- Provide airway management.
- Assist ventilation.
- Begin CPR.
- Control major bleeding.
- Seal sucking chest wounds.
- Stabilize flail chest.
- Decompress a tension pneumothorax.
- Stabilize impaled objects.

Consider whether or not the time delay in initiating these procedures outweighs the risks of delaying transportation. As mentioned elsewhere, the chance of survival decreases with a corresponding increase in the length of scene time. The same indications for immediate transport apply for the elderly as for younger patients (see Chapter 2), but remember that you may not have as dramatic a response to injury in the elderly, so you should have a low threshold for early transport. If one of the critical conditions is present, immediately transfer the patient to a long backboard (vacuum backboard is recommended) with appropriate padding, apply oxygen, load the patient into the ambulance, and transport rapidly to the nearest appropriate trauma facility.

Packaging and Transport

Package or prepare the elderly patient for transport as quickly and gently as possible. Take extra care when performing SMR on the geriatric trauma patient. This includes padding void areas that may be exaggerated due to the aging process. The elderly patient with kyphosis will require padding under the shoulders and head to maintain the neck in its usual alignment (Figure 18-1). Do not force the neck into a neutral position if it is painful to do so, or if the neck is obviously fused in a forward position. Remember to treat and transport the geriatric trauma patient, as you do all trauma patients, gently and quickly.

ITLS Secondary Survey and Ongoing Exams

Perform an ITLS Secondary Survey on scene if the patient is stable. If there is any question as to the patient's condition, you should transport and perform the ITLS Secondary Survey en route. Perform frequent ITLS Ongoing Exams. If IV therapy is to be started, it should be done en route to the hospital. If you start large-bore IV lines en route, monitor the patient's response to IV fluid infusion very closely. Volume infusion may precipitate congestive heart failure in patients with underlying cardiovascular disease. Frequently assess the patient's pulmonary status, including lung sounds and cardiac rhythm. All elderly patients should have cardiac monitoring, pulse oximetry, and capnography, if available.

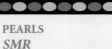

PEARLS
SMR

• When performing SMR on an elderly patient, take into consideration the fact that they might remain on a hard backboard for extended periods of time. You should use some extra padding, such as a folded blanket, for the entire body. The vacuum backboard is far superior to a hard backboard for use with the elderly patient.

• Extra padding may also be required under the head and shoulders in order to maintain the cervical spine in its normal alignment.

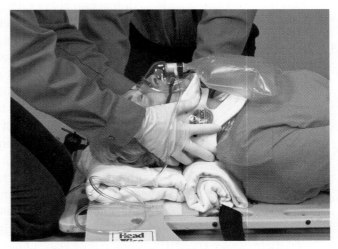

FIGURE 18-1 Elderly patients with kyphosis require padding under the shoulders and head to maintain the spine in its usual alignment.

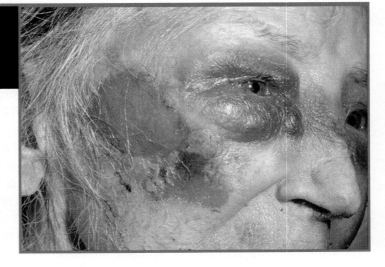

Case Study
continued

Dan, the team leader on this call, Joyce, and Buddy are dispatched to the home of an elderly woman whose neighbor called 9-1-1 and said she was hurt. The dispatcher asked the neighbor to remain with the patient until they arrived. On the way to the scene, they discuss common home injuries in the elderly. When they arrive, the neighbor meets them at the door and takes them to the patient's room. She is an 86-year-old woman (Mrs. Mary Higginbotham) who has bruises all over and appears to have been bed-bound for some time. She is confused and babbling. The room and bed linens are filthy. The sheets smell of urine and there are dried feces on the patient's legs. The neighbor states that the woman is usually alert and ambulatory and able to care for herself.

Because of Mary's failing eyesight, her grandson came to live with her about 6 months ago. The neighbor states that her grandson does not work but lives off her retirement (she's a retired college professor). "He drinks," she said. Mary's husband died 10 years ago and she has suffered from depression, but seemed to be doing better until her grandson came to live with her. She began having frequent bruises soon after he arrived, but she always explained them by saying, "I fall a lot." The neighbor (and long-time friend) said that Mrs. Higginbotham has a history of type II diabetes and mild hypertension, and takes medication for both. She said that Dexter (the grandson) had discouraged her visiting and lately would not let her talk to Mary on the phone. In response to this she had begun waiting until he went out and then coming over to visit and check on Mary. The neighbor (Mrs. Bixby) said that she had been away for a week and was anxious to see Mary. When she saw Dexter leave this morning, she came over and was appalled to see that Mary could not get out of bed and didn't even recognize her.

Dan began his exam while Buddy and Joyce looked for medicine bottles. Mrs. Bixby was not sure about allergies, but said that she did not know of any. Dan is still not sure if this is a medical or trauma call but decides to do a trauma survey. The airway is open and the respiratory rate is a little fast and shallow. The mucous membranes look dry. The breath sounds are present and equal and the peripheral pulse is weak and rapid. There is a large bruise and abrasion of the right cheek and periorbital area. The pupils are equal and reactive to light but there are obvious cataracts in both eyes. The pharynx is edentulous but Dan cannot find the dentures. The neck is nontender but there is marked dorsal kyphosis. There is equal expansion of the chest and no rales or wheezing is noted. The heart rate is fast but he hears no murmurs. The abdomen is thin and scaphoid with no obvious tenderness or masses. The pelvis is stable but she is tender over the left hip and the left leg is shortened and externally rotated. Peripheral pulses are present in both legs. There is very poor skin turgor. She moves all extremities but cries out when the left leg is moved.

By the time Dan is finished, Joyce has taken the vital signs and tells him that the blood pressure is 170/110, pulse 110, and respiration is 26 per minute. Pulse oximeter reading is 96 percent on room air. Buddy has found a half-empty bottle of Diabeta (oral diabetes medication) open by the bedside table and a full, unopened bottle of Tenormin (beta-blocker antihypertensive medication) in the kitchen on the counter. Both bottles were filled a week ago.

They carefully move Mrs. Higginbotham to a vacuum backboard and mold it to her to support her neck and hip. They then move her to the ambulance, where Dan applies nasal oxygen at 3 liters per minute. Buddy drives and Joyce does a finger-stick glucose, while Dan starts an IV with normal saline at a keep-vein-open rate. The glucose is 40. Dan gives 25 g IV glucose by protocol and soon Mrs. Higginbotham is alert and oriented. She complains of pain in her left hip. When asked how she hurt it, she lowers her eyes and says, "I fall a lot." She does not remember about her medicine but says that sometimes Dexter gives it to her and sometimes she takes it on her own. She has been unable to walk for 5 days. "Dexter has to be out a lot so I haven't been able to keep the place cleaned up. He is really a good boy but he is forgetful and he has to be gone on business a lot." (Mrs. Bixby had told them that his "business" is drinking at the local pub.) Mrs. Higginbotham denies allergies and cannot remember when she last ate. The ITLS Secondary Survey revealed no new findings.

At the hospital Mrs. Higginbotham is found to be dehydrated and malnourished with a fracture of her left hip and multiple bruises and abrasions. Dan reports their suspicion of abuse and neglect. An investigation later confirmed those suspicions. Mrs. Higginbotham survived her hip repair and upon recovery moved into an assisted living facility.

Case Study Wrap-up

Dealing with the very elderly can be challenging, especially if you are not already familiar with the patient. (Many are transported so regularly that responders are on a first-name basis.) If the patient has an altered mental status, it is always helpful if there are family members or friends who can give you pertinent history. In this case, the neighbor said that the patient was usually alert and ambulatory. She voiced accusations against the grandson that may or may not have been true, but the Scene Size-up suggested that the patient was at best being neglected, and at worst being physically abused. It became obvious that she had taken too much of her diabetes medication (hypoglycemic, with half of her tablets gone a week after the bottle was filled) and none of her blood pressure medication. (Tenormin is a beta-blocker that causes decrease in heart rate and blood pressure; she was hypertensive and tachycardic.) The team was misled by the evidence of trauma and mistakenly assumed that the altered level of consciousness was caused by age and head trauma. They correctly picked up the hypoglycemia when they started the IV and checked the blood glucose. No matter what the age, if the patient is not abusing alcohol or drugs, the most common cause of altered mental status is hypoglycemia. Just as for suspected abuse of children, you have a moral obligation to report suspicion of elderly abuse. You may be their last hope.

SUMMARY

You will be called upon to treat and transport an increasing number of geriatric trauma patients. Although the mechanisms of injury may be different from those of younger adults, the prioritized evaluation and treatment is the same. As a general rule, elderly patients have more serious injuries and more complications than younger patients. The physiologic processes of aging and frequent concurrent illnesses make evaluation and treatment more difficult. You must be aware of these differences to provide optimal care to the patient.

BIBLIOGRAPHY

1. Bergeron, E., et al. 2004. Elderly trauma patients with rib fractures are at greater risk of death and pneumonia. *The Journal of Trauma* 54(3): 478–85.
2. Diku, M., K. Newton. 1998. Geriatric trauma. *Emergency Medicine Clinics of North America* 16(1).
3. Jacobs, D. G. 2003. Special considerations in geriatric injury. *Current Opinions in Critical Care* 9(6): 535–39.
4. Patel, V. I., H. Thadepalli, P. Patel, A. Mandal. 2004. Thoracoabdominal injuries in the elderly: 25 years of experience. Journal of the National Medical Association 96(12): 1553–57.
5. Pudelek, B. 2002. Geriatric trauma: Special needs for a special population. *AACN Clinical Issues* 13(1): 61–72.
6. Stevenson, J. 2004. When the trauma patient is elderly. *J Perianesthesia Nursing* 19(6): 392–400.

Trauma in Pregnancy

Walter J. Bradley, MD, MBA, FACEP

OBJECTIVES

Upon completion of this chapter, you should be able to:

1. Understand the dual goals in managing the pregnant trauma patient.
2. Describe the physiological changes associated with pregnancy.
3. Understand the pregnant trauma patient's response to hypovolemia.
4. Describe the types of injuries most commonly associated with the pregnant trauma patient.
5. Describe the initial assessment and management of the pregnant trauma patient.
6. Discuss trauma prevention in pregnancy.

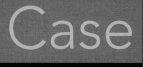

Case Study

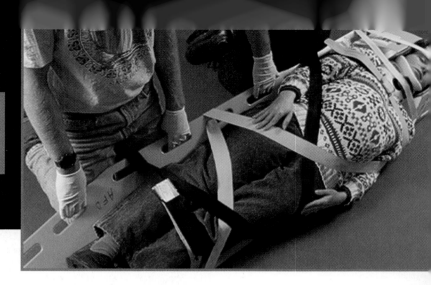

Joyce, Dan, and Buddy are dispatched to a single-auto crash. As they approach the scene, they decide that Buddy will be team leader. Upon arrival they find that the scene is safe. A local rescue squad has arrived and extricated the driver onto a long backboard. She is the only person involved. Her auto has run off the road and into a power pole. There are no downed wires. Since she is already packaged, Joyce, Dan, and Buddy move her into the ambulance and begin the exam. The young woman states she was talking on her cell phone and took her eyes off of the road. She was not restrained ("I heard that seat belts might kill the baby"), and the car was not equipped with airbags. She says that she is 25 years old and is 6 months pregnant. She denies any loss of consciousness. She complains of head, back, and lower abdominal pain. *What is different about caring for this patient? What sort of injuries should Buddy suspect?* Keep these questions in mind as you read the chapter. Then, at the end of the chapter, find out how the rescuers completed this call.

INTRODUCTION

When the crossroads of pregnancy and trauma meet, there are unique challenges. The vulnerability of the pregnant trauma patient and potential injuries to the unborn child serve as reminders of the dual roles of providing care to both mother and fetus. In addition, the pregnant patient is often at risk for a higher incidence of accidental trauma. The increase in fainting spells, hyperventilation, and excess fatigue that are commonly associated with early pregnancy, as well as the physiological changes that affect balance and coordination, add to risks.

Trauma is a leading cause of morbidity and mortality in pregnancy. Approximately 6 to 7 percent of all pregnant women experience some degree of trauma. Significant trauma occurs in approximately 1 in 12 patients who are injured. Injuries requiring ICU admission occur in 3 to 4 pregnancies per 100 deliveries. Motor-vehicle collisions account for 65 to 70 percent of trauma in pregnant patients. Falls, abuse and domestic violence, penetrating injuries, and burns follow.

Because minor injuries rarely present problems for EMS providers, the following discussion focuses on the more severe traumatic injuries to the pregnant patient.

PREGNANCY

Fetal Development

The fetus is formed during the first 3 months of pregnancy. After the third month of gestation, the fully formed fetus and uterus grow rapidly, reaching the umbilicus by the fifth month and the epigastrium by the seventh month (Figure 19-1 and Table 19-1). The fetus is considered viable at 24 weeks.

Physiological Changes During Pregnancy

During pregnancy, dramatic physiological changes occur. The changes that are unique to the pregnant state affect and sometimes alter the physiological response by both the mother and fetus. Changes include blood volume (increases), cardiac output (increases), and blood pressure (decreases) (Figure 19-2). The respiratory system also has significant changes due to an enlarging uterus that will elevate the diaphragm and decrease the overall volume of the thoracic cavity. This leads to a relative alkalosis and predisposes the patient to hyperventilation. There is, in addition, an increase in both red blood cells and plasma. With the increase of plasma greater than red blood cells, the patient will appear to be anemic (physiological anemia of pregnancy). However, many pregnant patients have poor nutritional intake during pregnancy and develop an absolute anemia. Gastric motility is also decreased; thus, always assume the stomach of a pregnant patient is full. Always guard against vomiting and aspiration. Table 19-2 illustrates changes during pregnancy.

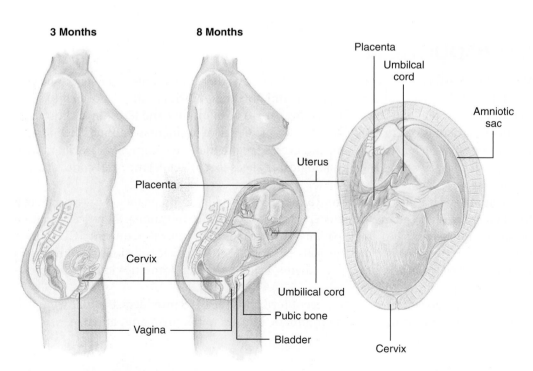

FIGURE 19-1 Anatomy of pregnancy: uterus at 3 months and at 8 months gestation.

TABLE 19-1 Assessment of a Pregnancy

	First Trimester (1–12 weeks)	Second Trimester (13–24 weeks)	Third Trimester (25–40 weeks)
Viability	Fetus not viable	Potential viability	Fetus viable
Vaginal bleeding	Potential for miscarriage	Potential miscarriage	Potential preterm birth
Fetal heart tones	Not obtainable	120–170 beats per minute	120–160 beats per minute
Height of fundus above symphysis pubis	Difficult to measure	Halfway to umbilicus equals 16 weeks; to the umbilicus equals 20 weeks	1 cm equals 1 week until 37 weeks, then uterus height decreases as the baby settles into the pelvis

Responses to Hypovolemia

Acute blood loss results in a decrease in circulating blood volume. The cardiac output decreases as the venous return falls. This hypovolemia causes the arterial blood pressure to fall, resulting in an inhibition of vagal tone and the release of catecholamines. The effect of this response is to produce vasoconstriction and tachycardia. This vasoconstriction profoundly affects the uterus. Uterine vasoconstriction leads to reduction in uterine blood flow by 20 to 30 percent. The pregnant patient may lose up to 1,500 cc of blood before any detectable change is noted in the blood pressure of the mother. The fetus reacts to this hypoperfusion by a drop in the arterial blood pressure and a decrease in heart rate. The fetus now begins to suffer from reduced oxygen concentration in the maternal circulation. Therefore, it is important to give 100 percent oxygen to the mother in order to provide sufficient oxygen to the fetus, who suffers from both oxygen starvation and inadequate blood supply. A shock state in the mother is associated with an 80 percent fetal mortality rate.

TABLE 19-2 Physiological Changes During Pregnancy

Parameter Monitored	Normal Female	Change
Blood volume	4000 mL	Increased 40%–50%
Heart rate	70	Increased 10%–15%
Blood pressure	110/70	Decreased 5–15 mmHg
Cardiac output	4–5 liters per minute	Increased 20%–30%
Hematocrit/hemoglobin	13/40	Decreased
PCO$_2$	38	Decreased
Gastric motility	Normal	Decreased

PEARLS
Hypovolemia

- Do not mistake normal vital signs in pregnant patients as signs of shock. The pregnant patient has a normal resting pulse that is 10 to 15 beats faster than usual and the blood pressure is 10 to 15 mmHg lower than usual. However, it is also important to realize that a blood loss of 30 to 35 percent can occur in these patients before there is a significant change in blood pressure. Therefore, be especially alert to all signs of shock, and monitor the vital signs with frequent ITLS Ongoing Exams.

- Cardiac arrest in the pregnant patient is treated the same as for other victims. Defibrillation settings and drug dosages are the same. For hypovolemic arrest, the volume of required fluid increases and 4 liters of normal saline should be given as fast as possible during transport.

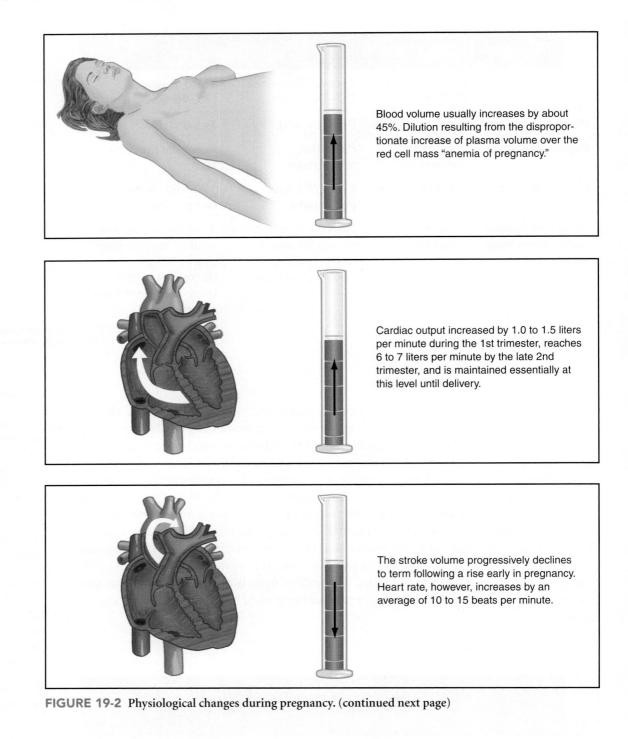

Blood volume usually increases by about 45%. Dilution resulting from the disproportionate increase of plasma volume over the red cell mass "anemia of pregnancy."

Cardiac output increased by 1.0 to 1.5 liters per minute during the 1st trimester, reaches 6 to 7 liters per minute by the late 2nd trimester, and is maintained essentially at this level until delivery.

The stroke volume progressively declines to term following a rise early in pregnancy. Heart rate, however, increases by an average of 10 to 15 beats per minute.

FIGURE 19-2 Physiological changes during pregnancy. (continued next page)

ASSESSMENT AND MANAGEMENT

Special Considerations

Major goals in caring for the pregnant trauma patient are evaluation and stabilization. The ITLS Primary Survey is the same for the pregnant patient as for other patients (see Chapter 2). All prehospital interventions are directed toward optimizing both fetal and maternal outcome. If the patient is pregnant, there are two patients being treated. Optimal care for the fetus is appropriate treatment of the mother. Oxygen administration (100 percent by nonrebreather mask or by endotracheal intubation) should be rapid. Promptly obtain venous access and begin administration of IV fluid. Monitoring of this patient

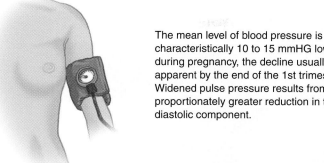

The mean level of blood pressure is characteristically 10 to 15 mmHG lower during pregnancy, the decline usually apparent by the end of the 1st trimester. Widened pulse pressure results from a proportionately greater reduction in the diastolic component.

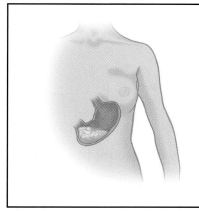

Peristalsis is slowed; thus, the stomach may still contain food hours after a meal. Be alert to the danger of vomiting and aspiration.

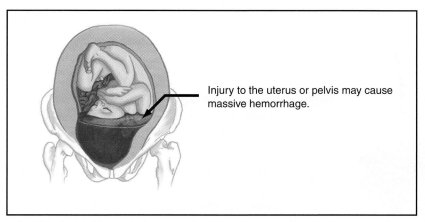

Injury to the uterus or pelvis may cause massive hemorrhage.

FIGURE 19-2 Continued.

should be immediate and constant because the anatomic and physiological changes of pregnancy make the trauma assessment more difficult.

Acute hypotension in the pregnant patient due to decreased venous return requires special mention. This "supine hypotension syndrome" usually occurs when the patient is in a supine position with a 20-week (uterus up to umbilicus) or larger uterus (Figure 19-3). This can lead to maternal hypotension, syncope, and fetal bradycardia.

Therefore, the transport of all pregnant trauma patients, if no contraindication exists, should be by one of the following methods to alleviate vena cava compression.

- Tilt or rotate the backboard 20 to 30 degrees to the patient's left.

- Elevate the right hip 4 to 6 inches with a towel and manually displace the uterus to the left.

PEARLS
Treatment

- You are treating two patients. However, the mortality of the fetus is related to the treatment provided to the mother. The goal of prehospital intervention is to maximize the chances of maternal survival, which will provide the fetus with the best chance for survival.

- If the mother dies, continue CPR and notify the hospital to be prepared for immediate cesarean section. Have them bring a sonogram machine to the emergency department for immediate evaluation of the fetus.

- Hypoxemia of the fetus may go unnoticed in the injured pregnant patient. Treatment should include high-flow oxygen.

PEARLS
Transport

Transport must include appropriate spinal motion restriction, extremity splints, and prevention of vena cava compression.

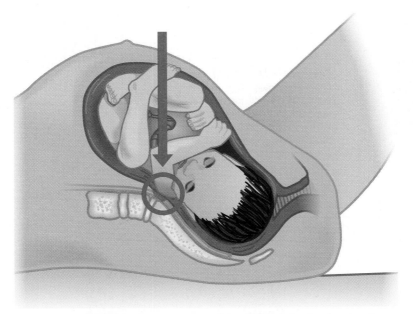

FIGURE 19-3 Venous return to the maternal heart may be decreased up to 30 percent because of vena cava compression by the fetus. Transport the patient on her left side or tilt the backboard to the left.

You must be very careful when strapping a third-trimester pregnant patient onto a long backboard and then tilting the backboard 15 to 30 degrees to the left. Many patients (and backboards) will roll right over onto the ambulance floor if the backboard is not secured to the stretcher. The vacuum backboard (Figure 19-4) is more comfortable and makes it easier to maintain SMR of the pregnant patient.

Table 19-3 illustrates evaluation of uterine size and its effect on management of the pregnant patient.

Types of Trauma

Motor-Vehicle Collisions: Though relatively minor abdominal trauma can cause fetal death, the most common cause of fetal death in trauma is maternal death. Motor-vehicle collisions account for 65 to 75 percent of pregnancy-related trauma. Fetal distress, fetal death, placental abruption, uterine rupture (Figure 19-5), and preterm labor are often seen in pregnant patients who have been in MVCs. A review of the literature indicates that less than 1 percent of pregnant patients will sustain injury when there is minor damage to the vehicle.

Head injury is the most common cause of death in pregnant patients involved in MVCs. This is closely followed by uncontrolled hemorrhage. Pregnant victims of MVCs have associated injuries, such as pelvic fractures, that often result in concealed hemorrhage within the retroperitoneal space. The retroperitoneal area, because of its low-pressure venous system, can accommodate the loss of 4 or more liters of blood into that area with few clinical signs. Seat-belt use with both a shoulder restraint and lap belt can significantly decrease patient mortality and has not shown any increase in uterine injuries.

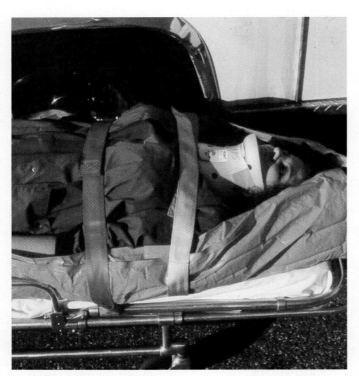

FIGURE 19-4 The pregnant patient is better stabilized and more comfortable in a vacuum backboard than a hard backboard.

TABLE 19-3 *ITLS Primary Survey Brief Evaluation of Uterine Size*

Uterine Size <20 Weeks	Uterine Size >20 Weeks
Uterus Not to Umbilicus	Uterus to Umbilicus or Higher
↓	↓
Pregnancy Management Unchanged	Lateral Displacement of Uterus
↓	↓
Maternal Stabilization	Brief Confirmation of Fetal Heart Activity (if possible)
	↓
	Maternal Stabilization
	Secondary Fetal Stabilization

Penetrating Injuries: Gunshot wounds and stabbings are the most common injuries encountered. If the path of entry is below the fundus, the uterus will often offer protection to the mother, absorbing the force of the bullet or knife. Upper abdominal wounds will often injure the bowel due to its compression in a smaller than normal space by the uterus.

Studies have shown that gunshot wounds to the pregnant abdomen carry a high mortality rate for the fetus (40–70 percent). They are lower for the mother (4–10 percent) because the large uterus usually protects vital organs. Stab wounds follow much the same pattern of outcome, with fetal mortality rates of about 40 percent. Definitive care will depend on several factors, involving degree of shock, associated organ injury, and time of gestation.

Domestic Violence: A large percentage of pregnant women experience domestic violence. The frequency appears to worsen as pregnancy progresses. Through the second and third trimesters, it is estimated that 1 in 10 pregnant women experiences abuse during pregnancy. Physical abuse is more likely to be manifest with proximal and midline injuries than the distal injuries of accidental trauma. The face and neck are most common. Domestic abuse has also been associated with low birth weight. The pregnant patient who is under great stress produces hormones (high circulating adrenaline levels, and so on) that are not good for her pregnancy. The "old wives' tale" that pregnant patients should be shielded from frightening or disturbing situations is probably true. Spouses and boyfriends are the perpetrators of the violence in 70 to 85 percent of cases.

Falls: The incidence of falls increases with the progression of pregnancy. This is in part due to an alteration in the patient's center of gravity. The incidence of significant injury is proportionate to the force of impact and the specific body part that sustains the impact. Pelvic injuries may result in placental separation and fetal fractures. Emergency department evaluation and monitoring is recommended for even minor abdominal trauma during pregnancy.

PEARLS
Abdominal Trauma
Trauma to the abdominal compartment can cause occult bleeding in either the intrauterine or retroperitoneal area. Keep in mind that gradual stretching of the abdominal wall during pregnancy, along with hormonal changes within the body, make the peritoneal surface less sensitive to irritable stimuli. Therefore, bleeding can occur intraperitoneally, and the signs of rebound, guarding, and rigidity may not be present.

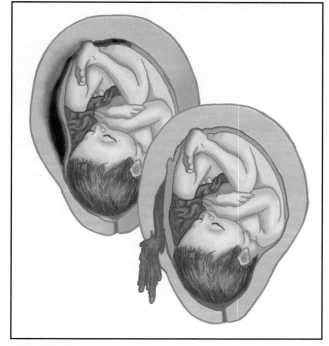

FIGURE 19-5 Blunt trauma to the uterus may cause separation of the placenta or rupture of the uterus. Massive bleeding may occur, but there may not be visible vaginal bleeding early.

Burns: Of the 2.2 million patients that suffer burn injuries in the United States annually, less than 4 percent are pregnant. The overall mortality and morbidity resulting from thermal injuries to the pregnant patient is not markedly different from the nonpregnant patient. However, it is important to remember that the fluid requirement for the pregnant patient is greater than that of the nonpregnant female. Fetal mortality increases when the maternal surface burn exceeds 20 percent.

TRAUMA PREVENTION IN PREGNANCY

Upon reviewing major causes of trauma in pregnancy, it is clear that specific recommendations such as proper seat-belt use in motor vehicles, reporting and counseling for domestic violence, as well as education of the multiple physiological, anatomical, and emotional changes associated with pregnancy will all serve to reduce trauma in pregnancy. Some patients get very little if any prenatal care, and even less prenatal education. If the situation is not critical, you should not hesitate to educate your pregnant patients when you are called to see them.

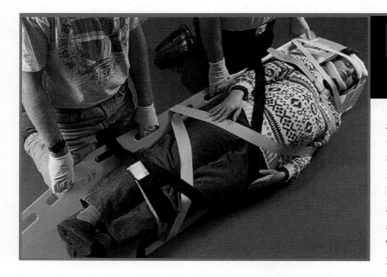

Case Study
continued

Joyce, Dan, and Buddy are dispatched to a single-auto crash. (Buddy is the team leader on this call.) Upon arrival they find that the scene is safe. A local rescue squad has arrived and extricated the driver onto a long backboard. She is the only person involved. Her auto has run off the road and into a power pole. There are no downed wires. Buddy notes that the windshield is starred and the steering wheel is bent. Since she is already packaged, they move the patient into the ambulance and begin the exam. Dan is told to transport to the hospital as soon as Buddy finishes the ITLS Primary Survey. The patient states she was talking on her cell phone and took her eyes off the road. She was not restrained and the car was not equipped with airbags. She says that she is 25 years old and is 6 months pregnant. She denies any loss of consciousness. She complains of head, back, and lower abdominal pain.

Buddy asks Joyce to tilt the backboard about 20 degrees to the left and strap it down well so it does not flip over onto the floor of the ambulance. The patient has an open airway and seems to be breathing normally. She has bruising and a laceration of the forehead where she struck the windshield. The cervical collar is opened to examine the neck. There is tenderness and spasm but no deformity noted. Neck veins are flat and the trachea is in the midline. The cervical collar is replaced. The chest has no obvious deformities but is tender over the sternum. Breath sounds are present and equal, heart sounds are easily heard, and she has a strong rapid peripheral pulse. The uterus is felt halfway between the umbilicus and the xyphoid, and it is hard and very tender. Buddy cannot hear fetal heart tones with his stethoscope and does not have a Doppler. The pelvis is stable and nontender. She has good PMS of the extremities. Joyce reports that the vital signs are BP 100/60, pulse 120, respiration 24, and the pulse oximeter reading is 95 percent on ambient air.

Joyce applies a nonrebreather oxygen mask while Buddy starts two large IVs. The patient says she feels as if she has wet herself but when Joyce checks there is a large bloodstain on her pants. Joyce notifies medical direction and asks her to have the emergency department send for a sonogram machine to assess the fetus on arrival. She also asks for the trauma team and the obstetrician on-call to be present on arrival. She then applies the cardiac monitor (sinus tachycardia) while Buddy does the ITLS Secondary Survey

The patient denies any medical problems or allergies and is taking only prenatal vitamins. She has not eaten today because she was a little nauseated. The Detail Exam reveals that the neurological status is normal but the abdomen is tender with obvious constant spasm of the uterus. The BP has dropped to 90/50 and the pulse is up to 130. Buddy gives a liter of normal saline as a bolus but the BP and pulse do not improve. He repeats the bolus, with the BP rising to 100/60 and the pulse dropping to 120.

When they arrive at the emergency department a sonogram reveals that the fetus is still alive but the abdomen is full of fluid. The patient is taken to surgery where a ruptured uterus is found. About 2,000 cc of blood is suctioned from the abdomen. The patient has to have a hysterectomy to stop the bleeding. The baby requires a month in the neonatal ICU, but both mother and child survive.

Case Study

Wrap-up

Because of the rapid treatment and transport, this patient survived what would have been a fatal injury. She was transported with the backboard tilted to the left to prevent compression of the inferior vena cava by the gravid uterus. Her shock was aggressively treated by oxygen and fluid resuscitation in the ambulance and by rapid evaluation and surgery at the hospital. If she had worn her seat belt, she would probably have had only minor injuries.

SUMMARY

Management of the pregnant trauma patient requires knowledge of the physiological changes that occur during pregnancy. Pregnant patients require rapid evaluation and also rapid interventions for stabilization, including aggressive oxygen administration and fluid resuscitation. They require special techniques in packaging and transport to prevent the vena cava compression syndrome. Because of the difficulty in early diagnosis, you should have a low threshold for load-and-go if there is any danger of the development of hemorrhagic shock. Pregnant patients with serious injuries should be directly transported to a facility (trauma center) capable of managing these complex patients. Optional fetal care is dependent on care of the mother.

BIBLIOGRAPHY

1. Chang, J., C. Berg, L. Saltzman, J. Herndon. 2005. Homicide: A leading cause of injury deaths among pregnant and postpartum women in the United States. *American Journal of Public Health* 95 (3): 471–77.

2. Coker, A., M. Sanderson, B. Dong. 2004. Partner violence during pregnancy and risk of adverse pregnancy outcomes. Paediatric and Perinatal Epidemiology 18 (4): 260–69.

3. El Kady, D., W. Gilbert, J. Anderson, et al. 2004. Trauma during pregnancy: An analysis of maternal and fetal outcomes in a large population. *American Journal of Obstetrics and Gynecology* 190 (6): 1661–68.

4. Esposito, T. J. 1994. Trauma during pregnancy. *Emergency Medicine Clinics of North America* 12: 167–99.

5. Fildes J., L. Reed, N. Jones, et al. 1992. Trauma: The leading cause of maternal death. *The Journal of Trauma* 32: 643.

6. Hill, D. A., J. J. Lense. 1996. Abdominal trauma in the pregnant patient. *American Family Physician* 53: 1269–74.

7. Maghsoudi, H., R. Samnia, et al. 2006. Burns in pregnancy. *Burns* 32 (2): 246–50.

8. Pons, P. T. 1994. Prehospital considerations in the pregnant patient. *Emergency Medical Clinics of North America* 12: 1–7.

9. Vaizey, C. J., M. J. Jacobson, F. W. Cross. 1994. Trauma in pregnancy. *British Journal of Surgery* 81: 1406–15.

10. Weiss, H., T. Songer, A. Fabio. 2001. Fetal deaths related to maternal injury. *JAMA* 286 (15): 1863–68.

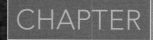
Patients Under the Influence of Alcohol or Drugs

Jonathan G. Newman, MD, MMM, FACEP, EMT-P

OBJECTIVES

Upon completion of this chapter, you should be able to:

1. List signs and symptoms of patients under the influence of alcohol and/or drugs.

2. Describe the five strategies you would use to best ensure cooperation during assessment and management of a patient under the influence of alcohol and/or drugs.

3. Describe situations in which you would restrain patients and tell how to handle an uncooperative patient.

4. List the special considerations for assessment and management of patients in whom substance abuse is suspected.

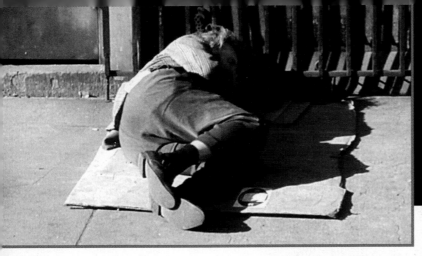

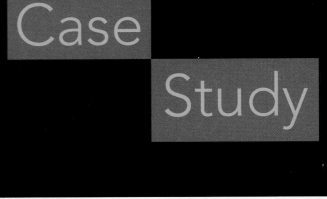

Joyce, Buddy, and Dan have been dispatched to a run-down section of town after the police called to report a man being stabbed. They have been to this area many times before to pick up patients after altercations over alcohol or drugs. They are told that the patient is covered in blood but is not cooperative. *What injuries would you expect in this situation? What strategies would you use to get the patient to cooperate with treatment?* Keep these questions in mind as you read the chapter. Then, at the end of the chapter, find out how the rescuers completed this call.

INTRODUCTION

The relationship between alcohol and trauma is well documented. For instance, it is reported that car crashes involving alcohol result in injuries to about 500,000 people a year. Studies of individuals who are substance abusers note that these persons are at greater risk to suffer an injury than the general population and that these individuals are more likely to have repeated injuries. Substance abuse includes individuals who have abused alcohol, drugs, or both. It has been associated with a number of traumatic events, often resulting from accidents, car crashes, suicides, homicides, and other violent crimes. Further, a study reported in the *Journal of the American College of Surgeons* found a high rate of alcohol and illicit drug use in patients who die from trauma. Therefore, it would not be surprising to find that a number of seriously injured trauma patients are under the influence of alcohol or some other substance. This group of trauma patients often presents with unique challenges that can require some special patient management techniques along with good ITLS care.

A high index of suspicion combined with the results of the physical exam, the history obtained from the patient or bystanders, and evidence at the scene can clue you into whether your patient is under the influence of alcohol or drugs. Table 20-1 includes commonly abused drugs, along with signs and symptoms of their use.

ASSESSMENT AND MANAGEMENT

While your ITLS Primary and Secondary Surveys should follow the ITLS guidelines that have been described in this book (see Chapter 2), there are some particular aspects to be aware of when conducting the exam when you suspect the patient has abused substances. Pay particular attention to mental status, pupils, speech, and respiration, and note any needle marks you may discover. An altered mental status can be seen in every form of substance abuse. However, remember that an altered level of consciousness is always due to a head injury, shock, or hypoglycemia until proven otherwise. Pupils are often constricted

TABLE 20-1 *Commonly Abused Drugs with Their Associated Signs and Symptoms*

Drug Category	Common Names	Signs and Symptoms of Use or Abuse
Alcohol	Beer, whiskey, wine	Altered mental function, confusion, polyuria, slurred speech, coma, hypertension, hyperthermia, tachycardia
Amphetamines/ Methamphetamine	Bennies, ice, speed, uppers, dexies, Ecstasy, MDMA	Excitement, hyperactivity, dilated pupils, hypertension, tachycardia, tremors, seizures, fever, paranoia, psychosis
Cocaine	Coke, crack, blow, rock	Same as amphetamines plus chest pain; lethal dysrhythmias
Hallucinogens	Acid, LSD, PCP	Hallucinations, dizziness, dilated pupils, nausea, rambling speech, psychosis, anxiety, panic
Marijuana	Grass, hash, pot, tea, weed	Euphoria, sleepiness, dilated pupils, dry mouth, increased appetite
Narcotics/Opiates	Heroin, horse, big H, Darvon, codeine, stuff, morphine, smack	Altered mental status, constricted pupils, bradycardia, hypotension, respiratory depression, hypothermia
Sedatives	Thorazine; GHB; barbiturates; benzodiazepines (e.g., Librium, Valium, Xanax, Ativan, Rohypnol)	Altered mental status, dilated pupils, bradycardia, hypotension, respiratory depression, hypothermia

in patients who have abused opiates. Dilated pupils are common in patients exposed to amphetamines, cocaine, hallucinogens, and marijuana. Patients who use barbiturates will have pupils that are constricted early on. However, if high doses have been consumed, the pupils can eventually become fixed and dilated. Speech can be slurred when patients use alcohol or sedatives, and patients who are under the influence of hallucinogens may seem to ramble when they talk. Respiration can be significantly depressed with opiates and sedatives.

The history supplied by the patient or bystanders can also help to establish whether substance abuse is involved. Try to find out what was used, when it was taken, and how much was taken. However, be aware that patients often deny that they have used or abused any substance. If possible, inspect the patient's surroundings for clues that drugs or alcohol may have been used. Note any alcoholic beverage bottles, pill containers, injection equipment, smoking paraphernalia, or unusual odors.

Trauma patients under the influence of alcohol or drugs can challenge the provider not only by their traumatic injuries but by their attitudes. The way in which you interact with patients who have abused substances can determine if the patient will be cooperative or uncooperative. How you speak to these patients can be as important as what you are doing for them. Your interaction style, if offensive, can make patients uncooperative and force you both to lose precious minutes of the Golden Hour. If your interactive style is positive

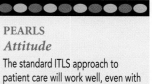

PEARLS
Attitude

The standard ITLS approach to patient care will work well, even with patients under the influence. Your attitude can help determine if your patient approach will be accepted or not. Be positive and nonjudgmental.

and nonjudgmental, the patient is more likely to be cooperative and to allow all the appropriate medical interventions, thus decreasing on-scene time. As noted before, all the substances that are abused can cause an altered mental state. When interacting with patients you must be prepared to deal with euphoria, psychosis, paranoia, or confusion and disorientation. Some strategies to help you gain your patient's cooperation follow:

- Identify yourself to patients and orient them to their surroundings. Tell them your name and your title, for example, "EMT, Paramedic." Ask them their name and how they would like to be addressed. Avoid using generic names like "Bub" or "Honey." With this patient population it may be necessary to orient them to place, date, and what is going on. These patients may need to be reoriented frequently.

- Treat the patient in a respectful manner and avoid being judgmental. Often a lack of respect can be heard in the tone of your voice or how you say things, not just in what you say. Never forget that you are there to save lives; this includes all patients. You are not a police officer (do not gather evidence) and you are not there to pass judgment on the patient's worth to society. Also take care not to destroy evidence.

- Acknowledge the patient's concerns and feelings. The patient who is scared or confused may be more comfortable with what is taking place if you recognize and address these feelings. Be gentle but firm. Explain all treatment interventions before they are performed. Be honest. Backboards and extrication collars are uncomfortable, and IV lines hurt.

- Let your patients know what will be required of them. For instance, they may be confused and not realize that they need to hold still while you are trying to stabilize them on a backboard.

- Ask closed-ended questions when getting your history from the patient. These are questions that can be answered with a yes or no. These patients may only be able to concentrate for short periods of time, and they may ramble when asked open-ended questions that require a full answer. Consider getting as much of the history as you can from relatives, friends, or bystanders. This may help improve the reliability of what you discover. Get as much relevant history as you can, but do not delay transport.

THE UNCOOPERATIVE PATIENT

A small percentage of your patients may be uncooperative. You must be firm with these patients. Set limits to their behavior, and let them know when their behavior is inappropriate. Consider physical restraint only if you are not able to secure enough cooperation to provide adequate care for your patient. Often a show of force may be enough to convince an uncooperative patient to allow medical care to be provided.

First, check with your local jurisdiction to determine what protocol you must use when restraining patients against their will. Most municipalities allow police officers to place people in custody if they are a threat to themselves or others. Severely injured trauma patients who refuse or will not cooperate with care can be considered a threat to themselves. Once the decision has been made to restrain the patient, it must be carried out with care. Securely strapping a patient to a backboard with use of a cervical collar and head motion-restriction device will serve to restrain most patients. Caution must be taken not to worsen any current injuries or to inflict any new ones. There is often no good solution to this predicament. Restrained patients may struggle so hard that spinal motion restriction is rendered ineffective. The Reeves sleeve is one of the few pieces of equipment that is very effective in providing both restraint and motion restriction (Figure 20-1).

Crews should plan and practice procedures for restraining patients. The trauma scene is not the place to learn new skills. Reassess restrained patients often. You don't want to be the one providing care for a drug-impaired patient who dies by asphyxiation during prehospital restraint.

The standard ITLS approach to patient care will work well, even with patients under the influence of alcohol or drugs. Ensure that the scene is safe, determine the number of injured, and discover the mechanism of injury. Use standard precautions. This patient population includes people who are at high risk for infection with hepatitis B, hepatitis C, and HIV. Follow the ITLS Primary and Secondary Surveys as recorded in Chapter 2. Remember to note any mental status changes that might be associated with substance abuse. When performing the ITLS Secondary Survey, be sure to include the specific areas that can provide clues to substance abuse. As with all trauma patients, treatment includes the consideration of oxygen, an IV line, cardiac monitoring, and O_2 saturation or expired CO_2 monitoring.

Table 20-2 lists drug categories and associated specific treatments or areas to pay close attention to when substance abuse is suspected.

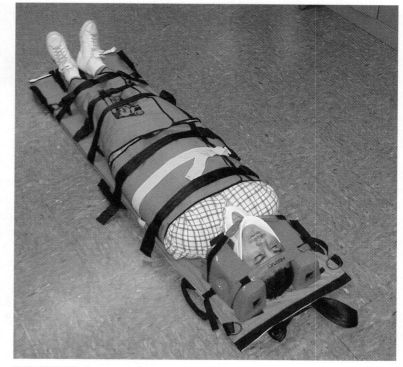

FIGURE 20-1 Reeves sleeve.

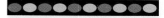

PEARLS
Management
- Check finger-stick glucose and provide EKG monitoring on every patient with altered mental status.
- In this population, hypothermia, hypotension, and respiratory depression are common and must be treated aggressively.

TABLE 20-2 *Drug Categories and Specific Treatments to Consider or Areas to Assess Closely*	
Drug Category	**Specific Treatments and Areas to Assess**
Alcohol	Administer IV thiamine and glucose; use $D_{50}W$ if indicated; watch for hypothermia.
Amphetamines/ Methamphetamine	Monitor for seizures and dysrhythmias; treat seizures with diazepam or lorazepam
Cocaine	Monitor for seizures and dysrhythmias; treat rhythm disorders
Hallucinogens	Provide reassurance.
Marijuana	Provide reassurance.
Nacotics/Opiates	Try naloxone*, watch for hypothermia, hypotension, and respiratory depression (CO_2 monitor).
Sedatives	Try naloxone* and consider flumazenil**, watch for hypothermia, hypotension, and respiratory depression (CO_2 monitor).

*Naloxone should be titrated to the patient's respirations. Repeated doses may be indicated as the narcotic may last longer than the effects of the naloxone.
**Flumazenil use is controversial; it can precipitate seizures in patients dependent on benzodiazepines. Further, flumazenil use may cause seizures in those who have been using benzodiazepines to prevent seizures and in those patients who have overdosed on tricyclic antidepressants. Flumazenil should only be given on direct order of medical direction.

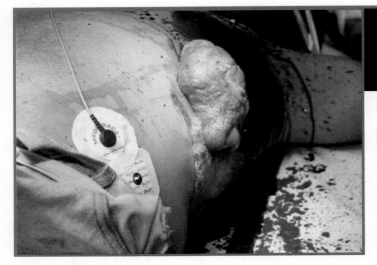

(Photo courtesy of
Roy Alson, MD)

Joyce, Buddy, and Dan have been dispatched to the scene of a stabbing. They have been to this area many times before to pick up patients after altercations over alcohol or drugs. They are told that the patient is covered in blood but is not cooperative. As they respond, they decide to have Joyce act as team leader since she is good at interacting with uncooperative patients. They carefully don personal protective equipment since the police described a lot of blood, and hepatitis and HIV were known to be present among the regulars they treat in this area.

When they arrive they see that the police have the scene under control and are putting a cursing, struggling, handcuffed man into a patrol car. There is a very unkempt man lying on a pallet on the sidewalk. He is actively bleeding from lacerations of the chest and abdomen. There is an impressive amount of blood on the front of his shirt and trousers. There are several empty wine bottles strewn about. Joyce introduces herself and asks him, "What happened?"

"We were drinking together and he hogged all of his wine down and then reached for my bottle. I told him to get his own wine and the SOB cut me!" Joyce asks him his name (Cuthbert Mulford), and assures him that he is not in any trouble and the police are only there to arrest the SOB who cut him. She explains that the paramedics are there to help him and take care of his wounds. She asks for permission to examine him and he grudgingly agrees. Since the patient denies any injury other than being cut, they do not apply spinal motion-restriction precautions.

He obviously has an open airway and seems to be in no respiratory difficulty (the odor of stale wine on his breath makes Joyce dyspneic), so she proceeds with the Rapid Trauma Survey. There are no apparent injuries of the head or face. His neck is nontender, the neck veins flat, and the trachea in the midline. There is equal expansion of the chest, with breath sounds present and equal. There are two 8–10 cm lacerations across his left anterior chest but they do not appear to go into the chest cavity. Heart sounds are heard and the rate is rapid, with a weak peripheral pulse. There is a deep laceration across the left upper quadrant of the abdomen with protruding intestines. As Joyce lifts his shirt, Cuthbert sees it and says, "He gutted me, didn't he?"

Joyce has Buddy apply a saline-moistened dressing and then an occlusive dressing. She continues her assessment. She finds no other injuries and so she explains to Cuthbert that they will have to take him to the hospital to fix his intestines. He seems markedly more sober after looking at his intestines and readily agrees. They carefully move him to the stretcher and transport immediately. During transport Joyce bandages his lacerations and starts a precautionary IV line while Buddy takes vital signs: BP 110/70, pulse 110, respiration 24, and oxygen saturation 96 percent. Cuthbert states his only medical history is seizures (alcohol withdrawal?) for which he takes no prescription medications, has no allergies, and has not eaten in the last 24 hours. "I get my nourishment from cigarettes and a bottle of Sly Fox." The ITLS Secondary Survey reveals no new findings. Cuthbert's recovery is complicated by delirium tremens and a wound infection, but he lives to ride with Joyce on many more occasions.

Because people who abuse alcohol and drugs frequently are the victims of trauma (and often the cause of trauma to people who do not abuse alcohol and drugs), you will treat them on almost a daily basis. A patient, caring attitude will save you much grief, but we all know that some people who are intoxicated are sociopathic and no matter what you do they will not cooperate. Many confrontations will not go as well as the case study above. The Reeves sleeve is invaluable for the patient that must be restrained for his own safety. It does not require placing the patient prone and it allows you to manage the airway and give medication and IV fluids. It can be carried rolled up in storage until you need it; slide a backboard into it, and you have a total body restraint system.

Whether or not the patient is sober enough to refuse treatment may be the hardest decision to make. Sometimes you, the police, and medical direction have to make the best decision based on the situation. As mentioned above, sometimes there is no good answer.

SUMMARY

Knowing the signs and symptoms of alcohol and drug abuse will allow you to recognize the patient who may be impaired from their use. Assessing the patient for signs and symptoms outlined in this section can help you confirm your suspicions. Determining that your patient has abused some substance will allow you to pay attention to specific areas for critical changes as well as provide life-saving interventions that may be indicated for individual substances. The five interaction strategies for improving patient cooperation are very important when dealing with the patient under the influence of alcohol or drugs, but these strategies should also be used with all patients. Remember that the patient's safety is a primary concern. If you must restrain a patient for his or her safety, do so in a preplanned manner that is most sensitive to your patient's needs.

BIBLIOGRAPHY

1. Bledsoe, B., R. Porter, R. Cherry. 2005. Paramedic care: principles and practice. 2nd ed. vol. 3. Upper Saddle River, NJ: Prentice Hall, pp. 414–57.
2. Demetriades D., G. Gkiokas, G. C. Velmahos, et al. 2004. Alcohol and illicit drugs in traumatic deaths: Prevalence and association with type and severity of injuries. *Journal of the American College of Surgeons* 199(5): 687–92.
3. Miller, T. R., D. C. Lestina, G. S. Smith. 2001. Injury risk among medically identified alcohol and drug abusers. *Alcoholism, Clinical and Experimental Research*, 25(1): 54–59.
4. Sanders, M. 2001. Mosby's paramedic textbook. 2nd ed., Saint Louis, MO: Mosby, Inc., 1011–36.

The Trauma Cardiopulmonary Arrest

John E. Campbell, MD, FACEP

OBJECTIVES

Upon completion of this chapter, you should be able to:

1. Identify patients in traumatic cardiac arrest for whom you should withhold resuscitation attempts.

2. Identify treatable causes of traumatic cardiopulmonary arrest.

3. Describe the proper evaluation and management of the patient in traumatic cardiopulmonary arrest.

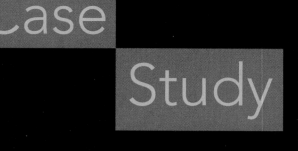

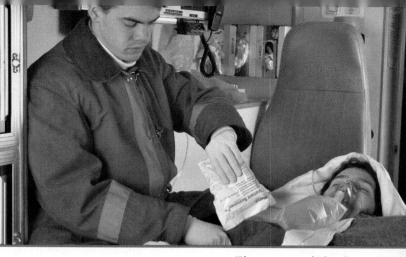

(Photo courtesy of Eduardo Romero Hicks, MD)

Joyce, Dan, and Buddy have been dispatched to an ice skating rink where a man has been injured in a fight. It's a cold, wet day. As they respond, they ponder what sort of injuries they will find. They decide to have Dan act as team leader. When they arrive they find a large group of teenagers gathered outside the rink. Police are on scene and have the crowd under control. Two boys have been in a fight and the injured one was winning until they fell down and he injured his wrist. The other got up and ran away when the police arrived.

The patient is an 18-year-old who complains of a broken wrist and some bruises on his face. He denies any other injuries. He is not very cooperative and is angry and belligerent. He admits to drinking "two beers." Dan's general impression is good, since the patient is ambulatory and talking loudly. Joyce coaxes the patient into the ambulance and he sits on the stretcher. He refuses to remove his coat ("I am too damn cold and my arm hurts!") but does let them strap him into the stretcher in a sitting position. Dan does a focused exam of the right wrist and sees a deformed distal forearm fracture with good pulse and sensation. He applies a splint to the wrist. When he is doing this, the patient begins to hyperventilate and then complains of dyspnea and tingling in his hands. He becomes very agitated. Dan is trying to attach a pulse oximeter and get him to accept a nonrebreather oxygen mask when he collapses. *What is going on here?*

Keep that question in mind as you read the chapter. Then, at the end of the chapter, find out how the rescuers completed this call.

INTRODUCTION

You will encounter trauma patients who are found pulseless or apneic on scene or who "crash" and develop those signs while under your care. While it is rare to save such a patient, it is possible in certain cases. The chance to save someone like this is why we chose this profession.

THE UNSALVAGEABLE PATIENT

Attempting to resuscitate the patient in traumatic cardiac arrest can put you and the public in danger (rapid transport and possible exposure to bloodborne pathogens). Do

TABLE 21-1 *Guidelines for Withholding or Termination of Resuscitation of Prehospital Traumatic Cardiopulmonary Arrest**

1. Resuscitation should be withheld in cases of:
   a. Blunt trauma with no breathing, pulse, or organized rhythm on EKG on EMS arrival at the scene.
   b. Penetrating trauma with no breathing, pulse, pupillary reflexes, spontaneous movement, or organized EKG activity.
   c. Any trauma with injuries obviously incompatible with life (e.g., decapitation).
   d. Any trauma with evidence of significant time lapse since pulselessness, including dependent lividity, rigor mortis, etc.
2. Cardiopulmonary arrest patients in whom the mechanism of injury does not correlate with the clinical condition, suggesting a nontraumatic cause of the arrest, should have standard resuscitation initiated.
3. Termination of resuscitation efforts should be considered (consult medical direction):
   a. With EMS-witnessed cardiopulmonary arrest and 15 minutes of unsuccessful resuscitation.
   b. When transport time to the ED is more than 15 minutes.
4. Special consideration should be given to victims of drowning, lightning strike, and hypothermia.

*Joint Position Statement of the National Association of EMS Physicians and the American College of Surgeons Committee on Trauma

not attempt resuscitation unless there is some chance of the patient's survival. One review of 195 trauma patients who presented unconscious, without palpable pulse or spontaneous respiration, found that patients with sinus rhythm and nondilated (<4 mm) reactive pupils had a good chance of survival; but of those with asystole, agonal rhythm, ventricular fibrillation, or ventricular tachycardia, there were no survivors (see Bibliography 2). The National Association of EMS Physicians and the American College of Surgeons Committee on Trauma have jointly developed guidelines for withholding or terminating resuscitation in prehospital traumatic cardiopulmonary arrest (Table 21-1).

Advanced cardiopulmonary resuscitation has always been directed toward dealing with a cardiac cause for the pulseless patient. In the trauma situation cardiopulmonary arrest is usually not due to primary cardiac disease such as coronary artery disease with acute myocardial infarction. You must direct treatment by identifying the underlying cause of the arrest, or you will almost never be successful in resuscitation. Use the ITLS Primary Survey to identify the cause of the arrest and those patients for whom you should attempt resuscitation.

PEARLS
Cardiac Arrest
Cardiac arrest following trauma is usually not due to cardiac disease.

HYPOXEMIA

Hypoxemia is the most common cause of traumatic cardiopulmonary arrest. Acute airway obstruction or ineffective breathing will be clinically manifested as hypoxemia. Carbon dioxide accumulation from inadequate breathing will play a role in your being unable to resuscitate the patient. Airway problems such as those listed in Table 21-2 lead to hypoxemia by preventing the flow of oxygen to the lungs. Drugs and/or alcohol, often

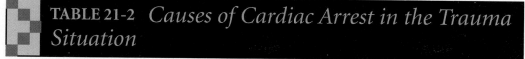

TABLE 21-2 *Causes of Cardiac Arrest in the Trauma Situation*

1. Airway Problems
   a. Foreign body
   b. Tongue prolapse
   c. Swelling
2. Breathing Problems
   a. Tension pneumothorax
   b. Sucking chest wound
   c. Flail chest
   d. High spinal-cord injury
   e. Carbon monoxide inhalation
   f. Smoke inhalation
   g. Aspiration
   h. Near-drowning
   i. Central nervous system depression from drugs/alcohol
   j. Apnea secondary to electric shock or lightning strike
3. Circulatory Problems
   a. Hemorrhagic shock (empty heart syndrome)
   b. Tension pneumothorax
   c. Pericardial tamponade
   d. Myocardial contusion
   e. Acute myocardial infarction
   f. Cardiac arrest secondary to electric shock

in conjunction with minor head trauma, can result in airway obstruction by the tongue as well as by respiratory depression.

Careful monitoring of the intoxicated patient may prevent an arrest situation. The same is true of the patient who is unconscious from a head injury. The lax muscles in the pharynx allow the tongue to fall back and obstruct the airway. Obtaining and maintaining an open airway by jaw thrust along with an oral or nasopharyngeal airway is paramount for patients without a gag reflex. You may need to use a blind insertion airway device (Combitube, LMA, and so on) but insertion of an endotracheal tube is even better, since it will also decrease the chance of aspiration if the patient vomits. Patients with cardiorespiratory arrest caused by airway obstruction will respond to Advanced Life Support if the anoxic period was not prolonged.

Patients with hypoxia secondary to a breathing problem have an adequate airway, but are unable to oxygenate their blood because they cannot get oxygen and blood together at the alveolar capillary membrane of the lungs. This could be from the following:

■ Inability to ventilate, as in a tension pneumothorax, sucking chest wound, flail chest, or high spinal-cord (C-3 or above) injury.

■ Lung tissue filled with fluid, as in the patient with aspiration of blood or vomitus or adult respiratory distress syndrome (ARDS). Near-drowning patients have hypoxemia early from lack of oxygen, but later their lungs are full of water (like pulmonary edema or ARDS).

■ Lungs filled with gas (smoke inhalation) that does not contain the appropriate amount of oxygen but instead contains harmful gases such as carbon monoxide or cyanide. In addition, the hot vapor can result in pulmonary edema, further preventing oxygenation by increasing the distance (by alveolar capillary membrane swelling) between the red blood cells and oxygen.

■ Hypoventilation caused by head injury, lightning strike, and/or drugs and alcohol.

Patients with breathing problems should have aggressive airway management and ventilation with high-flow oxygen. Many of these patients will respond quickly if they have not been anoxic for too long. A significant number (19 percent, in one study) of near-drowning patients who appear lifeless in the field will eventually have a complete recovery.

CIRCULATORY PROBLEMS

Patients with tissue hypoxia because of inadequate blood flow will have one of the causes listed in Table 21-2. Hemorrhagic shock (hypovolemic or empty heart syndrome) is the most common circulatory cause of the trauma cardiopulmonary arrest.

The patient with cardiac arrest secondary to pericardial tamponade will present as a pulseless patient who may or may not have an electrical complex on the cardiac monitor—pulseless electrical activity (PEA). The patient with pericardial tamponade may rapidly deteriorate from shock to PEA to, finally, asystole. In pericardial tamponade the cardiac output may be so low that you cannot feel a pulse. The heart is squeezed by the blood in the pericardial sac and cannot fill with blood before each beat because the pressure inside the sac (and thus in the heart chambers) is higher than the pressure in the venous system returning the blood to the heart. Thus there is a rapid, weak pulse that will continue to diminish as the tamponade worsens. The radial pulse may disappear with inspiration (pulsus paradoxus) as the condition worsens. Early in the pericardial tamponade syndrome a tiny amount of blood flows from the heart with each beat. The main clinical features in isolated tamponade are profound shock with distended neck veins and normal bilateral breath sounds. In the more typical multiple-trauma situation, the patient will have associated blood loss and the neck veins will not be distended. Patients without distended neck veins may appear to be in PEA but will not respond to Advanced Cardiac Life Support (ACLS) protocols.

Acute myocardial infarction and myocardial contusion can produce inadequate blood flow (circulation) by either one or a combination of three mechanisms. These mechanisms are dysrhythmias, acute pump failure, or pericardial tamponade. The patient with a myocardial contusion has usually been in a deceleration accident. There may be a chest wall or sternal contusion.

A full arrest from an electric shock usually presents as ventricular fibrillation. It responds readily to ACLS protocols if you arrive in time. The cardiac arrest is frequently due to the prolonged apnea that may follow electrocution or lightning strike. The victim of an electrical shock has suffered severe muscle spasm and may well have been thrown down or fallen a great distance. Thus the same systematic approach to the patient is required to identify all associated injuries and to give the patient the best chance for a good outcome. Be sure the patient is no longer in contact with the electricity source. Do not become a victim yourself!

Patients with cardiopulmonary arrest related to inadequate circulation have either of the following:

■ Inadequate return of blood to the heart because of
  • Increased pressure in the chest causing increased resistance to the venous return to the heart, as in tension pneumothorax or pericardial tamponade
  • Hemorrhagic shock with inadequate blood volume to be returned to the heart

■ Inadequate pumping of the heart because of
- Rhythm disturbances as in myocardial contusion, acute myocardial infarction, or electrical shock
- Acute heart failure with pulmonary edema, as in large myocardial contusion or acute myocardial infarction

APPROACH TO TRAUMA PATIENTS IN CARDIAC ARREST

Trauma patients in cardiac arrest are a special group. Most are young and do not have preexisting cardiac conditions or coronary disease. Ensuring a complete Scene Size-up is important as some involve criminal activity (stabbings, shootings), so carefully record (after the run) your observations of the scene. Some of these patients may be resuscitated if you arrive soon enough and you pay attention to the differences from the usual medical cardiac arrest.

The extremely poor resuscitation rate for trauma patients in cardiac arrest is probably due to the fact that many of them have been hypoxic for a prolonged period of time before the arrest occurred. Prolonged hypoxia causes such severe acidosis that the patient will not respond to attempted resuscitation.

Patients who suffer cardiorespiratory arrest from isolated head injury usually do not survive, but these patients should be aggressively resuscitated because the extent of injury cannot always be determined in the field and, therefore, you cannot predict the outcome for the individual patient. (They are also potential organ donors.) Patients who are found in asystole after massive blunt trauma are dead; they may be pronounced dead in the field.

Children are a special case. While some reports show the same dismal results for resuscitation of children in cardiac arrest in the field as for adults, one review of over 700 cases of children who received CPR in the field found that 25 percent survived to discharge. This may be in part because sometimes the pulse is difficult to find in a child, but is still present. In any case, you should be especially aggressive in attempting to resuscitate children with no palpable pulse.

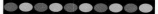

PEARLS
Pregnant Patients
Cardiac arrest in the pregnant patient is treated the same as in other patients. Defibrillation settings and drug dosages are exactly the same. The volume of fluid needed increases and 4 liters of normal saline should be given as fast as possible during transport.

GENERAL PLAN OF ACTION

After determining unresponsiveness, restrict the motion of the cervical spine and secure the patient's airway. Open the airway with the modified jaw thrust. If there are no respirations, give two full breaths. If the airway is obstructed, repeat the jaw thrust and try ventilation again. If the airway is still obstructed by a foreign body, attempt to clear the airway with your fingers or a laryngoscope and suction. You will need assistance to maintain cervical motion restriction. If this is unsuccessful, do abdominal thrusts (the patient must be on a firm surface). There is a chance of injuring the spine if there is an associated vertebral injury, but this is of less concern if the patient is dying of an airway obstruction. (Desperate situations often require desperate measures.) If still unsuccessful, you may attempt cricothyroidotomy or translaryngeal jet ventilation (if you are trained and protocols allow).

If the airway is not obstructed, give two full breaths and then check the pulse. If no pulse is palpable, you must begin cardiopulmonary resuscitation and prepare for immediate transport. Allow two of your teammates to do the cardiopulmonary resuscitation while you get the monitor and check the cardiac rhythm. If ventricular fibrillation is present, go ahead and defibrillate at 360 watts/sec (or use the manufacturer's recommended setting on biphasic defibrillator). Immediately resume CPR.

If asystole or PEA is present or if the ventricular fibrillation persists, you should evaluate the patient for the cause of the arrest. If the patient is a victim of blunt trauma, consider

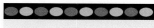

PEARLS
Proper Response
An adequate number of rescuers are required to handle this situation well: one to drive the ambulance, one to ventilate, one to do chest compressions, and one to diagnose and treat the cause of the arrest.

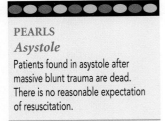

termination of resuscitation. If the patient has penetrating trauma, check the pupils. If the pupils are dilated and nonreactive you should consider termination of resuscitation. Resuscitation efforts for patients with injuries incompatible with life or those who have evidence of prolonged time since the arrest (Table 21-1) should not be initiated or should have termination of resuscitation efforts as directed by your local medical direction.

For patients with an organized rhythm on EKG, you must quickly evaluate and treat for the cause of the arrest. This should be done in the ambulance during transport, if possible. Follow the ITLS Primary Survey that you follow for every trauma patient.

PROCEDURE
✣ Initial Assessment and Critical Actions

1. Establish and control the airway (with an endotracheal tube if possible) and ventilate with 100 percent oxygen. While the other two rescuers are ventilating and performing chest compressions, you must systematically look for the correctable cause(s) of the arrest.

2. Look for breathing problems as a cause of the arrest. Answering the following questions will allow you to identify any breathing problems that may be the cause or a contributing factor.

   a. Look at the neck:
      (1) Are the neck veins flat or distended?
      (2) Is the trachea midline?
      (3) Is there evidence of soft-tissue trauma to the neck?

   b. Look at the chest:
      (1) Does the chest move symmetrically each time you ventilate?
      (2) Are there chest injuries (penetrations, bruising, flail segment)?
      (3) If there is spontaneous respiration, is there any paradoxical motion noted?

   c. Feel the chest:
      (1) Is there any instability?
      (2) Is there any crepitation?
      (3) Is there any subcutaneous emphysema?

   d. Listen to the chest:
      (1) Are breath sounds present on both sides?
      (2) Are the breath sounds equal?

If breath sounds are not equal, percuss the chest. Is the side with the absent or decreased breath sounds hyperresonant or dull? If intubated, is the endotracheal tube inserted too far?

If there are distended neck veins, decreased breath sounds on one side of the chest, with the trachea deviated away from the side of the injury, and hyperresonance to percussion of the chest on the affected side, then the patient probably has a tension pneumothorax. An improperly positioned endotracheal tube can cause unequal breath sounds and will be harmful to the patient, since only one lung can be ventilated. You should always recheck the position of the endotracheal tube before you make a diagnosis of tension pneumothorax. It is much more common to have a poorly positioned endotracheal tube than to have a tension pneumothorax. A tension pneumothorax requires needle decompression (if you are trained, and protocols allow). If required, call medical direction immediately for permission to decompress. Continue ventilation with 100 percent oxygen.

Do not discontinue chest compressions until there is a palpable pulse. Even though you have found a cause, there may be other causes for the patient's arrest. Other breathing problems (sucking chest wound, flail chest, simple pneumothorax) will be adequately treated by endotracheal intubation and ventilation with high-flow oxygen. Once you have intubated the patient, you no longer have to seal sucking chest wounds or apply external stabilization to flails. Remember that positive pressure ventilation can convert a simple pneumothorax to a tension pneumothorax.

Now that the patient has both an adequate airway and is being ventilated, you may concentrate on the circulatory system. As soon as IV access is obtained, rapidly give 2 liters of normal saline. Once again, do not delay at the scene. All treatment past establishing the airway should be done during transport.

Hemorrhagic shock is the most common circulatory cause of traumatic cardiopulmonary arrest. If there is no external bleeding, the patient must be carefully examined for evidence of internal bleeding. Reexamine the neck veins. Flat neck veins with sinus tachycardia favor the presence of hypovolemic shock (empty heart syndrome). Attempt to start two large-bore IV lines while en route.

If during the chest exam there are decreased breath sounds on one side with percussion dullness on the same side, this confirms a hemothorax of such degree that shock will be present. Obvious bleeding, distended abdomen, multiple fractures, or an unstable pelvis also confirm inadequate volume. If any of these situations exist, assume the arrest is secondary to hemorrhagic shock. Transport rapidly with rapid infusion of 2 to 4 liters of normal saline.

If the neck veins are distended but the trachea is midline and breath sounds are equal, you must suspect pericardial tamponade. Penetrating wounds of the chest or upper abdomen, or contusions of the anterior chest, are associated with pericardial and/or myocardial contusion. Attempt to start two large-bore IV lines while proceeding with all possible haste to the emergency department.

Electrical shock creates a special situation. It usually presents as ventricular fibrillation. Cardiorespiratory arrest secondary to electric shock responds readily to ACLS protocols if you arrive before the acidosis is too severe. Severe acidosis can develop rapidly, making resuscitation more difficult. Do not forget to restrict the motion of the spine. A victim of high-voltage electrical shock will often have fallen from a power line or have been thrown several feet by the violent muscle spasm associated with the shock. Be sure the patient is no longer in contact with the electrical source. Do not become a victim!

> **PEARLS**
> *Transport*
> Rapid transport to a surgical facility is necessary. Perform procedures in the ambulance during transport. Do not waste valuable time.

Case Study

continued

Joyce, Dan, and Buddy have been transporting an 18-year-old boy who seemed to be drunk and have a focused injury to the right wrist until he began hyperventilating and then collapsed during transport to the hospital. As soon as the patient becomes unresponsive, Dan begins an Initial Assessment, while Joyce cuts off his clothes. His airway is open but he is not breathing. There is no peripheral or carotid pulse and the neck veins are very distended. The trachea appears to be in the midline. Joyce (Buddy is driving) immediately begins bag-valve mask ventilation. Dan hears breath sounds only on the right side, and he now sees a stab wound in the left posterior chest. It is not a

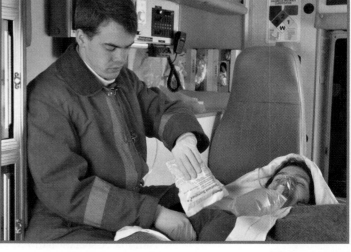

(Photo courtesy of Eduardo Romero Hicks, MD)

sucking wound and there is almost no bleeding. The chest is hyperresonant to percussion on the left side. Dan tells Buddy to call medical direction and tell her that they have a young male who has been stabbed in the chest and has a trauma arrest from a tension pneumothorax. While Buddy is talking to medical direction, Dan is getting a large-bore over-the-needle catheter and an Asherman chest seal. With medical direction's permission he inserts the catheter over the third rib in the midclavicular line anteriorly and there is an immediate rush of air. He applies the Asherman chest seal over the needle to act as a one-way valve.

The patient now develops a rapid pulse and his blood pressure is 110/70. Dan now has time to apply monitor leads, and the patient is seen to have a sinus tachycardia. The pulse oximeter reading is 98 percent. Dan quickly inserts a large-bore IV in the left arm. The patient begins to breathe on his own and make some purposeful movement by the time they get to the hospital.

Case Study Wrap-up

This case is loosely based on a real case in which a young man died of a tension pneumothorax after having been allowed to go to jail from the scene of a fight. It was winter and the paramedics did not remove his coat, since he did not complain of a chest injury. The young man did not realize he had been stabbed at the time. When he collapsed in jail it was too late to save him. This is a good example of how an intoxicated patient can throw you off of your usual exam. Luckily for Dan, he observed the collapse and rapidly repeated the Initial Assessment. He quickly found the cause of the arrest and performed the correct life-saving treatment. Doing a disorganized survey at this time would have been a fatal error.

SUMMARY

The trauma patient in cardiopulmonary arrest is usually suffering from a breathing or circulatory problem. If you are to save this patient, you must identify the cause of the arrest with the ITLS Primary Survey, and then rapidly transport the patient while performing those procedures that specifically address the cause of the arrest. While it is very rare to successfully resuscitate a patient suffering from a trauma arrest secondary to hemorrhagic shock, attention to detail will allow you the best chance to "bring one back from the dead," which is the greatest challenge and greatest satisfaction in EMS.

BIBLIOGRAPHY

1. American Heart Association. 2005. International Consensus on Cardiopulmonary Resuscitation (CPR) and Emergency Cardiovascualar Care (ECC) Science with Treatment Recommendations. *Circulation* 112 (22): III-1 to III-136.
2. Cera, S., G. Mostafa, R. Sing, et al. 2003. Physiologic predictors of survival in post-traumatic arrest. *The American Surgeon* 69: 140–44.
3. Hopson, L., E. Hirsh, J. Delgado, et al. 2003. Guidelines for withholding or termination of resuscitation in prehospital traumatic cardiopulmonary arrest: Joint position statement of the National Association of EMS Physicians and the American College of Surgeons Committee on Trauma. *Journal of the American College of Surgeons* 196: 106–12.
4. Perron, A. D., R. Sing, et al. 1997. Research forum abstracts. Predicting survival in pediatric trauma patients receiving CPR in the prehospital setting. *Annals of Emergency Medicine* 30: 381.

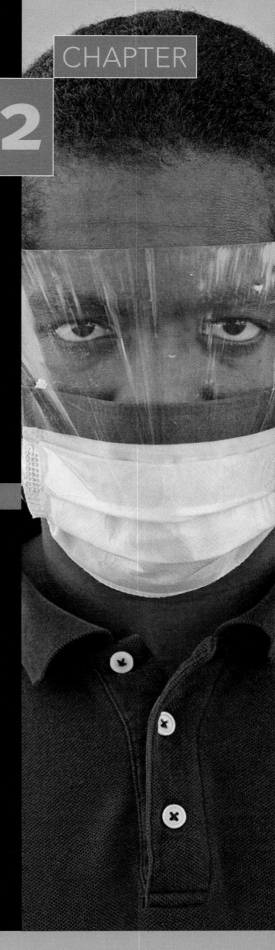

Standard Precautions in the Prehospital Setting

Howard Werman, MD, FACEP

Richard N. Nelson, MD, FACEP

Katherine West, BSN, MSEd, CIC

OBJECTIVES

Upon completion of this chapter, you should be able to:

1. Discuss the three most common bloodborne viral illnesses to which EMS providers are likely to be exposed in the provision of patient care.

2. Discuss the signs and symptoms of tuberculosis and describe protective measures to reduce possible exposure to TB.

3. Describe precautions EMS providers can take to prevent exposure to blood and other potentially infectious materials (CSF, synovial fluid, amniotic fluid, pericardial fluid, pleural fluid, or any fluid with gross visible blood).

4. Identify appropriate use of personal protective equipment.

5. Describe procedures for EMS providers to follow if they are accidentally exposed.

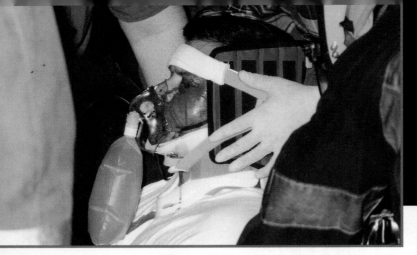

Joyce, Buddy, and Dan have been dispatched to a bar where a man has been injured in a fight. As they respond, they decide that Buddy will be team leader, and they don personal protective equipment, since they expect the patient to be bloody. When they arrive they find that the police are already there and have the scene under control. Sitting in a chair is a young man who has been beaten and "stomped" by motorcycle gang members. As they approach, Buddy's initial impression is not good. The patient is bloody and is struggling to breathe.

The patient answers them appropriately when they introduce themselves. They ask him not to move until they finish examining him. Joyce stabilizes his neck with her hands and asks Dan to apply a nonrebreather oxygen mask. The airway is open but there is poor movement of air. There is a rapid, weak peripheral pulse and an obvious large flail segment on the left side of the chest. Buddy instructs Dan to get the backboard and the Kendrick extrication device (KED) to use to splint the flail chest. He begins the Rapid Trauma Survey. The face has bruises and abrasions all over and there is dried blood in the nose, but the active bleeding has stopped. He appears to have facial fractures but the airway is not compromised. The neck is bruised and tender but with no obvious deformities. Neck veins are flat and the trachea is midline. The breath sounds are decreased on the left side but heart sounds are normal. The abdomen is tender to palpation but not distended, and there are no masses felt. The pelvis is stable and nontender. The extremities are bruised but there is good PMS. The patient has good sensation and movement in his fingers and toes.

The KED is applied to stabilize the flail chest. The patient says the pain is much improved. The team then moves the patient onto the long backboard and transports immediately. Joyce drives. Vital signs taken en route are BP 90/50, pulse 140, respiration 36, and pulse oximeter reading 95 percent on 100 percent oxygen. The cardiac monitor shows sinus tachycardia. Buddy starts an IV with a large-bore catheter. Before the safety device is set, the patient becomes combative, causing Buddy to stick his hand with the bloody needle. *What should he do now? What tests will need to be done? What sort of information should be recorded? What is the worst that can happen?* Keep these questions in mind as you read the chapter. Then, at the end of the chapter, find out how the rescuers completed this call.

INTRODUCTION

EMS personnel have always faced risks when carrying out their jobs. These risks have mostly involved highway hazards, fires, downed electrical wires, toxic substances, and scene security problems. The provision of patient care may present the possibility of exposure to bloodborne and other diseases. Fortunately, there are precautions that may be taken to markedly reduce these risks. Additionally, if personal protective equipment could not be used or failed, treatment is available to reduce the risk of acquiring these diseases following an exposure event. Exposure does not mean infection; exposure can be treated.

The spectrum of diseases to which you are potentially exposed is beyond the scope of this book. However, the three most common types of viral infections are appropriate to discuss in conjunction with trauma management, since their modes of spread are primarily by contaminated blood and other potentially infectious materials (OPIM). They are hepatitis B (HBV), hepatitis C (HBC), and HIV infection. **Body fluids that do not pose a risk for HBV, HBC, and HIV are tears, sweat, saliva, urine, stool, vomitus, nasal secretions, and sputum unless they contain visible blood contamination.**

> **PEARLS**
> *An EMS Standard*
> All patients are potential carriers of infectious disease. That is why standard precautions are the EMS standard for practice.

HEPATITIS B

The term *viral hepatitis* is used to describe a group of viral infections involving the liver. At least five types of viruses have been described: hepatitis A, B, C, D, and E. Hepatitis A and E are spread primarily through contact with contaminated fecal material and are not bloodborne. Hepatitis D is transmitted through blood and body fluid exposure to patients already infected with hepatitis B. Because of their frequent contact with blood and needles, healthcare workers are considered at risk of becoming infected with the hepatitis B virus (HBV). Fortunately, hepatitis B is the one form of hepatitis for which there is an effective vaccine.

> **PEARLS**
> *Immunizations*
> Be prepared! Stay up to date on all of your immunizations.

HBV is a major cause of acute and chronic hepatitis, cirrhosis, and liver cancer. An estimated 3,000 people in the United States are infected each year. In 1995, OSHA reported that about 800 health-care workers acquired the disease through occupational exposure. Because of the universal vaccination program, these numbers have decreased by almost 90 percent since 1992. Following acute infection, 5 to 10 percent of these patients continue to be chronic carriers of the virus. These carriers are potentially infectious.

HBV is spread by contact with contaminated blood or OPIM (other potentially infectious material), sexual transmission, and direct contact with a contaminated item and nonintact skin. Infection usually occurs from contaminated needle sticks or through sexual contact. There is an estimated 6 to 30 percent chance that health-care workers who are exposed to a needlestick by HBV-contaminated blood will develop hepatitis B infection if they have not received their vaccine or have not developed an appropriate immune response to the vaccine.

Passage of the Needlestick Safety and Prevention Act of 2000 by the U.S. Congress requires the use of needle-safe or needleless devices. This legislation has cut the number of sharps injuries by more than half since 2003. Infection can also occur by contacting infectious bloody secretions with open skin lesions or mucosal surfaces. Routine testing of donor blood for HBV makes transmission from blood transfusion very rare.

Although HBV infection is uncommon in the general population, members of certain groups are considered much more likely to harbor the virus. High-risk groups are immigrants from areas where HBV is prevalent (Asia, Pacific Islands), incarcerated individuals, institutionalized patients, intravenous drug users, male homosexuals, hemophiliacs, household contacts of HBV patients, and hemodialysis patients.

In the United States, the Occupational Safety and Health Administration (OSHA) mandated in 1991 that all employers of health-care workers are required to offer HBV vaccine to any health-care worker who is at risk of occupational exposure to blood and OPIM. This must occur within 10 days of being hired. This vaccine offers lifelong protection. Vaccines available today are recombinant; they contain no human components. A titer (blood test) is performed 1 to 2 months after completion of the vaccine series to document response to the vaccine. If positive, no further titer testing is needed or recommended. The vaccine is safe and produces immunity in over 90 percent of people vaccinated.

The second form of protection is hepatitis B immunoglobulin (HBIG). This preparation contains antibodies to HBV and provides temporary, passive protection against HBV. HBIG is only 70 percent effective and when effective, provides protection for only 6 months. HBIG is used only when there has been a significant exposure to HBV in an unimmunized person but is given in conjunction with vaccine to offer full coverage postexposure.

HEPATITIS C

The hepatitis C virus (HCV) was identified in 1988–1989. This virus is thought to be responsible for the majority of what had been identified as non-A, non-B hepatitis infections. The incubation period is 6 to 7 weeks. Antibodies to the HCV have been used to identify patients with previous HCV infection. Those exposed to HCV are test-positive 5 to 6 weeks after exposure.

Prior to 1992, HCV was the leading cause of hepatitis resulting from blood transfusions. In addition to being spread by blood transfusion, the virus also appears to be spread by sharing of intravenous needles, sexual contact, tattooing, and body piercing, much like HBV. Health-care workers can acquire infection through hollow-bore needlesticks with contaminated needles. The likelihood of becoming infected with HCV after a single high-risk needlestick is estimated at 1.8 percent. This risk is further reduced by the use of needle-safe devices.

HCV infection tends to be less severe than HBV during the initial infection. However, there appears to be a greater likelihood of becoming a chronic carrier of HCV following infection. Liver failure and cirrhosis occur in 10 to 20 percent of chronic HCV carriers.

There is currently no vaccine available to protect against HCV infection. Evidence suggests that there is no protective effect provided by administering immune globulin following exposure to HCV. Now, rapid HCV testing can be performed on the source patient and if positive, the exposed provider can be offered a follow-up test (HCV-RNA) in 4 to 6 weeks postexposure. This latter test detects the virus itself. This reduces the concern about having acquired the disease to 4 to 6 weeks instead of 6 months of follow-up. Treatment is available for people who acquire the disease. Current treatment is with Pegasys, a combination of long-acting interferon and another antiviral agent, ribavirin. Together, this treatment has resulted in 56 percent of persons clearing their infection.

HUMAN IMMUNODEFICIENCY VIRUS INFECTION

HIV infection is caused by the human immunodeficiency virus (HIV). Patients with HIV infection develop a defect in their immune system. This predisposes the HIV-infected patient to a variety of unusual infections not generally seen in healthy patients of similar age. Patients infected with HIV can present with a wide spectrum of clinical manifestations. Many patients with HIV infection are asymptomatic. However, any patient who carries HIV, whether he manifests symptoms of AIDS or not, can transmit the virus. HIV patients being treated with current drugs may be virus negative and as such, pose a minute risk.

HIV appears to be transmitted in a manner similar to HBV. Although the virus has been cultured from a variety of body fluids, only blood has been implicated in the transmission of the virus in the workplace. This is because other body fluids do not carry enough virus particles to transmit the disease. Semen and vaginal secretions have been shown to transmit the virus during sexual activity, but this should be of no concern in the workplace. There is no evidence to suggest that the HIV is transmitted by casual contact. Transmission to health-care workers has been documented only after accidental parenteral exposure (needlestick) or exposure of mucous membranes and open wounds to large amounts of infected blood. Measurable risk data for occupational exposure is 0.3 percent for needlestick injuries and 0.09 percent for mucous membrane exposure. There is one documented case of transmission from infected blood on nonintact skin. This case was reported in 2002 and involved a health-care worker with extensive dermatitis who did not always use gloves appropriate when caring for a patient coinfected with HIV and HCV.

HIV appears to be different from the hepatitis B virus in two ways.

■ HIV does not survive outside the body. No special cleaning agents are required.

■ HIV is transmitted far less efficiently than HBV.

Several groups have been identified as having a high risk of HIV infection. These include male homosexuals or bisexuals, intravenous drug abusers, patients who have received blood transfusions or pooled-plasma products (such as hemophiliacs), and heterosexual contacts of HIV-positive people. However, because of the difficulty in identifying HIV-infected patients, all contacts with blood and OPIM should be considered a potential HIV exposure. This concept (all patients are potentially infective) is why standard precautions are "universally" applied.

There is currently no available vaccine to protect against HIV infection. Antiretroviral drug regimens, though not a cure, have been shown to prolong the life of HIV/AIDS patients. Some studies have suggested that antiretroviral agents may reduce the risk of HIV transmission in health-care workers if administered immediately following a significant exposure to HIV-infected blood and OPIM. The decision to administer such agents should be based on the nature of the exposure, the likelihood that the patient is infected with HIV, and the duration of time following exposure (Figure 22-1). In general, hollow-needle exposures are more significant than solid instruments (such as a scalpel).

If the exposure meets the CDC criteria for offering drugs postexposure to the health-care worker, they can be administered within "hours but not days." Employees need to be counseled about the side effects and the unknown issues involving the use of these drugs before they are started. Baseline lab work also needs to be drawn. This can all be avoided by performing rapid HIV testing on the source patient. This is the standard of care and prevents a health-care provider from being placed on these drugs awaiting blood work on the source. Remember, all postexposure medical follow-up begins with testing the source, not the exposed employee.

TUBERCULOSIS

From 1985 to 1993, the incidence of active tuberculosis increased significantly to over 25,000 cases in the United States. This was the result of an increase in cases among people infected with HIV and an increase in immigration of people from areas where tuberculosis infection is endemic (Asia, Latin America, the Caribbean, Africa). Because of better

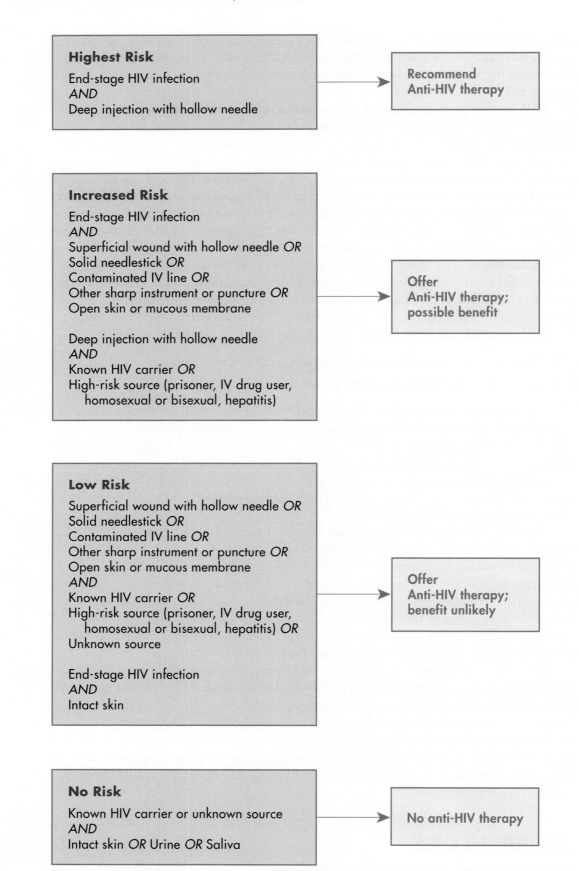

FIGURE 22-1 Risk assessment for anti-HIV therapy following blood and body fluid exposure.

public health measures, tuberculosis has been declining in the last several years. Cases decreased by 58.8 percent from 1997 to 2004. In fact, the number of cases in 2004 was the lowest ever reported in the United States. Risk factors for tuberculosis include homeless patients, certain immigrant populations, patients at risk for HIV infection, and people who live in congregate settings (correction facilities, nursing homes, homeless shelters). On a global perspective, tuberculosis is still the deadliest infectious disease with 8 million new infections annually and 3 million deaths.

Tuberculosis is caused by a bacterium, *Mycobacterium tuberculosis*, which is spread from an infected person to susceptible people through the air, especially by coughing or sneezing. This is *not* a highly communicable disease. Contracting tuberculosis requires prolonged direct contact, as in a family living situation. Only persons with active infection of the lung or throat spread tuberculosis. It is estimated that up to 5 percent of health-care workers will test positive for tuberculosis when working in high-prevalence environments.

Clinical manifestations of the disease become apparent only when the patient's immune system fails to keep the bacteria in check. The bacteria then begins to infect the lungs and may spread to other portions of the body, particularly the kidneys, spine, or brain. These cases are termed "extrapulmonary" and are not communicable to the care provider. Symptoms of active tuberculosis are most prominent in the lungs and include a bad cough that lasts longer than 3 weeks in conjunction with two or more of the following: pain in the chest, coughing up bloody sputum, weakness or fatigue, unexplained weight loss, loss of appetite, fever, chills, night sweats, or hoarseness.

> **PEARLS**
> *TB*
> If your patient has a persistent cough plus other symptoms suggestive of TB, place a mask on the patient, not on yourself. You should wear a mask if the patient requires oxygen and cannot wear a mask.

Treatment of tuberculosis includes antibiotic agents. TB infection means a positive skin test. This means no active disease. *TB disease* is the term for active disease. If there is a positive skin test but no symptoms of active TB, isoniazid (INH) or rifampin is used for a period of 6 to 9 months to eradicate the infection. Three to four antibiotic agents are used when TB disease is confirmed. Although some strains of TB are developing resistance to many of the agents used to treat the disease, multidrug-resistant TB is still treatable and is rare (121 cases in the United States in 2004).

Since 1995, the U.S. Center for Disease Control and Prevention has recommended placing a surgical mask on any patient suspected of having TB. Thus the care provider does not need to wear a mask of any kind. Health-care workers should receive tuberculin skin testing prior to employment and periodically thereafter, depending on the TB risk assessment in their work area, to ensure that tuberculosis has not been acquired. This is in keeping with the CDC guidelines published on December 30, 2005, which OSHA is enforcing.

PRECAUTIONS FOR PREVENTION OF TRANSMISSION OF INFECTIOUS AGENTS

"Standard precautions" refer to treating everyone (including you) as if they are infectious. Your goal is to prevent the spread of infection from you to the patient and from the patient to you. In today's environment, you must use precautions for each and every patient. Equipment used is task based (Table 22-1).

PROCEDURE

✴ General Considerations

1. Be knowledgeable about infection from hepatitis B, hepatitis C, and HIV. Understand their etiologies, signs and symptoms, routes of transmission, and epidemiology

TABLE 22-1 *Recommended Personal Protective Equipment for Worker Protection Against HIV and HBV Transmission in Prehospital Settings**

Task or Activity	Disposable Gloves	Gown	Mask	Protective Eyewear
Bleeding control with spurting blood	Yes	Yes	Yes	Yes
Bleeding control with minimal bleeding	Yes	No	No	No
Emergency childbirth	Yes	Yes	Yes	Yes
Blood drawing	Yes	No	No	No
Starting IV line	Yes	No	No	No
ET intubation or use of BIAD	Yes	No	No, unless splashing is likely	No, unless splashing is likely
Oral/nasal suctioning, manually cleaning airway	Yes	No	No, unless splashing is likely	No, unless splashing is likely
Handling and cleaning instruments with microbial contamination	Yes	No, unless soiling is likely	No	No
Measuring blood pressure	No	No	No	No
Measuring temperature	No	No	No	No
Giving an injection	No	No	No	No

*From U.S. OSHA Guidelines

(relationships of the various factors determining the frequency and distribution of a disease).

2. If you have open or weeping lesions, take special precautions to prevent exposure of these areas to blood or OPIM. Lesions should be covered with a bandage. If these lesions cannot be adequately protected, avoid invasive procedures, other direct patient care activities, or handling of equipment used for patient care. You are placed on work restriction.

3. Perform routine handwashing before and after all patient contact. Wash hands as soon as possible following exposure to blood or OPIM. Alcohol-based foam or gel is best for in-field use. No artificial nails or extensions for patient care providers (see reference 2 at the end of this chapter).

4. Become immunized against the hepatitis B virus.

5. Report any exposure event to your designated infection control officer.

PROCEDURE

❋ Personal Protection During Patient Exposures

1. Wear gloves if exposure to blood or OPIM is anticipated. This precaution should be taken when performing an invasive procedure or handling any item soiled with blood or body fluids. Almost all trauma patients are risks for exposure to blood or body fluids.

2. Disposable gowns, masks, and eye coverings are necessary only when extensive contact with blood or body fluids is anticipated. These precautions are advised when spraying, or airborne spread of blood or body fluids is likely (such as with endotracheal intubation, blind insertion airway device, vaginal deliveries, and major trauma).

3. When treating any patient with respiratory complaints, mask the patient with a surgical mask or nonrebreather oxygen mask. It is also important to get a travel history.

4. Direct mouth-to-mouth ventilation of patients during CPR is discouraged. Use disposable mouthpieces when artificial ventilation is indicated. However, if not available or not working, mouth-to-mouth is to be performed. Do not let the patient die because you were not prepared.

> **PEARLS**
> *Artificial Ventilation*
> Be prepared! Have appropriate barrier devices with you so you are not required to do mouth-to-mouth breathing. However, you have an obligation to perform mouth-to-mouth resuscitation if your patient needs it and you forgot your equipment.

PROCEDURE

❋ Handling and Cleaning of Items Exposed to Blood or OPIM

1. Prevent sharps injuries by using needle-safe or needle-less devices. It is the law and in your best interest.

2. Any disposable equipment such as masks, gowns, gloves, mouthpieces, and airways that have been contaminated by blood or OPIM should be collected in an impervious plastic bag. These plastic bags should then be disposed of according to state definitions of medical waste, in proper waste containers available in hospital emergency departments or other health-care locations. Nondisposable gowns can be laundered using simple laundry procedures. Your hospital should have linen bags or linen containers designated for contaminated gowns, etc.

3. With a low-sudsing detergent with a neutral pH, wash any surface spills on nondisposable equipment that does not usually come in contact with skin or mucous membranes. The equipment should then be wet down or soaked for 10 minutes in a 1:100 dilution of household bleach (or 70 percent isopropyl alcohol). In this concentration, bleach will not cause corrosion of metal objects (U.S. Center for Disease Control and Prevention, 1989).

4. Using a low-sudsing detergent with a neutral pH, wash nondisposable medical devices that will frequently contact skin or mucous membranes. Then soak them for 30 to 40 minutes or more in 2 percent alkaline glutaraldehyde (e.g., Cidex) or similar solution in a well-ventilated area, rinse in sterile water, and package until reuse.

PROCEDURE

❋ Reporting Accidental Exposure to Blood or OPIM

1. Thoroughly wash or irrigate the exposed area immediately following an exposure to blood or contaminated body fluids. In the United States, you must contact your designated officer (mandated by federal law, March 1994). All employers of health-care

REPORT OF EXPOSURE TO BLOOD OR OPIM

NAME OF EMS PERSONNEL _____

NAME OF EMS SERVICE _____

SSI _____

ADDRESS OF EMS SERVICE _____

PHONE NUMBER (HOME)_____ (WORK) _____

DATE OF EXPOSURE _____ TIME OF EXPOSURE _____

NAME OF PATIENT_____

HOSPITAL ID NUMBER _____

PATIENT ADDRESS_____

PHONE NUMBER (WORK) _____ (HOME) _____

ROUTE OF EXPOSURE: _____

( ) Parenteral exposure (needlestick or sharp instrument)

( ) Mucous membrane

( ) Open skin

( ) Intact skin

( ) Other_____

TYPE OF FLUID:

( ) blood   ( ) emesis   ( ) saliva

( ) stool   ( ) urine   ( ) other_____

SOURCE OF EXPOSURE:

HIV:	( ) Yes	( ) No	( ) Unknown
Hepatitis B:	( ) No	( ) Acute	( ) Chronic Carrier ( ) Unknown
Hepatitis C:	( ) No	( ) Acute	( ) Chronic Carrier ( ) Unknown
Tuberculosis:	( ) No	( ) Yes	

RISK FACTORS:

( ) Homosexual   ( ) IV Drug Abuser

( ) Hemophilia   ( ) Dialysis Patient

( ) Sexual Contact of the Above

( ) Other_____

HIV Test: ( ) Pos.   ( ) Neg.   ( ) Unknown

Date of HIV Test: _____

HBsAg: ( ) Pos.   ( ) Neg.   ( ) Unknown

Date of HBsAg Test _____

Description of Circumstances Surrounding the Exposure, Including Measures Taken After Exposure:

_____

_____

_____

INSTITUTION NOTIFIED:_____

PHYSICIAN OR RESPONSIBLE PERSON: _____

DATE OF NOTIFICATION: _____TIME OF NOTIFICATION: _____

NAME OF EXPOSED PERSONNEL _____DATE _____

SIGNATURE _____

FIGURE 22-2 Sample report form.

workers must have a designated officer (DO). The designated officer will deal with the incident and the medical facility from this point.

2. The DO will make the first determination regarding whether or not an exposure occurred. The DO will notify the receiving facility of the possible exposure at the time of the incident. The DO will ask the facility to cooperate in determining the serologic status of the source. In some areas, informed consent need not be obtained to determine serologic status of the source. Know your local laws.

3. Write a report of the incident as soon as possible. The minimum information that should be recorded on the report is included in Figure 22-2. The written ambulance report may be used to supplement, but not replace, the incident report. In the United States, you will fill out a confidential exposure report form. Only the exposed employee, the DO, and the treating physician are allowed to see the form. An exposed employee has become a patient and has a right to privacy.

4. Blood tests (if any) to be done on the exposed employee depend on reports of testing of the source patient. If the results of rapid HIV testing are negative, then no further testing of the employee is needed. If the source patient is positive for HIV, then the exposed employee should undergo HIV serology determination at the time of the incident. Repeat testing should be done at 1 month, 3 months, and 6 months. If the source patient is HCV positive, the exposed employee can be tested for HCV in 4 to 6 weeks. If the source patient is HBV positive and the exposed care provider has not already been immunized, hepatitis B vaccine should be administered. The administration of HBIG should be determined by the serologic testing of both the source (where possible) and the exposed health-care provider, as well as by the assessment of the risk of the exposure.

PEARLS
Reporting an Exposure
Immediately report to your designated officer (know who this is) any possible exposure to blood or OPIM or an airborne transmissible disease.

Case Study

continued

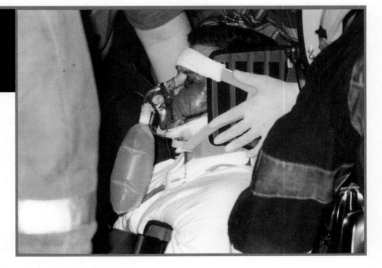

Joyce, Dan, and Buddy are transporting a male patient who was beaten severely and has a flail chest. As he is starting the IV, Buddy accidentally sticks himself with the catheter needle. He finishes connecting the IV fluids and tapes the IV in place and immediately washes his hand thoroughly. He continues his care of the patient. The SAMPLE history reveals that the patient was beaten by a gang of men but did not lose consciousness. He complains of pain "all over." He has a history of HIV infection but has never been told that he has AIDS. He also had "hepatitis," but does not know which kind. He takes several medications for his HIV but does not know their names and does not have them with him. He last ate an hour ago. He has no known allergies. An ITLS Secondary Survey reveals that the abdomen is becoming distended and more tender. The blood pressure has dropped to 70/40.

Buddy reports all of this to medical direction, who instructs him to give enough IV fluids to maintain a blood pressure of 80–90 systolic. The patient does not improve with 2 liters normal saline en route and is taken directly to surgery when they arrive at the hospital. The patient has a fractured liver and a hemothorax as well as the flail chest. He requires 10 units of blood and survives surgery but later dies of pneumonia. His blood is positive for HIV and for hepatitis B.

Buddy has already been immunized for hepatitis B. He is offered anti-HIV therapy but he declines and signs a declination form. He is counseled by the medical director of infectious disease and is followed by him for a year. Buddy has HIV tests done immediately and at 1, 3, and 6 months afterwards. He remains seronegative.

Case Study

Wrap-up

All health-care workers should be immunized against hepatitis B since the immunization is very effective and without it there is one chance in four of contracting hepatitis B if exposed. In contrast, there is no immunization for HIV but there are only three chances in 1,000 of contracting the disease if exposed to a large hollow-needle stick with visible blood, and the source has a high titer of virus in the blood. This patient was a low risk for transmission because he was taking his anti-HIV medications and thus should not have had a viral load in his blood. Buddy's refusal of anti-HIV medication was based on his consideration of the toxicity of the antiviral drugs being offered and also the low risk of infection in this situation.

SUMMARY

Like most health-care workers, you are at risk of exposure to many contagious diseases. Because of the presence of blood and contaminated secretions in many trauma victims, you must take extra precautions to avoid exposure to the viruses that cause hepatitis B, hepatitis C, and HIV and to the bacteria that cause tuberculosis. Knowledge of the modes of exposure, as well as adherence to barrier precautions, or postexposure medical follow-up will reduce your risk of contracting any of these infections. In the United States, the recent standards released by OSHA make adherence to these precautions mandatory for health-care workers at risk for exposure to contaminated blood or OPIM with the exception of not delaying care if personal protective equipment is not readily available.

BIBLIOGRAPHY

1. NIOSH Alert. 1997, June. Latex allergy.
2. U.S. Centers for Disease Control and Prevention. 2002, October 25. Hand hygiene guidelines.
3. U.S. Centers for Disease Control and Prevention. 2001. Updated U.S. Public Health Service guidelines for the management of occupational exposures to HBV, HCV, and HIV and recommendations for postexposure prophylaxis. *Morbidity and Mortality Weekly Report* 50(RR11): 1–42.
4. U.S. Center for Disease Control and Prevention. 1989. Guidelines for Public Safety.
5. U.S. Congress. 2000. Needlestick Safety and Prevention Act.
6. U.S. Department of Labor. 2001, November 27. *Compliance directive for occupational exposure to bloodborne pathogens* (CPL 2-2.69).
7. U.S. Public Health Service. 2005, December 30. Guidelines for the prevention of transmission of *Mycobacterium tuberculosis* in health-care settings.

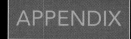
Optional Skills

Donna Hastings, EMT-P (Optional Skills 1–8)

Roy L. Alson, PhD, MD, FACEP (Optional Skill 9)

OPTIONAL SKILL 1: Digital Intubation

Objectives

Upon completion of this Skill Station, you should be able to:

1. Recite the indications for performing digital intubation.
2. Perform digital intubation.

The original method of endotracheal intubation, quite widely known in the 18th century, was the "tactile" or "digital" technique. The intubator merely felt the epiglottis with the fingers and slipped the endotracheal tube distally through the glottic opening. Recently, the technique has been refined and demonstrated to be of use for a wide variety of patients.

INDICATIONS

Digital orotracheal intubation is particularly useful for deeply comatose or cardiac arrest patients who:

- Are difficult to position properly.
- Are somewhat inaccessible to the full view of the rescuer.
- May be at risk for cervical-spine injury.
- Have facial injuries that distort anatomy.
- Have copious oropharyngeal bleeding or secretions that render visualization difficult.

You may prefer to perform digital intubation when you are confident of your ability with this technique or when a laryngoscope fails or is not immediately available. The technique is most valuable in those patients in difficult positions such as extrications and in those who have copious secretions despite adequate attempts at suctioning.

EQUIPMENT

This method of intubation requires the following:

- Endotracheal tube, 7.0-, 7.5-, or 8.0-mm internal diameter
- Malleable stylet (Note: Some prefer to perform the procedure without a stylet.)

■ Water-soluble lubricant
■ 12-cc syringe
■ Dental prod, mouth gag, and so on for placing between the teeth
■ Rubber gloves

TECHNIQUE

1. Perform routine preparation procedures as taught in Chapter 5.
2. Prepare the tube by inserting the lubricated stylet and bending the tube into an "open J" configuration. The stylet should not protrude beyond the tip of the tube, but it should come to at least the side hole.
3. Apply a water-soluble lubricant liberally to the tip and cuff of the tube.
4. Wear gloves for protection.
5. Kneel at the patient's left shoulder facing the patient, and place a dental prod or mouth gag between the patient's molars (Figure A-1).
6. "Walk" the index and middle fingers of your left hand down the midline of the tongue, all the while pulling forward on the tongue and jaw. This is a most important maneuver and serves to lift the epiglottis up within reach of the probing fingers.
7. Palpate the epiglottis with your middle finger; it feels much like the tragus of the ear.
8. Press forward on the epiglottis and slip the tube into the mouth at the left corner of the mouth (Figure A-2). Use the index finger to keep the tube tip against the side of the middle finger (that is still palpating the epiglottis). This guides the tip to the epiglottis. You can also use the side hole of the tube as a landmark to ensure that you are always aware of the position of the tip of the endotracheal tube. This is a crucial principle of this technique.

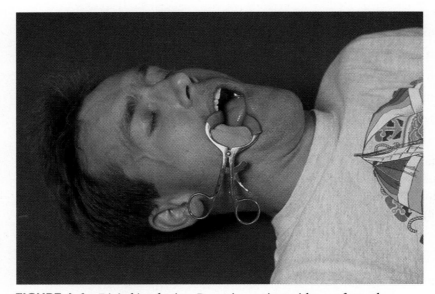

FIGURE A-1   Digital intubation. Preparing patient with use of mouth (dental) prod to protect the intubator against being bitten.

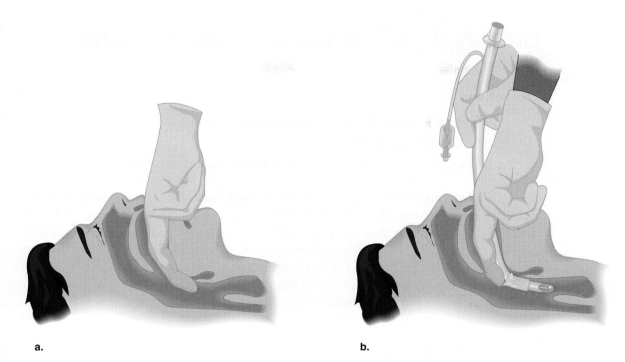

a.   b.

FIGURE A-2 (a) Insert your index and middle finger into the patient's mouth. Elevate the epiglottis with your middle finger. (b) Guide the tube forward and into the glottic opening with your index and middle fingers.

9. Guide the tube tip to lie against the epiglottis using the middle and index fingers. The epiglottis is in front and the fingers behind. Advance the tube distally through the cords using the right hand. Press forward with the index and middle fingers of the left hand to prevent the tube from slipping posteriorly into the esophagus. Note: At this point the tube-stylet combination may encounter resistance, especially if the distal curve of the tube is sharp. This usually means that the tube tip is pressing on the anterior wall of the thyroid cartilage. Pulling back slightly on the stylet will allow the tube to conform to the anatomy, and the tube should slip into the trachea.

10. Confirm placement by the confirmation protocol taught in Chapter 5.

OPTIONAL SKILL 2: Transillumination (Lighted Stylet)

Objectives

Upon completion of this Skill Station, you should be able to:

1. Describe the advantages of this technique.
2. Perform endotracheal intubation by the transillumination method.

The transillumination or lighted stylet method of endotracheal intubation is based on the fact that a bright light inserted inside the upper airway can be seen through the soft tissues of the neck when inside the larynx or trachea. This permits you to guide the tube tip through the glottic opening without directly visualizing the cords. It has been called the "indirect visual" method and has been shown in several studies to be reliable, quick, and atraumatic. It is particularly attractive in trauma patients because it appears to move the head and neck less than conventional orotracheal methods.

EQUIPMENT

■ *Stylet.* The lighted stylet (Figure A-3) is a malleable wire connecting a proximal battery housing to a distal lightbulb, covered with a tough plastic coating that prevents the light from being separated from the wire. An on/off switch is located at the proximal end of the battery housing.

■ *Endotracheal tubes.* All tubes should have an internal diameter of 7.5 to 8.5 mm.

■ *Other equipment* will be standard to any intubation procedure: suction, oxygen, gloves, lubricant, and so on.

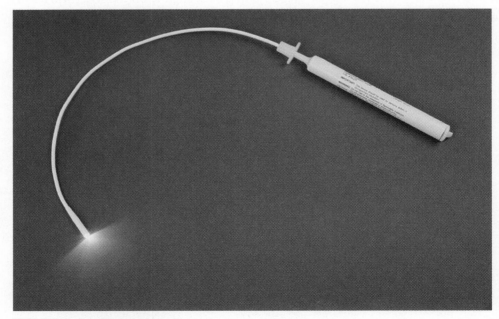

FIGURE A-3 The lighted stylet.

TECHNIQUE

The success of this intubation method depends upon several factors.

- *Level of the ambient light.* The light should be cut down to about 10 percent of normal, or the patient's neck should be shielded from direct sun or bright daylight. While the transilluminated light can be seen in thin patients even in daylight, success will be more likely in darker surroundings.

- *Pulling forward on the tongue*—or tongue and jaw—lifts the epiglottis up out of the way. This is essential to this method (Figure A-4).

- *Bend of the tube-stylet.* Bend the tube-stylet combination just proximal to the cuff. A bend that is too far proximal will cause the tube to strike against the posterior pharyngeal wall and prevent the tube advancing anteriorly through the glottic opening (Figure A-4). Slip the lubricated stylet into the tube and hold firmly against the battery housing while bending the tube-stylet. Bend the tube-stylet more sharply if the patient is not in the sniffing position.

To perform the transillumination or lighted stylet method of endotracheal intubation, follow these steps.

1. Perform routine preparation procedures taught in Chapter 5.

2. Stand or kneel on either side facing the patient's head. Wear gloves for the procedure. Switch on the light.

3. Grasp the patient's tongue—or more easily, the tongue and jaw—and lift gently forward while slipping the liberally lubricated tube-stylet combination down the tongue.

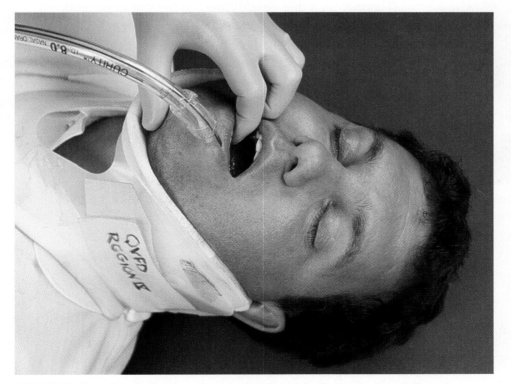

FIGURE A-4 Pulling forward on the tongue and jaw lifts the epiglottis and allows for intubation with the stylet. The bend in the stylet must not be too far proximal so that it will not strike against the posterior pharyngeal wall. Note gloves are worn.

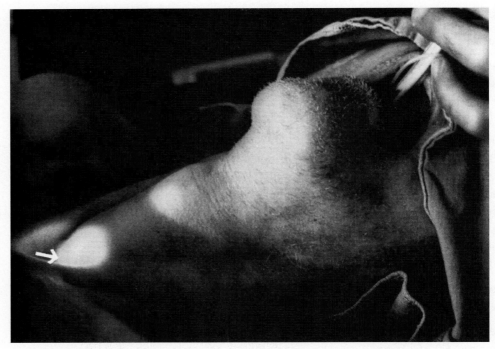

FIGURE A-5   Correct placement of tube. Bright circumscribed glow seen when the tip of the stylet is at or beyond the cords.

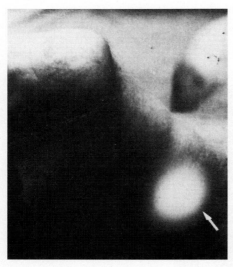

4. Using a "soup ladle" motion, "hook" up the epiglottis by the tube-stylet. The transilluminated light can then be seen in the midline. Correct placement at or beyond the cords is indicated by the appearance of a circumscribed area of light at the level of the laryngeal prominence (Figure A-5). A dull glow, diffuse and difficult to see, indicates esophageal placement (Figure A-6).

5. When you see the light, hold the stylet firmly in place and use the fingers of the other hand to support the tube as you advance the tube off the stylet and more distally into the larynx.

6. Confirm placement of the tube with the confirmation protocol taught in Chapter 5.

FIGURE A-6   Incorrect placement of tube. Clearly seen light transilluminated from the right pyriform fossa.

OPTIONAL SKILL 3: Translaryngeal Jet Ventilation

Objectives

Upon completion of this Skill Station, you should be able to:

1. Discuss the indications for this procedure.
2. Perform translaryngeal jet ventilation (TLJV).

When the airway cannot be maintained because of obstruction or partial obstruction above the cords, access below the level of the cords is needed. Translaryngeal jet ventilation (TLJV) provides a quick, reliable, and relatively safe method of adequate oxygenation and ventilation, especially in the trauma patient. Many misconceptions and erroneous impressions persist about this technique, and the medical literature is in a state of confusion on the subject. Clinical experience and studies done using appropriate equipment in both animals and patients clearly indicate the following:

■ Patients can be both oxygenated and ventilated with this technique, which delivers 100 percent oxygen in volumes exceeding 1 L per second.

■ Ventilation can proceed indefinitely, providing the correct size cannula is used with the proper driving pressure.

■ Cannula of 14 gauge or larger with side holes must be used.

■ Driving pressures of at least 50 psi (30 psi in a small child) must be used to deliver sufficient volumes to ensure adequate ventilation.

You cannot ventilate patients using small-bore cannulae with continuous flow oxygen attached. The foregoing principles must be adhered to if you are to safely and effectively use this technique.

EQUIPMENT

The tools needed for TLJV should be prepared well in advance and stored in a small bag or kit.

■ *No. 14 or 13-gauge cannula,* with side holes (Figure A-7). These sizes are the minimum necessary for adequate ventilation. Side holes are especially important, since they prevent the cannula from remaining against the tracheal wall and subjecting it to sudden pressures that could rupture it.

■ *Manual jet ventilator device.* These are commercially available and are merely valves that allow high-pressure oxygen to flow through them when a button is pushed. They should have high-pressure tubing attached solidly with special fasteners and tape.

■ *Wrench.* A small wrench should be attached to the jet ventilator tubing so that you lose no time looking for a way to tap into the oxygen tank or turn it on.

TECHNIQUE

Identification of the cricothyroid membrane is essential to this technique, although placement between the tracheal rings probably would not result in major complications.

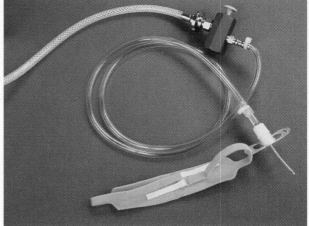

FIGURE A-7 A specially designed 13-gauge cannula for translaryngeal jet ventilation. This is hooked into a 50-psi oxygen source for adequate ventilation and oxygenation.

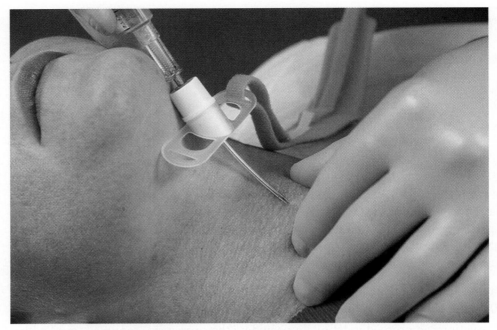

FIGURE A-8 Puncture of cricothyroid membrane with jet ventilator cannula. Note syringe in place filled with saline. Bubbles on aspiration indicate correct intratracheal placement.

1. While continuing attempts at ventilation and oxygenation, puncture the cricothyroid membrane with the cannula to which is attached a 5-cc syringe filled with 1 to 2 cc of saline (Figure A-8). Note: Several cubic centimeters of 2 percent lidocaine can be used instead of saline to produce local anesthesia of the mucosa in the area of the distal port of the cannula.

2. Direct the cannula downward, continually aspirating to promptly demonstrate entry into the larynx, identified when you aspirate bubbles of air. At this point, if lidocaine is contained in the syringe, you can inject it into the larynx to provide some anesthesia and to prevent the coughing that sometimes occurs.

3. When the cannula enters the larynx, slide cannula off the needle trochar and hold it in place while the TLJV is connected to the proximal port of the cannula (Figure A-9).

4. Immediately ventilate the patient using 1- to 5-second bursts of oxygen from the 50-psi manual source. Ventilate at a rate of at least 20 per minute, that is, an inspiratory/expiratory ratio of 1:2 (Figure A-10).

5. If a tie is available, fix the cannula in place. Tape can also be used, but you must fasten it firmly to the cannula and then around the patient's neck. Apply firm pressure at the site of insertion to reduce the small amount of subcutaneous emphysema that usually occurs with this technique.

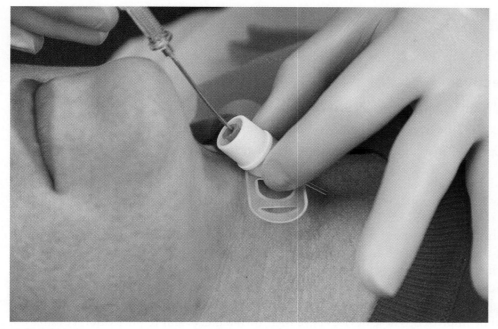

FIGURE A-9 Cannula is distally slid off the needle when membrane is punctured.

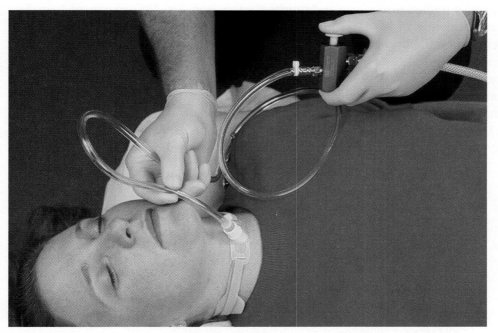

FIGURE A-10 Patient is ventilated indefinitely with 1- to 5-second bursts of oxygen from a 50-psi source at a rate of 20/min.

OPTIONAL SKILL 4: Pharyngotracheal Lumen Airway

Objectives

Upon completion of this Skill Station, you should be able to:

1. Explain the five essential points about use of this airway.
2. Correctly insert the pharyngotracheal lumen airway (PtL).

Introduced in the early 1970s, blind insertion airway devices (BIADs) were designed for use by EMS personnel who were not trained to intubate the trachea. All of these devices (PtL, Combitube, Rusch Easy Tube, and KING LT-D airway) are designed to be inserted into the pharynx without the need for a laryngoscope to visualize where the tube is going. All of these devices have a tube with an inflatable cuff that is designed to seal the esophagus, thus preventing vomiting and aspiration of stomach contents as well as preventing gastric distention during bag-valve mask or demand-valve mask ventilation. It was also thought that by sealing the esophagus, more air would enter the lungs and ventilation would be improved. These devices have their own dangers and require careful evaluation to be sure that they are in the correct position. None of the BIADs are equal to the endotracheal tube, which has become the invasive airway of choice for advanced EMS providers.

The pharyngotracheal lumen (PtL) airway is an airway developed for EMS providers who are not trained to perform endotracheal intubation. The PtL consists of a smaller-diameter long tube inside of a short large-diameter tube (Figure A-11). The longer tube goes either into the trachea or the esophagus, while the shorter tube opens into the lower pharynx. Each tube has a cuff; the longer tube's cuff seals the esophagus or trachea, and the shorter tube's cuff seals the oropharynx so that there is no air leak when you ventilate the patient. You insert the PtL blindly into the pharynx, and then you must carefully determine whether the longer tube is in the esophagus or the trachea. If the long tube is in the trachea, you ventilate through it. If the tube is in the esophagus, you ventilate through the larger tube in the pharynx. The PtL has advantages over the obsolete EOA and EGTA in

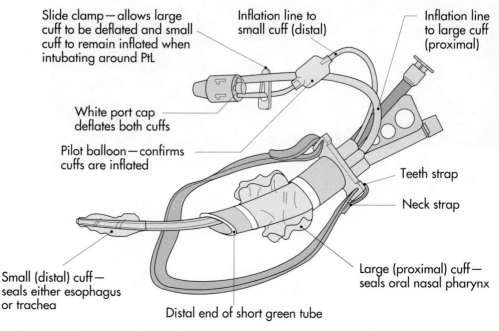

Slide clamp—allows large cuff to be deflated and small cuff to remain inflated when intubating around PtL

Inflation line to small cuff (distal)

Inflation line to large cuff (proximal)

White port cap deflates both cuffs

Pilot balloon—confirms cuffs are inflated

Teeth strap

Neck strap

Small (distal) cuff— seals either esophagus or trachea

Distal end of short green tube

Large (proximal) cuff— seals oral nasal pharynx

FIGURE A-11 Parts of the PtL airway.

that you don't require extra hands to keep a seal with a face mask; also, the cuff in the pharynx prevents blood and mucus from entering the airway from above.

ESSENTIAL POINTS

You must remember five essential points about the PtL.

- Use the PtL only in patients who are unresponsive and without protective reflexes.
- Do not use it in any patient with injury to the esophagus (e.g., caustic ingestions) or in children who are below the age of 15 and of average height and weight.
- Pay careful attention to proper placement. Unrecognized intratracheal placement of the long tube is a lethal complication that produces complete airway obstruction. Such an occurrence is not always easy to detect, and the results are catastrophic. One of the great disadvantages of this airway is that you can determine correct placement only by auscultation and observation of chest movement and both may be quite unreliable in the prehospital setting. Use of capnography to confirm airway placement and monitor position of the airway is recommended.
- You must insert gently and without force.
- If the patient regains consciousness, you must remove the PtL, as it will cause retching and vomiting.

TECHNIQUE

The airway is relatively easily inserted and must never be forced. In the supine patient the following procedure is used.

1. Ventilate with mouth-to-mask or bag-valve mask and suction the pharynx before insertion of the airway.
2. Prepare the airway by checking to be sure that both cuffs are fully deflated, that the long no. 3 tube (Figure A-12) has a bend in the middle, and that the white cap is securely in place over the deflation port located under the no. 1 inflation valve.
3. After liberal lubrication, slide the airway into the oropharynx while the tongue and jaw are pulled forward.
4. Holding the PtL in your free hand so that it curves in the same direction as the natural curvature of the pharynx, advance the airway behind the tongue until the teeth strap contacts the lips and teeth. On very small patients you may have to withdraw the airway so that the teeth strap is up an inch from the teeth. Conversely, on very large patients you may have to insert the teeth strap into the mouth, past the teeth.
5. Immediately inflate both cuffs. Make sure that the white cap is in place over the deflation port located under the inflation valve. Deliver a sustained ventilation into the inflation valve. You can detect failure of the cuffs to inflate properly by failure of the external pilot balloon to inflate or by hearing or feeling air escape from the patient's mouth and nose. This usually means that one of the cuffs is torn and that the airway must be removed and replaced. When you determine that the cuffs are inflating, continue inflation until you get a good seal.
6. Immediately determine whether the long no. 3 tube is in the esophagus or the trachea. First ventilate through the short no. 2 tube. If you see the chest rise, hear breath sounds, feel good compliance, and hear no breath sounds over the epigastrium, the long no. 3 tube is in the esophagus, and you should continue ventilating through the no. 2 tube.

A

B

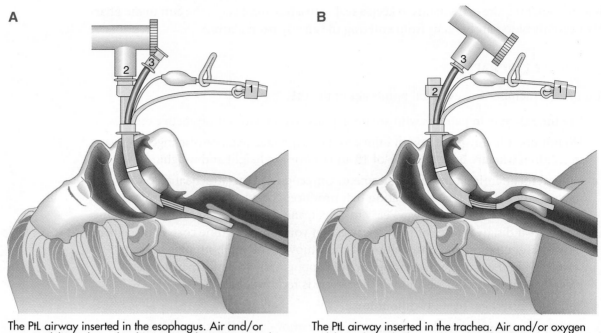

The PtL airway inserted in the esophagus. Air and/or oxygen delivered into the short no. 2 tube passes into the lungs. An inflated cuff at the end of the long no. 3 tube seals the esophagus, while another inflated cuff seals the oropharynx and prevents air loss from the mouth and nose.

The PtL airway inserted in the trachea. Air and/or oxygen is delivered into the long no. 3 tube after the stylet is removed. The inflated cuff at the end of the long tube keeps air from leaking from the trachea into the esophagus. The large cuff that is sealing the oropharynx serves as a secondary seal.

FIGURE A-12 The PtL in place in (a) the esophagus or (b) the trachea.

7. If you do not see the chest rise, hear breath sounds, and feel good compliance when the no. 2 tube is ventilated, the no. 3 tube is probably in the trachea. In this case, remove the stylet from the no. 3 tube and ventilate through the no. 3 tube. If you see the chest rise, hear breath sounds, feel good compliance, and hear no breath sounds over the epigastrium, the no. 3 tube is in the trachea, and you should continue ventilating through the no. 3 tube.

8. When you are sure that the patient is being adequately ventilated, carry the neck strap over the patent's head and tighten it in place. Continually monitor the appearance of the pilot balloon during ventilation. Loss of pressure in the balloon signals a loss of pressure in the cuffs. If you suspect a cuff is leaking, increase pressure by blowing into the no. 1 inflation valve or replace the airway.

If the patient becomes conscious, you must remove the PtL. Remove the white cap from the deflation port to simultaneously deflate both cuffs. Extubation is likely to cause vomiting, so be prepared to suction the pharynx and turn the backboard.

Optional Skill 5: Esophageal Tracheal Combitube

Objectives

Upon completion of this Skill Station, you should be able to:

1. Explain the five essential points about use of this airway.
2. Correctly insert the Combitube.

Introduced in the early 1970s, blind insertion airway devices (BIADs) were designed for use by EMS personnel who were not trained to intubate the trachea. All of these devices (PtL, Combitube, Rusch Easy Tube, and KING LT-D airway) were designed to be inserted into the pharynx without the need for a laryngoscope to visualize where the tube is going. All of these devices have a tube with an inflatable cuff that is designed to seal the esophagus, thus preventing vomiting and aspiration of stomach contents, as well as preventing gastric distention during bag-valve mask or demand-valve mask ventilation. It was also thought that by sealing the esophagus, more air would enter the lungs and ventilation would be improved. These devices have their own dangers and require careful evaluation to be sure that they are in the correct position. None of the BIADs are equal to the endotracheal tube, which has become the invasive airway of choice for advanced EMS providers.

The Combitube is like the PtL airway in that it has a double lumen. However, in the Combitube the two lumens are separated by a partition rather than one being inside of the other (see Figure A-13). One tube is sealed at the distal end, and there are perforations in the area of the tube that would be in the pharynx. When the long tube is in the esophagus, the patient is ventilated through this short tube. The long tube is open at the distal end, and it has a cuff that is blown up to seal the esophagus or the trachea, depending on which it has entered. When inserted, if the long tube goes into the esophagus, the cuff is inflated and the patient is ventilated through the short tube. If the long tube goes into the trachea, the cuff is inflated and the patient is ventilated through the long tube. Like the PtL airway, this device has a pharyngeal balloon that seals the pharynx and prevents blood and mucus from entering the airway from above. The Combitube is somewhat quicker and easier to insert than the PtL airway but, as with the other BIADs, you must be sure that you are ventilating the lungs and not the stomach.

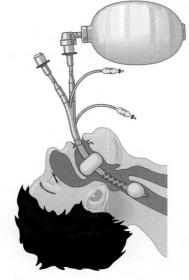

FIGURE A-13 Esophageal placement of the Combitube—ventilate through tube 1.

ESSENTIAL POINTS

You must remember five essential points about the Combitube.

- Use the Combitube only in patients who are unresponsive and without protective reflexes.

- Do not use it in any patient with injury to the esophagus (e.g., caustic ingestions) or in children who are below the age of 15 and of average height and weight.

- Pay careful attention to proper placement. Unrecognized intratracheal placement of the long tube is a lethal complication that produces complete airway obstruction. Such an occurrence is not always easy to detect, and the results are catastrophic. Like the PtL, one of the great disadvantages of this airway is the fact that you can determine correct placement only by auscultation and observation of chest movement and both may be quite unreliable in the prehospital setting. Use of capnography to confirm airway placement and monitor position of the airway is recommended.

- You must insert gently and without force.
- If the patient regains consciousness, you must remove the Combitube, as it will cause retching and vomiting.

TECHNIQUE

1. Insert the tube blindly, watching for the two black rings on the Combitube that are used for measuring the depth of insertion. These rings should be positioned between the teeth and the lips (Figure A-13).

2. Use the large syringe to inflate the pharyngeal cuff with 100 cc of air. When inflated, the Combitube will seat itself in the posterior pharynx behind the hard palate.

3. Use the small syringe to fill the distal cuff with 10 to 15 cc of air.

4. The long tube will usually go into the esophagus. Ventilate through the esophageal connector. It is the external tube that is the longer of the two and is marked no. 1. As with the PtL airway, you must see the chest rise, hear breath sounds, feel good compliance, and hear no breath sounds over the epigastrium to be sure that the long tube is in the esophagus.

5. If you do not see the chest rise, hear breath sounds, feel good compliance, and you hear breath sounds over the epigastrium, the tube has been placed in the trachea (see Figure A-14). In this case, change the ventilator to the shorter tracheal connector, which is marked no. 2. Again you must check to see the chest rise, hear breath sounds, feel good compliance, and hear no breath sounds over the epigastrium in order to be sure that you are ventilating the lungs.

Like the other BIADs, if the patient becomes conscious, you must remove the Combitube. Extubation is likely to cause vomiting, so be prepared to suction the pharynx and turn the backboard.

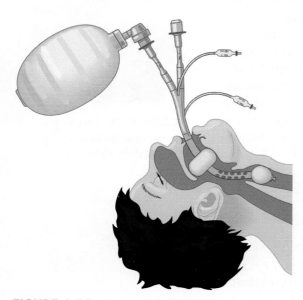

FIGURE A-14 Tracheal placement of the Combitube—ventilate through tube 2.

OPTIONAL SKILL 6: KING LT-D Airway

Objectives

Upon completion of this Skill Station, you should be able to:

1. Explain the six essential points about use of this airway.
2. Correctly insert the KING LT-D airway.

Introduced in the early 1970s, blind insertion airway devices (BIADs) were designed for use by EMS personnel who were not trained to intubate the trachea. All of these devices (PtL, Combitube, Rusch Easy Tube, and KING LT-D airway) were designed to be inserted into the pharynx without the need for a laryngoscope to visualize where the tube is going. All of these devices have a tube with an inflatable cuff that is designed to seal the esophagus, thus helping to prevent vomiting and aspiration of stomach contents, as well as preventing gastric distention during bag-valve mask or demand-valve mask ventilation. It was also thought that by sealing the esophagus, more air would enter the lungs and ventilation would be improved. These devices have their own dangers and require careful evaluation to be sure that they are in the correct position. None of the BIADs are equal to the endotracheal tube, which has become the invasive airway of choice for advanced EMS providers.

The KING LT-D airway differs from the Combitube and the PtL airways in that it has a single lumen (Figure A-15). Once the tube is inserted into the esophagus, both the esophageal and pharyngeal cuffs are inflated and the patient is ventilated through the single tube. With the airway in place you may insert a bougie or a fiberoptic bronchoscope through the ventilating tube and swap the airway for an endotracheal tube. There is also an LTS-D airway that has a port through which you can insert a gastric tube to decompress the stomach. It is inserted exactly the same as the LT-D airway. The KING LT-D airway is quicker and easier to insert than either the PtL airway or the Combitube but, as with the other BIADs, you must be sure that you are ventilating the lungs and not the stomach.

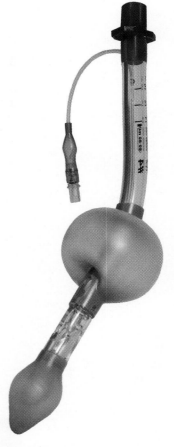

FIGURE A-15 KING LT-D airway.

ESSENTIAL POINTS

You must remember six essential points about the KING LT-D airway.

- Use the KING LT-D airway only in patients who are unresponsive and without protective reflexes.
- Do not use it in any patient with injury to the esophagus (e.g., caustic ingestions) or in children who are below the age of 15 and of average height and weight.
- Do not use in patients who are less than 4 feet tall.
- Pay careful attention to proper placement. Unrecognized intratracheal placement of the tube is a lethal complication that produces complete airway obstruction. Such an occurrence is not always easy to detect, and the results are catastrophic. Capnography is recommended for confirmation of tube placement.
- You must insert gently and without force.
- If the patient regains consciousness, you must remove the airway, as it will cause retching and vomiting.

TECHNIQUE

1. Select the correct size KING LT-D airway.
   - Size 3 (yellow connector color) is for adults 4 to 5 feet in height.
   - Size 4 (red connector color) is for adults 5 to 6 feet in height.
   - Size 5 (purple connector color) is for adults greater than 6 feet in height.

2. Test cuff inflation system for air leak.

3. Apply water-soluble lubricant to the distal tip.

4. Hold the airway at the connector with your dominant hand. With your nondominant hand, hold the mouth open and apply a chin lift. Using a lateral approach, introduce the tip into the mouth (Figure A-16).

5. Advance the tip behind the base of the tongue while rotating the tube back to the midline so that the blue orientation line faces the chin of the patient (Figure A-17).

6. Without exerting excessive force, advance tube until base of connector is aligned with teeth or gums (Figure A-18).

7. Hold the KLT 900 Cuff Pressure Gauge in nondominant hand, inflate the cuffs of the KING LT-D with air to a pressure of 60 cm H_2O (Figure A-19). If a cuff pressure gauge is not available and a syringe is being used to inflate the KING LT-D, inflate cuffs with the minimum volume necessary to seal the airway at the peak ventilatory pressure employed (just seal volume). Typical inflation volumes are as follows:
   - Size 3 (yellow) = 45–60 mL
   - Size 4 (red) = 60–80 mL
   - Size 5 (purple) = 70–90 mL

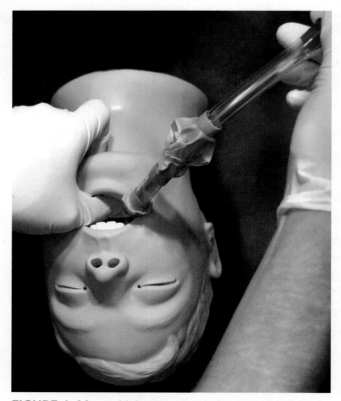

FIGURE A-16   Hold the KLT-D with dominant hand. With nondominant hand, open mouth and apply chin lift. Using a lateral approach, introduce tip into mouth.

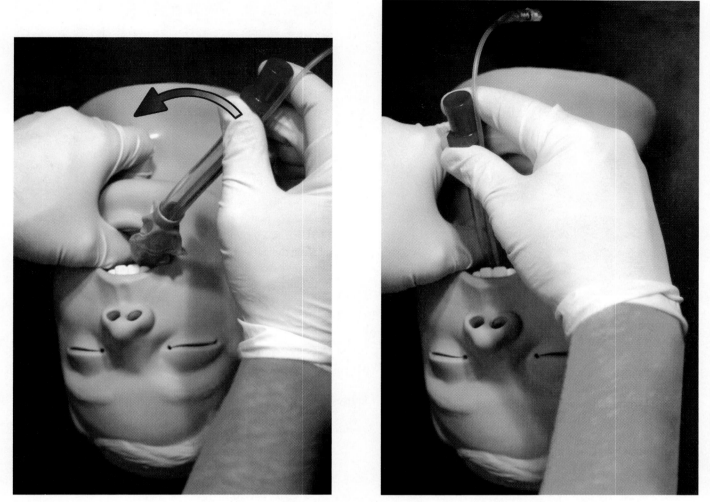

FIGURE A-17 Advance the tip behind the base of the tongue while rotating the tube back to the midline so that the blue orientation line faces the chin of the patient.

8. Attach the resuscitator bag to the airway. While bagging the patient, gently withdraw the tube until ventilation becomes easy and free flowing (Figure A-20). Adjust cuff inflation if necessary to obtain a seal of the airway at the peak ventilatory pressure employed. You must see the chest rise, hear breath sounds, feel good compliance, and hear no breath sounds over the epigastrium to be sure that the KING LT-D airway is correctly placed. However, this method is unreliable and thus capnography is recommended for confirming and monitoring the position of the tube.

Like the other BIADs, if the patient becomes conscious, you must remove the airway. Extubation is likely to cause vomiting, so be prepared to suction the pharynx and turn the backboard.

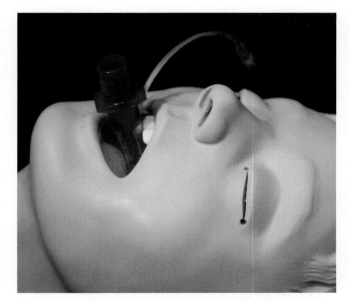

FIGURE A-18 Gently advance the tube until the base of connector is aligned with teeth or gums.

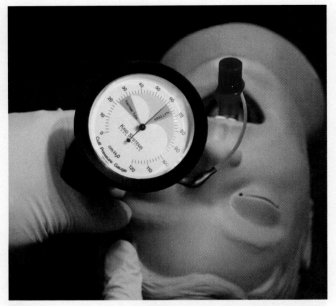

FIGURE A-19 Holding the KLT 900 Cuff Pressure Gauge in nondominant hand, inflate the cuffs of the KING LT-D with air to a pressure of 60 cm H$_2$O. If a cuff pressure gauge is not available and a syringe is being used to inflate the KING LT-D, inflate cuffs with the minimum volume necessary to seal the airway at the peak ventilatory pressure employed (just seal volume). Typical inflation volumes are as follows:
– Size 3 (yellow) = 45–60 mL
– Size 4 (red) = 60–80 mL
– Size 5 (purple) = 70–90 mL

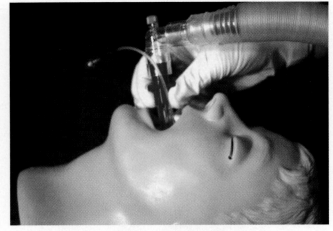

FIGURE A-20 Attach the BVM to the airway. While bagging the patient, gently withdraw the tube until ventilation becomes easy. Adjust cuff inflation if necessary to obtain a seal of the airway.

OPTIONAL SKILL 7: Laryngeal Mask Airway

Objectives

Upon completion of this Skill Station, you should be able to:

1. Explain the five essential points about use of the airway.
2. Correctly insert the laryngeal mask airway (LMA).

The laryngeal mask airway (LMA) was developed for use as an alternative to the face mask for achieving and maintaining control of the airway during routine anesthetic procedures in the operating room. Since it does not protect the airway against vomiting and aspiration, it was meant to be used in patients who had been fasting and thus had an empty stomach. It was later found to be useful in the emergency situation when intubation is not possible and you cannot ventilate with a bag-valve mask. It may prevent having to do a surgical procedure to open the airway. The LMA is another BIAD but differs from the others in that it was never designed to seal the esophagus and was not originally meant for emergency use. It is not equal to the endotracheal tube, and should only be used when efforts to intubate the trachea have been unsuccessful and ventilation is compromised.

WARNINGS

- Use the LMA only in patients who are unresponsive and without protective reflexes. If the patient still has a gag reflex, the LMA may cause laryngospasm or vomiting.
- Do not use it in any patient with injury to the esophagus (e.g., caustic ingestions) or in children who are less than 30 kg.
- Lubricate only the posterior surface of the LMA to avoid blockage of the aperture or aspiration of the lubricant.
- Patients should be adequately monitored (constant visual monitoring, cardiac monitor, and if possible, pulse oximeter) at all times during LMA use.
- To avoid trauma to the airway, force should never be used during LMA insertion.
- Never overinflate the cuff after insertion. Overinflation may cause malposition, loss of seal, or trauma. Cuff pressure should be checked periodically, especially if nitrous oxide is used.
- If airway problems persist or ventilation is inadequate, the LMA should be removed and reinserted or an airway established by other means.
- The LMA does not prevent aspiration if the patient vomits. The presence of a nasogastric tube does not rule out the possibility of regurgitation and may even make regurgitation more likely because the tube makes the esophageal sphincter incompetent.
- If the patient regains consciousness, you must remove the LMA, as it will cause retching and vomiting.

TABLE A-1 *Cuff Volumes for LMA*

LMA Size	Patient Size	Maximum Cuff Volumes (Air Only)
3	Children >30 kg and small adults	20 mL
4	Normal and large adults	30 mL
5	Large adults	40 mL

TECHNIQUE

1. Ventilate with mouth-to-mask or bag-valve mask and suction the pharynx before insertion of the airway.

2. Remove the valve tab and check the integrity of the LMA cuff by inflating with the maximum volume of air (Table A-1).

3. The cuff of the LMA should be tightly deflated using the enclosed syringe so that it forms a flat oval disk with the rim facing away from the aperture. This can be accomplished by pressing the mask with its hollow side down on a sterile flat surface (Figure A-21a). Use the fingers to guide the cuff into an oval shape and attempt to eliminate any wrinkles on the distal edge of the cuff. A completely flat and smooth leading edge facilitates insertion, avoids contact with the epiglottis, and is important to ensure success when positioning the device (Figure A-21b).

4. Lubricate the posterior surface of the LMA with a water-soluble lubricant just before insertion.

5. Preoxygenate (do not hyperventilate) the patient.

6. If there is no danger of spinal injury, position the patient with the neck flexed and the head extended. If the mechanism of injury suggests the potential for spinal injury, the head and neck must be maintained in a neutral position.

7. Hold the LMA like a pen, with the index finger placed at the junction of the cuff and the tube (Figure A-21c). Under direct vision, press the tip of the cuff upward against the hard palate and flatten the cuff against it (Figure A-21d). The black line on the airway tube should be oriented anteriorly toward the upper lip.

8. Use the index finger to guide the LMA, pressing upward and backward toward the ears in one smooth movement (Figure A-21e). Advance the LMA into the hypopharynx until definite resistance is felt (Figure A-21f).

9. Before removing the index finger, gently press down on the tube with the other hand to prevent the LMA from being pulled out of place (Figure A-21g).

10. Without holding the tube, inflate the cuff with just enough air to obtain a seal. The maximum volumes are shown in Table A-1.

11. Connect the LMA to the bag-valve mask and employ manual ventilation of less than 20 cm H_2O (this precludes use of a FROPVD unless you use one that allows you to set the pressure). As with the BIADs, you must see the chest rise, hear breath sounds, feel good compliance, and hear no breath sounds over the epigastrium to be sure that the LMA is correctly placed. However, this method is unreliable, so use of capnography to confirm and monitor tube position is recommended.

12. Insert a bite block (not an oropharyngeal airway) and secure the LMA with tape (Figure A-21h). Remember that the LMA does not protect the airway from aspiration. If the patient becomes conscious, the LMA must be removed. Extubation is likely to cause vomiting; be prepared to suction the pharynx and turn the backboard.

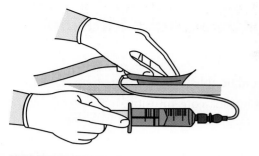

FIGURE A-21A

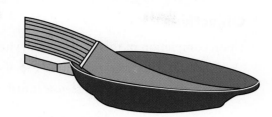

FIGURE A-21B

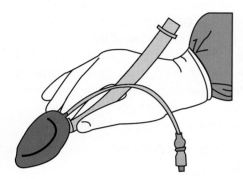

FIGURE A-21C

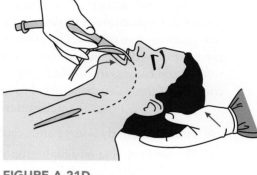

FIGURE A-21D

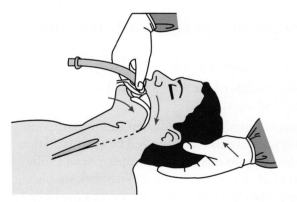

FIGURE A-21E

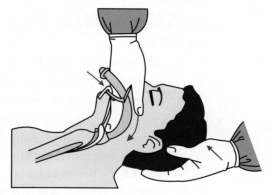

FIGURE A-21F

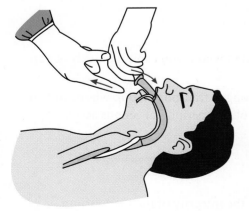

FIGURE A-21G

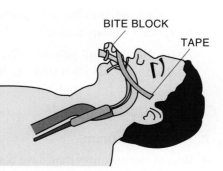

BITE BLOCK

TAPE

FIGURE A-21H

FIGURE A-21 Insertion of the laryngeal mask airway.

OPTIONAL SKILL 8: Adult Intraosseous Infusion

Objectives

Upon completion of this Skill Station, you should be able to:

1. Explain the indications for the use of adult intraosseous infusion.
2. Perform an adult intraosseous infusion.

Standard vascular access in the adult patient involves the peripheral venous system. Under conditions common in trauma, the peripheral veins often collapse. In the past, adult intraosseous infusion was used in some cases to give medications, but the flow rate was too slow to be used for fluid resuscitation of adult trauma patients. Now devices are available that allow adult intraosseous infusion to be used for fluid resuscitation and for administration of medications. The first of these devices (F.A.S.T. 1) makes use of the sternum but now there are two other devices that use the proximal tibia. They are not included here but can be reviewed by going to their respective websites: the EZ-IO (battery-powered drill) at www.vitaid.com/usa/ez-io/index/htm and BIG (Bone Injection Gun) at www.waismed.com. All of these devices may fail to reach the marrow cavity in very obese persons.

The F.A.S.T. 1 uses the sternum for the intraosseous site because of the following:

- The sternal body is large and relatively flat, and can be readily located.
- The sternum retains a high proportion of red marrow.
- It has a thinner, more uniform cortical bone overlying a relatively uniform marrow space.
- It is less likely to be fractured than the extremities, particularly at the level of the manubrium.
- It is usually exposed, or easy to expose, in a trauma patient.
- The recommended infusion site on the midline of the manubrium, 15 mm below the sternal notch, is easy to locate and landmark.
- There is no appreciable time lag between central venous infusion and intraosseous infusion of most substances. For adult trauma patients who need fluid resuscitation or medications and for whom you are unable to quickly obtain a peripheral IV line, this device may be the vascular access of choice. It is fast (60–90 seconds), simple (failure rate <5 percent), safe (the device positions the infusion tube at a controlled depth), and has adequate flow rates (30 mL/min by gravity, 125 mL/min by pressure cuffed IV bag, and 250 mL/min by syringe).

INDICATIONS

- The adult patient who is in cardiac arrest and in whom you cannot quickly obtain peripheral venous access
- Hypovolemic adult patients who have a prolonged transport and in whom you are unable to quickly (two sticks or 90 seconds) obtain peripheral venous access

CONTRAINDICATIONS

- Fractured sternum
- Recent sternotomy (may have compromised the integrity of the manubrium or its vascularization)
- Severe osteoporosis or bone-softening conditions

ESSENTIAL POINTS ON ADULT INTRAOSSEOUS INFUSION

- As with all advanced procedures, this technique must be accepted local protocol, and you must obtain medical direction orally or by protocol before performing.

- If infiltration occurs (rare), you must abort the procedure. This is the only bone in which this device is used.

- Potential complications are subperiostial infusion due to improper placement, osteomyelitis, sepsis, fat embolism, and marrow damage. Studies have shown these complications to be rare. However, good aseptic technique is important, just as with IV therapy.

TECHNIQUE

1. Place the target patch at the site. The single recommended site of insertion is the adult manubrium, on the midline and 1.5 cm (5/80) below the sternal notch. The site is prepped with aseptic technique, and the index finger is used to align the target patch with the patient's sternal notch (Figure A-22a).

2. With the patch securely attached to the patient's skin, the introducer is placed in the target zone, perpendicular to the skin. A firm push on the introducer releases the infusion tube into the correct site and to the right penetration depth. The introducer is pulled straight back, exposing the infusion tube and a two-part support sleeve that falls away (Figure A-22b).

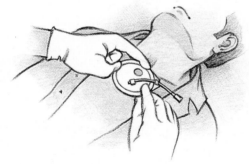

a. Placing the target patch at the site

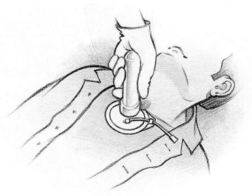

b. Inserting the infusion tube

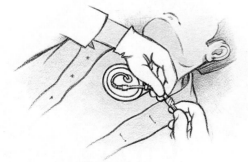

c. Connecting the fluid source

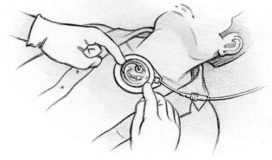

d. Applying the protector dome

FIGURE A-22 Insertion of the F.A.S.T. 1 adult intraosseous infusion device. *(Courtesy of Pyng Medical Corporation)*

3. Correct placement is verified by observation of marrow entering the infusion tube. The infusion tube is joined to tubing on the patch, which is connected to a purged source of fluid. Fluid can now flow to the patient (Figure A-22c).

4. The protector dome is pressed down firmly over the target patch to engage the Velcro fastening. The site is clearly visible through the dome, the infusion tube and connection tubing move easily with any strain on the skin, and the site requires no further stabilization while the patient is transported (Figure A-22d).

OPTIONAL SKILL 9: Rapid Sequence Intubation

Objectives

Upon completion of this Skill Station, you should be able to:

1. Discuss the situations where rapid sequence intubation (RSI) can be of benefit to the patient.
2. Discuss the situations were RSI can be detrimental to the patient.
3. Correctly perform RSI.

The importance in appropriately managing the airway of the trauma patient cannot be overemphasized. Loss of airway remains the leading cause of early preventable trauma deaths, and hypoxia has been shown to worsen outcomes for trauma patients, especially those with closed head injury. The indications for active airway management and the options managing the airway are well covered in Chapter 4 and the skills for managing the airway are detailed in Chapter 5 of the text. All responders should be familiar with the materials in these two chapters and be able to apply this care.

When EMS first obtained ability to perform endotracheal intubation, it was essentially performed on "dead" patients: unresponsive and apneic. Not all patients fit this situation and airway management of patients who were agitated, combative, or had airway trauma had to wait until they deteriorated and became unresponsive.

It is important to remember that all airways managed in the field meet the American Society of Anesthesiology's definition of a "difficult airway." Thus the responder must have many "tools" in the toolbox, available to manage the airway of the trauma patient. Popular in EMS circles, one tool in the toolbox for airway management (one that addresses the problem above) is rapid sequence intubation (actually *rapid sequence induction*). The term *rapid sequence intubation* is a misnomer because this procedure is certainly not rapid (Figure A-23). Because of this, it can adversely affect patient outcome by prolonging scene time. Unless there is a critical need, this procedure should be performed during transport. In the urban setting where there are short transport times there are almost no indications for this procedure.

A variant of the practice of rapid sequence induction used by anesthesiologists when confronted with a nonfasting patient, the technique allows the intubator to achieve conditions that improve the likelihood of intubating the patient, while minimizing the risks of aspiration, by rapidly administering a sedative and paralytic to improve intubating conditions. Numerous studies have shown that EMS personnel can be effectively taught to use this technique and apply it in the field setting. Other studies have shown the real danger in the patient having prolonged hypoxia during this procedure, so constant recording of pulse oximetry reading should be done and there should be a strict Quality Improvement program that monitors intubation time, oxygenation of the patient, and scene time.

The actual technique of RSI is quite simple. The difficult part for EMS personnel is to recognize the patient who should not undergo RSI. The worst thing you can do in airway management is take a spontaneously breathing patient and place her into a "can't intubate and can't ventilate" situation. All personnel who utilize RSI should be familiar with and able to use one of the many blind insertion airway devices (BIAD) and also should be able to perform a cricothyrotomy if unable to ventilate or intubate the patient. Lastly (but most important of all), all EMS personnel should be able to manage an airway using a BVM. Remember BLS comes before ALS. Lastly, many EMS providers erroneously see use of RSI and even intubation as a measure of "prestige." It is simply one of many tools available to us to manage an airway. The real trick is to choose the right one for your patient and correctly apply it.

Rapid Sequence Intubation

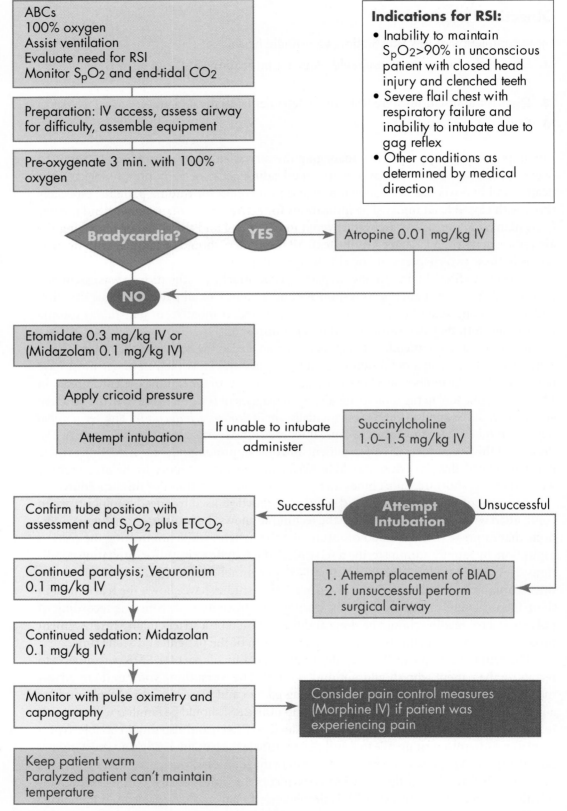

FIGURE A-23 Steps in rapid sequence intubation.

At the time of publication, several studies have called into question the utility of this skill in the field setting. The decision to implement the use of RSI by an EMS system should be carefully reviewed, especially with respect to issues of skill retention, transport times, and the availability of alternative airway methods. Any system using RSI must have in place a strong educational and quality improvement program.

TECHNIQUE

The ideal approach uses the six Ps: Preparation, Preoxygenation, Premedicate, Paralyze, Pass the tube, confirm Position.

1. *Preparation.*   First, evaluate the difficulty you may experience when you try to intubate. Do this by using the Mallampati score (see Chapter 4). If the patient appears to be particularly difficult to intubate, you would be better served using a BIAD or BVM than struggling with a paralyzed, apneic, hypoxic patient. If you decide to perform RSI, you should have a plan for an escape airway should intubation be unsuccessful. All necessary equipment, including suction, should be readily available and checked.

    Proper positioning is an important part of preparation. While the EMS environment often precludes placing the patient at a good height, on a stretcher, in the sniffing position, any steps we can take to better position ourselves so that we have the best view are helpful. Given that many of our patients are in spinal motion restriction, one "positioning step" we can take, just prior to intubation, is to remove or loosen the cervical collar and apply in-line stabilization. This will allow you to move the jaw forward and improve visualization of the cords.

2. *Preoxygenation.*   Since the patient will be rendered apneic, hypoxia will rapidly follow. To extend the time for intubation, nitrogen in the lungs is "washed out" by having the patient breathe 100 percent oxygen for 2–3 minutes. Washout of the nitrogen allows the patient to tolerate up to 5 minutes of apnea (only 2–3 minutes in children) during intubation without becoming hypoxic. In patients with airway compromise or other problems, ventilations can be assisted, though care should be made not to ventilate with too much force, thus reducing the risk of insufflating air into the stomach and thus regurgitation of stomach contents leading to aspiration. Application of cricoid pressure (Sellick's maneuver) will help reduce this, as well as reduce risk of aspiration as the lower esophageal sphincter relaxes after administration of paralytic. All patients should be placed on a cardiac monitor, a pulse oximeter, and a capnometer at this time, if not previously done.

3. *Premedicate.*   Both the act of intubation and some paralytics can raise intracranial pressure. Though advocated in the past, use of IV lidocaine prior to intubation has been found to be of no benefit in the field setting. Pediatric patients given succinylcholine may develop bradycardia. Most experts feel that pediatric patients and those adults receiving a repeat dose of succinylcholine should receive 0.1 mg/kg of atropine. Remember also in the pediatric patient that the use of a length-based system, such as the Broselow tape or similar, can decrease dosing errors. Depolarizing paralytic agents like succinylcholine can cause fasiculations, which can cause a rise in both intracranial pressure and intraocular pressure as well as be uncomfortable for the patient. A nondepolarizing blocking agent such as vecuronium at 0.01 mg/kg can be given at 3 minutes prior to administering the paralytic agent. Because it adds time to the process in what is often a time-critical situation, many field providers omit this step.

    The last premedication is the sedative. This ensures that the patient is not awake while paralyzed. Benzodiazepines such as versed at 0.1 mg/kg can be used, though

TABLE A-2 *Contraindications for Use of Succinylcholine*

Absolute
- History of Malignant Hyperthermia
- Burns over 24 hours old
- Crush Injury over 48 hours old
- Stroke, Cord Injury > 7 days < 6 months
- Sepsis over 7 days
- Myopathies, Denervating Diseases

etomidate (0.3 mg/kg) is a more common sedative agent and has the advantages in that it has minimal effects on hemodynamics. Some trauma surgeons do not support use of etomidate due to reported adrenal suppression, with even a single dose.

4. *Paralyze.* Two types of paralytics are available. A depolarizing agent, such as succinylcholine is the preferred agent due to rapid onset of action and rapid degradation. At a dose of 1 to 1.5 mg/kg (2 mg/kg in children), intubating conditions are achieved within 90 seconds of administration and is cleared within 5 minutes. Contraindications to use of depolarizing agents are listed in Table A-2.

   Nondepolarizing agents have a longer onset and paralysis lasts longer. The fastest acting agent is rocuronium (0.5 mg/kg adult; 0.75 mg/kg in children). Vecuronium 0.1 mg/kg can be used to maintain paralysis after intubation is successful.

5. *Pass the Tube.* Once intubating conditions are achieved, pass the tube. Aids in the process include the use of a stylet, the gum elastic bougie, and external laryngeal manipulation.

6. *Confirm Position.* Use techniques described in Chapter 5. Use of capnography is mandatory so that inadvertent tube dislodgement can be detected. See ideal timeline for RSI in Table A-3.

TABLE A-3 *Suggested Rapid Sequence Intubation Timeline*

Time	Action
	Identify need for intubation
	Brief history if possible to rule out contraindications
−7 minutes	Prepare equipment and patient
−5 minutes	Preoxygenate
−3 minutes	Pretreat and sedate
0	Paralyze
3/4 to 1.5 minutes	Pass the tube
1.5 to 2 minutes	Confirm position
> 2 minutes	Postintubation care

BIBLIOGRAPHY

1. Davis, D. P., D. Hoyt, M. Ochs, et al. 2003. The effect of paramedic rapid sequence intubation on outcome in patients with severe traumatic brain injury. *Journal of Trauma* 54(3): 444–53.

2. Nowicki, T., S. London. 2005. Management of the difficult airway. EM Reports, American Health Consultants 26: 208–22.

3. Robinson, N., M. Clancy. 2001. In patients with head injury undergoing rapid sequence intubation, does pretreatment with intravenous lignocaine/lidocaine lead to an improved neurological outcome? A review of the literature. *Emergency Medicine Journal* 18(6): 453–57.

4. Sivestri, S., G. Ralls, B. Krauss, et al. 2005. The effectiveness of out-of-hospital use of continuous end-tidal carbon dioxide monitoring on the rate of unrecognized misplaced intubation within a regional emergency medical services system. *Annals of Emergency Medicine* 45(5): 497–503.

5. Stewart, C. 2002. *Advanced airway management.* Upper Saddle River, NJ: Brady-Pearson Education.

6. Walls, R., et al. 2004. *Manual of emergency airway management,* 2nd ed. Philadelphia: Lippincott Williams and Wilkins.

7. Wang, H., et al. 2005. Procedural experience with out-of-hospital endotracheal intubation. *Critical Care Medicine* 33(8): 1718–21.

8. Wang, H. E., D. Davis, R. O'Connor, R. Domeier. 2006. Drug assisted intubation in the prehospital setting. *Prehospital Emergency Care,* 10(2): 261–71.

9. Wang H. E., J. Li, B. Dannenberg. 2006. Managing the airway of the pediatric trauma patient: Meeting the challenge. Trauma Reports, American Health Consultants 7(2).

Communications with the Receiving Hospital

Corey M. Slovis, MD, FACP, FACEP

Objectives

Upon completion of this appendix, you should be able to:

1. Discuss the four-phase communications policy.
2. Discuss the 12 steps that make up those phases.
3. Provide accurate and succinct patient care reports to your receiving hospital.

COMMUNICATION BASICS

It is imperative that you provide your receiving hospital or base station physician with an accurate, succinct radio (or telephone) report. This is an essential skill to develop. In general, the physician or nurse at the other end of the radio transmission will not be able to focus on more than three to five key bits of information. Thus, before beginning your call, spend a few moments thinking about what specifics of the history and physical exam need to be transmitted. The purpose of receiving hospital/base station communication is not to give all of the available findings to the physician, but to transmit only that information needed for appropriate care in the field, and to ready the emergency department for patient arrival. If you are requesting medications or procedures, then your report should focus on the information that justifies your request.

When giving your report, no matter how emergent the situation, speak clearly and avoid speaking rapidly or in an emotional, high-pitched voice. However, using a slow monotone voice in reporting a cardiac arrest would be inappropriate as well. You should try to convey the urgency of the situation in a professional manner. The radio microphone should be held a few inches from your mouth to allow accurate voice transmission but not so far (more than 6 inches) as to allow interference from other noises at the scene.

The following format for communications is designed to maximize the efficient transfer of information (see Tables B-1 and B-2). It may also be used for calls not involving trauma.

FOUR-PHASE COMMUNICATIONS POLICY

The ITLS communications policy is divided into four parts, having a total of 12 steps. The first of these phases is devoted to the EMS unit confirming radio contact with a specific hospital or base station.

TABLE B-1 *ITLS Communications Format*

Phase I: Establishing Contact

1. **Initiation of call**
   EMS service
   Level of function (basic, paramedic, etc.)
   Unit number
   Medical direction facility being contacted

2. **Receiving facility response**
   Name of facility
   Name and title of radio operator
   Renaming of calling EMS service

Phase II: In-the-Field Report

3. **Reidentification**
   EMS service
   Level of function (basic, paramedic, etc.)
   Unit number

4. **Chief complaint/on-scene report**
   One brief sentence
   Includes age, sex, complaint, and/or mechanism of injury

5. **Life-saving resuscitation**
   Patient's response to life-saving maneuvers

6. **Vital signs/primary survey abnormalities**
   Vital signs in stable patient
   or
   Primary Survey in unstable patient

7. **ETA**
   State ETA

8. **Request for orders**
   State what is desired
   or
   State "no orders requested"

Phase III: Base Station (Hospital) Directed Activity

9. **Physician response**
   Agree or deny or state desired orders
   Request for additional history and/or information

10. **Rescuer response**
    Clarification or response to requested maneuver or therapy

Phase IV: Sign-Off

11. **EMS unit sign-off**

12. **Base station sign-off**

TABLE B-2 *Do's and Don'ts of Successful Radio Communications*

Do's
- Think about your report before making radio contact.
- Be brief and concise.
- Talk calmly and clearly.
- Relate only the key points of the history—don't give every single fact you've learned about the patient.
- State the patient's primary problem and what you are requesting early in the call.
- Ask questions if you are unsure of the base station's reply.
- Ask for clarification on therapies you think are wrong or dangerous.
- Call your supervisor for "unresolvable" problems.

Don'ts
- Don't make a speech.
- Don't ramble.
- Don't use jargon, codes, or abbreviations.
- Don't significantly alter how you normally talk.
- Don't assume anything.
- Never give a therapy you think is dangerous BEFORE further clarification.
- Don't make unprofessional comments that will embarrass you when the tape is replayed.
- Don't argue over the radio.

Phase I: Contact Phase

Step 1—Identification In attempting to establish radio contact, state what EMS service is calling, the unit's level of function (e.g., basic, paramedic), and the unit's identification number. For example:

> "This is county paramedic unit 501 calling county hospital."

It is important for you to identify your level of function so the physician knows which procedures and medications to consider. The EMS service should be identified, because different services operating in the same area may function with different protocols. The EMS unit's own identification number needs to be included for potential recontacting and for audit purposes. As different hospitals may have the same radio frequency, the specific facility being called should be stated by the caller each time contact is initiated.

Step 2—Facility Response The base station or receiving hospital should now respond by identifying their facility, the person speaking on the radio (including their professional title), and then the call sign of the EMS unit they are addressing. An example might be:

> "This is Dr. Thomas Smith at county hospital. Go ahead county paramedic unit 501."

By restating the EMS unit's service and number, confusion will be minimized when multiple units are communicating with a single receiving facility. It is recommended that hospital-based radio operators identify themselves. This is important because the initial response to an EMS radio call is often not by a physician. It is also important that physicians identify themselves so that you may document who is giving you orders.

Phase II: In-the-Field Report

The second phase of communications is the most important. Here you should give the all-important Primary Survey information and request appropriate orders. If a physician is not on the radio and you will be requiring one for orders or advice, then specifically request that a physician come to the radio console. This phase of communication is divided into the six steps that follow.

Step 3—Reidentification Once contact has been confirmed, the in-the-field report begins by you reidentifying the EMS service, its level of function, and unit number:

> "This is county paramedic unit 501 calling county hospital."

This information may not yet have been recorded or even heard by a physician, if she has just arrived at the radio console.

Step 4—Chief Complaint/On-Scene Report After you have identified your level of function and unit number, the next sentence should provide the receiving facility with the most complete picture of the patient possible. This sentence should include the patient's approximate age, sex, complaint, and/or mechanism of injury. Having information such as the victim's approximate age and sex allows the physician and/or other listeners to form a mental picture of the patient. Similarly, by knowing the chief complaint and/or type of injury, the physician has an idea of the type of emergency she will be handling. Examples of this part of communication might be:

> "We are on the scene with a 23-year-old female restrained driver involved in a deceleration motor-vehicle collision. She is complaining of chest pain."

> "We are on the scene with a 23-year-old female who has a gunshot wound to the chest."

The patient's medications, additional complaints, or more complete description of injuries should not be given at this time.

Step 5—Life-Saving Resuscitation If any emergency maneuvers or life-saving therapy has been performed during the Primary Survey, then it should be reported next. Thus, if an airway maneuver has been performed or CPR started, it should be reported at this point. Examples of this include:

> "The patient's sucking chest wound has been sealed."

> "We have begun CPR and defibrillated the patient."

The result of a finger-stick glucose, if already performed on a comatose patient, should be reported during this phase.

Step 6—Vital Signs/Primary Survey Abnormalities In the next sentence, give vital signs and/or Primary Survey abnormalities. In stable patients with a normal Primary Survey, a complete set of vital signs are blood pressure, pulse, respiratory rate, skin temperature (if pertinent), and oxygen saturation by pulse oximetry (if available; see Chapter 5). A typical communication might be:

> "The patient has a normal Primary Survey with vital signs of blood pressure 130/90, pulse 90, respiration 16, and oxygen saturation of 98 percent on room air."

If, however, there is an abnormal Primary Survey, as many of the specified vital signs as could be obtained should be reported. In this type of unstable patient, problems with airway, breathing, cardiovascular stability, and neurologic disability would be reported to the physician. In this so-called load-and-go type of call, unimportant physical findings, historical facts, or medication usage do not need to be reported at this time. Two examples of typical communication would be:

> "Primary Survey as follows: no palpable pulses present, respiration is 40, chest exam reveals a sucking chest wound; patient is confused and combative, no O_2 saturation can be obtained."

> "Blood pressure is 70 by palpation, pulse is 130 and weak, and patient is very hot and dry. We found him in a warm, enclosed room. Finger-stick blood glucose is 100."

Step 7—Estimated Time of Arrival You should now state how much time it will take to get to the hospital from the present location. If you are en route, this should be reported. If, however, significant additional time is required to extricate or load the patient into the EMS vehicle, this should be specifically stated. Examples of the estimated time of arrival (ETA) phase of communication include:

> "We are en route to your location; our ETA is less than 4 minutes."

> "We are still on-scene and will require 10 to 15 minutes before we begin transport to the hospital."

Step 8—Request for Orders Before relinquishing radio/telephone control to the base station, state what orders are desired, or that no orders are desired, or that the base station physician's help is needed to determine what to do for the patient. Examples of these respective situations include:

> "Requesting two large-bore IVs of normal saline to maintain blood pressure."

> "No orders requested."

> "Base station, how do you advise?"

Phase III: Base Station (Hospital) Directed Activity

In this phase of communication you are no longer in charge of directing the conversation. You should now respond to the physician's approval or denial of orders. In other cases there may be talk back and forth between you and the physician.

Step 9—Physician's Response It is now up to the physician to determine how to proceed with management of the patient. The physician may merely agree with your request by stating:

> "Go ahead with your requested therapy of 0.5 mgs of atropine."

Or the physician may disagree completely:

> "Orders denied. Transport the patient as soon as possible."

Physicians should always try to repeat the specifics of the order to minimize any chance of confusion. With complicated patients, the physician may need more information than you have transmitted. This is not a criticism of the rescuer's radio abilities, but merely a need for the physician to obtain additional information. Examples:

> "Are the patient's neck veins flat or distended?"

> "Does the patient seem to improve in the Trendelenburg position?"

You should be prepared to answer routine questions readily and to perform requested maneuvers.

Step 10—Your Response You should confirm any given orders by repeating them. If the base station has given orders that are incomplete or with which you disagree, it is now appropriate to give additional history or request an order. Examples of these problems include:

"Be advised that the patient has a long history of cardiac problems and is on multiple medications."

"Base Station, did you copy that the patient is hypotensive and that we are requesting an IV of normal saline wide open?"

If you cannot answer a question asked by the base station, then tell the physician. Examples of this type of exchange would be:

"We do not have any available information on downtime."

"We are unable to attempt this. The patient is still trapped inside the vehicle."

Phase IV: Sign-off

The final phase of EMS–base station communications is the sign-off. You should make it very clear that the unit is leaving the medical frequency and returning to dispatch frequency.

Step 11—EMS Unit Sign-off You should now advise the base station that you are ending communications. Although everyone seems to favor a different ending phrase, each EMS service should agree on a common sign-off phrase. The use of a time signal at the end of a comment is recommended but optional. Acceptable closings include:

"Paramedic unit 501 is clear."

"Unit 501 is out at 13:59 hours."

Avoid using code numbers, as many physicians do not understand them or may use similar codes for different purposes; thus "Unit 501 is 10-8 your location code 3" is not recommended, nor is "501, 10-8, 1359."

Step 12—Base Station Closing The base station physician should similarly end communication with the same agreed-upon phrase, for example:

"County hospital clear."

You should try to concentrate on transmitting the most information with the least amount of words.

BIBLIOGRAPHY

1. Browner, B., A. Pollak, C. Gupton (editors). 2002. *Emergency care and transportation of the sick and injured.* 8th ed. Boston: Jones and Bartlett, 280–303.
2. Limmer, D., M. O'Keefe, et al. 2001. *Emergency care.* 9th ed. Upper Saddle River, NJ: Prentice Hall, 279–89.

Documentation: The Patient Care Record

Arlo F. Weltge, MD, MPH, FACEP

Objectives

Upon completion of this appendix, you should be able to:

1. Create a patient care record that chronicles the medical care given, communicates medical information, and provides a permanent record that can be used as evidence that the standard of care was delivered.
2. Discuss when to use an addendum to the record.
3. Discuss what to do if there is a complication or bad result and you did not record pertinent information on the run report.

INTRODUCTION

With the recognition of the important and increasing role of the prehospital care provider has come deserved respect. However, with this recognition comes the expectation of a standard of care and resultant liability when the care does not meet that standard. This appendix shows how to create a record that chronicles the medical care given, communicates medical information, and provides a permanent record that can be used as evidence that the standard of care was delivered. This record also can become the basis for third-party billing and quality improvement efforts.

THE NARRATIVE REPORT

The EMS system narrative report can vary dramatically from being primarily a billing form to an excellent narrative medical record. In most EMS systems the narrative report usually provides enough space for medical documentation to be adequate for the majority of transports, since most runs do not require much more than basic skills and a simple transport. This report can be effective whether based upon paper records or electronic templates, but it does require knowledge and practice.

It is important to use the system narrative report effectively. There should be enough space for a chief complaint, simple history and assessment, and other comments. All narrative reports should be filled out completely for the level of service. Even though the transport may have been "simple," failure to document vital signs, to complete checkoff boxes for the history and physical, and to enter times, events, and other simple information may reflect poorly on the care delivered if the report is ever reviewed.

If the system report does not provide adequate space for a reasonable history and assessment, or if the case is more difficult, for example, requiring intervention or long transport times, or involving potential patient complications, then it may be necessary to include an addendum. The addendum can be a simple form. It requires basic information, including the patient's name, date, identification of the EMS system, and the run identification number. The report should be written at or near the time of the run, and the original must be signed and kept as a regular part of the system's medical records and attached to the regular written report. An example of a simple addendum is shown in Figure C-1.

An addendum can be used for almost any situation or problem. The narrative report, using an addendum, requires more effort, however, since there is not a host of fill-in-the-blank or checkoff boxes to use when creating the report. To document a complex case adequately using the continuation sheet, one needs to be familiar with the general form or sequence of a narrative report. The form is dictated by convention (or otherwise known in

THIS MUST BE ATTACHED TO CORRESPONDING EMS REPORT

DATE _____   HO NO: _____

NAME _____

ATTENDANT: _____

EMT REPORT:	TIME	B.P.	PULSE	RESP. RATE	TEMP.

SIGNATURE X

EMT CONTINUATION

P & S AMBULANCE TEXAS, INC.
7849 ALMEDA
HOUSTON, TEXAS 77054

WHITE - FINANCE, CANARY - HOSPITAL, PINK - SUPERVISOR

FIGURE C-1 Example of an addendum.

the medical community as a generally agreed-upon habit or standard). Effective documentation requires using this convention as well as skill and practice. It is also recognized that a patient care record cannot be comprehensive for all aspects of the patient encounter, so it can be helpful at times to record events or items that might help one recall specific events.

The narrative report should be brief, yet, like the verbal report, relevant and focused. There are times when the clinical problem is confusing and the report must be lengthier, but length does not necessarily reflect accuracy or relevancy. The record should document relevant events and discrepancies and should be created so another reader can reconstruct the events. The report should also justify the action, even if one's impression at the time was wrong. A "mistake" may have been entirely justified given the circumstances at the time, but it often can be justified only if the circumstances are clearly and honestly documented as part of the record.

The report contains the following information, but rarely will include all the information. In fact, it is more important to effectively treat the patient and document that treatment than it is to get all the information while the patient suffers because of lack of treatment or delay in transport. It is reasonable to take brief notes and to fill out the patient care record at the hospital before returning to service. Care of the patient is the provider's first goal.

Contents of the Narrative Report

Contents of a narrative report include: description of the run call, scene description, patient's chief complaint, history of the present illness/injury or symptoms, patient's medical history, findings from the physical exam, any procedures performed, findings from the Ongoing Exams, impression, and priorities (Table C-1).

Run Call Note how the call was dispatched, particularly if there is discrepancy between the dispatch description and the actual findings. It is helpful, for example, to explain delays in transport if a call came in as a routine sick party when actually it was a motor-vehicle collision with multiple victims. Document time whenever possible. The dispatch time is important because, realistically, it may be the last reliable documented time until arrival at the hospital.

Scene Description Document any scene hazards that delay or affect patient treatment or transport. It is easy to forget scene hazards, but delays may affect patient outcomes and the mention of scene hazards may help jog the memory of the run when reading the report at a later time.

TABLE C-1 *Components of the Narrative Report*
1. Run call
2. Scene description
3. Chief complaint
4. History of the present illness/injury or symptoms
5. Past medical history
6. Physical exam
7. Procedures
8. Ongoing Exam
9. Impression
10. Documenting the priorities

The mechanisms should be noted as well. Often this is most effectively done by stick figures (Figure C-2). The EMS personnel are often the only source of the mechanism of injury for subsequent treatment providers. Clear, simple drawings of mechanisms are quick and easy, useful for communicating mechanism and suspicion of occult injuries, and can help jog the memory of the event at a later time.

Chief Complaint Record age, sex, mechanism, chief complaint or injury, and the onset or time of occurrence. These identifiers focus the thought process. If previously mentioned, mechanism does not have to be documented here.

History of the Present Illness/Injury or Symptoms Record relevant positives and negatives. Document any relevant history that you obtain from the patient. If the history does not come from the patient but from another witness, note the source and the specific information from that person, especially when it conflicts with other history.

Additional useful information includes the patient's recollection of the events immediately prior to the incident (such as did the patient faint first and then fall?), prior injuries to the same location (fractured the same leg last year, for example), and any treatment given before your arrival (such as patient pulled from car by bystanders).

Past Medical History Record previous illness, medications, recent surgery, allergies, and when the patient last ate a meal. You are usually not responsible for getting a complete medical history. However, in acutely sick and injured victims, you may be the last person able to get this information before the patient loses consciousness. Again, treating the patient is the most important priority, but gaining useful information may save a number of complications. Other information that can be useful may include relevant family history (any diseases that run in the family) and social history (use of alcohol, tobacco, or other drugs). This should be documented as the SAMPLE history.

S — *Symptoms*

A — *Allergies*

M — *Medications*

P — *Past medical history (other illnesses)*

L — *Last meal*

E — *Events preceding incident*

Physical Exam Record appearance, vital signs, level of consciousness, Primary Survey, and Secondary Survey. A general statement of the appearance helps focus the reader on urgencies (e.g., the patient appeared alert and in no distress or appeared in extreme pain and was ashen and short of breath). The level of consciousness should be documented with the vital signs. This is best done using stimulus and response (responds to voice/pain with moan,

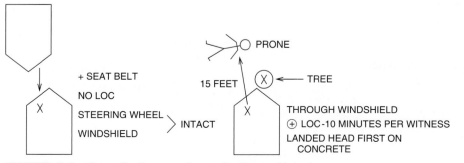

FIGURE C-2 Example diagrams for mechanisms of injuries.

decerebrate posturing). The shorthand method is to note the stimulus that provokes a response using the AVPU scale:

A — *Alert*
V — *Responds to verbal stimuli*
P — *Responds to pain*
U — *Unresponsive*

Document that a complete exam was done. Simply stating the body part (back, abdomen, upper extremity) with a zero or slash afterward can indicate that the part was examined and that there were no significant findings.

One of the easiest and best ways to document the exam in a seriously injured patient is to sequentially note the findings and procedures as one does the Primary and Secondary Surveys. It can be helpful to write "Primary Survey," note findings, describe the resuscitation, and then start the rest of the exam with "Secondary Survey." By doing this, anyone reviewing the record can immediately recognize that you are oriented to trauma assessment, and by assumption, have performed an organized Primary Survey.

One picture is worth a thousand words and may aid the memory at a later date. Diagrams of injuries for locations or for severity (like cuts) should be simple yet contain enough detail to locate site of injury; that is, identify if it is right or left, volar (palmar) or dorsal, part of an extremity, or front or back trunk (Figure C-3).

Procedures (Indication, Procedure, Result) Document the need, describe the procedure, and note the time and patient response when performing an invasive procedure (Table C-2). Any procedure potentially can have a harmful effect, sometimes delayed. All procedures should be documented (for example, stating an IV was started in the right forearm on the second stick protects you from charges of improper technique when the patient later develops a thrombophlebitis from an IV in the left arm). It may not be possible to document every IV attempt. However, when performing invasive treatment procedures such as needle decompressions and needle cricothyroidotomies, you should document the need, the confirming evidence, the procedure, and the effect, even if the effect is a negative result.

Ongoing Exam (Recheck, Changes, Condition on Arrival) Documenting the initial findings establishes a baseline, but Ongoing Exams during long transports, changes while the patient is still in your care, and condition on or just prior to arrival should be recorded as necessary to establish that decompensation did or did not occur while in your care. It is important to remember that as soon as the patient arrives, other people will perform an exam

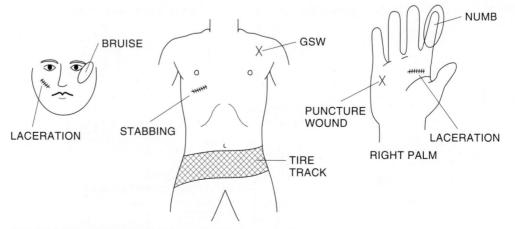

FIGURE C-3 Example diagrams of injuries.

> **TABLE C-2** *Example of Properly Documented Prehospital Procedure*
>
> Patient was pale, short of breath, lost the radial pulse (hypotensive), and had decreased breath sounds on right side (the suspicion). The right chest was tympanic and the trachea was deviated to the left, but neck veins were not distended (confirming findings present or absent). A 14-gauge needle was inserted over the top of the third rib in the midclavicular line with a rush of air. The patient's radial pulse returned and color improved, but respirations were still labored.

and record their findings. Any discrepancies or findings documented in their report will be presumed to have occurred while in your care unless documented by you as not having existed prior to your arrival. Discrepancies place the burden for documentation on you to show that complications did not occur while in transport but at the scene prior to your arrival. This is not to suggest that patients will not decompensate while in your care, but you should notice such decompensation and document that you responded to it.

Impression Your impression may be included to summarize the significant findings. However, care must be taken not to overdiagnose. A tender forearm does not necessarily mean fracture any more than shortness of breath must mean a tension pneumothorax. Impressions should be as "generic" as possible, noting the actual finding, such as pain or bruising (not the diagnosis, such as fracture or pulmonary contusion), and should include relevant information such as distal pulse. Suspicions should be noted (for example, shortness of breath, decreased breath sounds on right, and tender right chest; or tender right forearm, possible fracture, sensation/pulse intact).

Documenting the Priorities The detailed description is designed for the occasion when events allow time for gathering of the information and completion of the Secondary Survey (Table C-3). There are times when urgent priorities limit the evaluation to treating the immediate complications and the exam never gets past the Primary Survey. Care of the

> **TABLE C-3** *Example of Properly Documented Priorities (Just the Facts)*
>
> **Call:** Single MVC.
>
> **Scene:** One victim in roadway, car head-on into pole, patient through windshield supine in roadway.
>
> **Diagram:** See diagram attached.
>
> **Primary Survey:** Mid-twenties, unresponsive male, ashen, grunting respiration with contusions to face, neck, and anterior chest. Absent radial pulse, rapid, thready carotid pulse, sucking wound right chest. Abdomen distended and tender, pelvis stable, extremities appeared to have no major injuries.
>
> Cervical spine controlled manually, no change in respiration with jaw thrust, chest wound covered with an Asherman Chest Seal. Patient log-rolled onto long board. No obvious back injuries. Loaded and transported.
>
> **Ongoing Exam:** Patient's right pupil fixed and dilated, left midposition. Respiration remained rapid and shallow. Patient given oxygen and ventilated by BVM. One 14-gauge IV RL right anticubital started, arrived at city hospital in 3 minutes, patient still with rapid thready carotid pulse.

patient is the first priority. Often the best way to document this is to describe the sequence as it occurs, using the Primary Survey and Secondary Survey and/or Ongoing Exams.

IMPROVING DOCUMENTATION SKILLS

Documentation reflects on the quality of clinical practice. Like clinical care, one can improve skills by practice as well as by observing the better qualities of others. Following are suggestions to help improve the quality of documentation.

- *Practice documentation with critique.* Have somebody else try to reconstruct the events based on your narrative and evaluate what comments were useful and what comments were left out. Sometimes the most obvious events are the easiest to forget to document.
- *Read others' narrative reports* and try to reconstruct the events.
- *Practice anticipating problems and criticisms.* A fractured bone needs to have distal pulse and sensation checked and documented. Invasive procedures, complications, unusual events, or anticipated patient complaints can be noted and justification written. Many complications of invasive procedures, such as infections, may not be discovered for days or weeks. Anticipation of these delayed complications can be an important part of the documentation process.
- *Write to remind yourself.* If there are specific events unique to this run or which will help you distinguish this run from other similar runs, note it in the record.
- *Be professional.* People's lives depend on your care. Your records should reflect that you take your responsibility seriously. The medical record is not a place for humorous or derogatory comments. Use caution when describing the patient. Do not use words that could indicate your care was prejudiced by the patient's presentation. Words such as "the patient was hysterical" would be better written as "the patient was very excited and upset."
- *Be concise.* Longer is not necessarily better. If it is of interest, write it down, but get to the point and write what is important.
- *Review your own records.* Can you reconstruct the events and were complications anticipated? Would this record be a friend in court?
- *Practice quality care,* including caring for the patient. A patient is a potential adversary or advocate. The excitement of the minute often results in a brusque attitude. Ask yourself if you would have been happy with the way you were treated if you had been the patient.

IMPORTANT POINTS ABOUT THE WRITTEN REPORT

The narrative report should be kept as a regular part of the patient's record and should be considered a legal document (Figure C-4). There are some basic rules to follow.

- *Keep the report legible* if handwritten and attempt to be thorough if using an electronic template.
- *Fill in the blanks* as much as possible. Empty boxes imply that the question was not asked. Open spaces imply that information might be added after the fact. However, relevant boxes should be completed only if based upon your assessment. Do not document actions as having been done, if they were not done.
- *Never alter a medical record.* If there is an error on the record, note the error or in a paper record draw a single line through the error and make a note that it was an error and why.

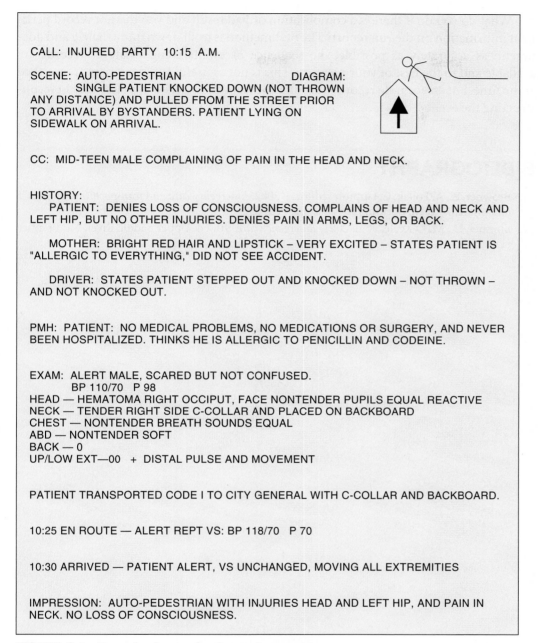

CALL: INJURED PARTY 10:15 A.M.

SCENE: AUTO-PEDESTRIAN   DIAGRAM:
        SINGLE PATIENT KNOCKED DOWN (NOT THROWN
ANY DISTANCE) AND PULLED FROM THE STREET PRIOR
TO ARRIVAL BY BYSTANDERS. PATIENT LYING ON
SIDEWALK ON ARRIVAL.

CC: MID-TEEN MALE COMPLAINING OF PAIN IN THE HEAD AND NECK.

HISTORY:
    PATIENT: DENIES LOSS OF CONSCIOUSNESS. COMPLAINS OF HEAD AND NECK AND
LEFT HIP, BUT NO OTHER INJURIES. DENIES PAIN IN ARMS, LEGS, OR BACK.

    MOTHER: BRIGHT RED HAIR AND LIPSTICK – VERY EXCITED – STATES PATIENT IS
"ALLERGIC TO EVERYTHING," DID NOT SEE ACCIDENT.

    DRIVER: STATES PATIENT STEPPED OUT AND KNOCKED DOWN – NOT THROWN –
AND NOT KNOCKED OUT.

PMH: PATIENT: NO MEDICAL PROBLEMS, NO MEDICATIONS OR SURGERY, AND NEVER
BEEN HOSPITALIZED. THINKS HE IS ALLERGIC TO PENICILLIN AND CODEINE.

EXAM: ALERT MALE, SCARED BUT NOT CONFUSED.
      BP 110/70   P 98
HEAD — HEMATOMA RIGHT OCCIPUT, FACE NONTENDER PUPILS EQUAL REACTIVE
NECK — TENDER RIGHT SIDE C-COLLAR AND PLACED ON BACKBOARD
CHEST — NONTENDER BREATH SOUNDS EQUAL
ABD — NONTENDER SOFT
BACK — 0
UP/LOW EXT—00 + DISTAL PULSE AND MOVEMENT

PATIENT TRANSPORTED CODE I TO CITY GENERAL WITH C-COLLAR AND BACKBOARD.

10:25 EN ROUTE — ALERT REPT VS: BP 118/70   P 70

10:30 ARRIVED — PATIENT ALERT, VS UNCHANGED, MOVING ALL EXTREMITIES

IMPRESSION: AUTO-PEDESTRIAN WITH INJURIES HEAD AND LEFT HIP, AND PAIN IN
NECK. NO LOSS OF CONSCIOUSNESS.

FIGURE C-4   Example of a completed narrative report.

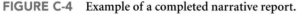

- *Document the call in a timely manner.* Events fade and memory can be challenged. Write the chart as soon as possible after the event. If there is some delay, note the reason.

- *Always be honest on the chart.* Never record observations not made. Never try to cover up actions. (We cannot always be right, but we must always be honest.) The record, your primary source of support, may be discredited if any of your observations are shown not to be accurate.

- *Always clearly distinguish, time, and date any changes or additions to the record.* Changes after the fact may be used against you if the appearance is that you were trying to alter the record in your favor. Such alterations give the appearance of lying.

What do you do if there is a complication or bad result and you did not record pertinent information on the run report? The best method is to sit down immediately and document, as accurately as possible, the sequence of events using whatever records are available and to the best of your memory. This is not as useful as a document transcribed at the time, but an accurate record even after the fact can be useful at a later date in reconstructing the events.

BIBLIOGRAPHY

1. Browner, B., A. Pollak, C. Gupton (editors). 2002. *Emergency care and transportation of the sick and injured.* 8th ed. Boston: Jones and Bartlett, 297–301.
2. Limmer, D., M. O'Keefe, et al. 2001. *Emergency care.* 9th ed. Upper Saddle River, NJ: Prentice Hall, 290–305.

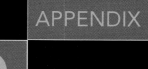

Trauma Care in the Cold

Jere F. Baldwin, MD, FACEP, FAAFP

Objectives

Upon completion of this appendix, you should be able to:

1. Modify the principles of trauma care to the cold environment.

2. Discuss general principles of the management of hypothermia.

INTRODUCTION

One evening during the winter of 1998 it was reported that 24 of the U.S. and all of the Canadian provinces had temperatures below freezing. In a multihospital study done in the United States, of 400 reported cases of frostbite, 69 came from the sunny state of Florida. Thus, for many if not most prehospital EMS providers, thought needs to be given to the application of ITLS principles to trauma care in the cold environment.

This appendix addresses the basics of managing a hypothermic trauma patient (core temperature less than 95 degrees Fahrenheit or 35 degrees Celsius) and describes how a cold environment changes the assessment and treatment of trauma patients. Managing trauma patients in the cold is both challenging and rewarding. You need a thorough understanding of the principles of ITLS and knowledge of the conditions and limitations imposed by the cold environment. You also must always be aware that your patient may be hypothermic. The signs and symptoms of hypothermia are listed in Table D-1.

COLD WEATHER TRAUMA CARE

Six Stages of an Ambulance Call

There are six stages of an ambulance call (Figure D-1). The predispatch stage is the most important in the successful application of the principles of ITLS in the cold environment. Effective cold weather response is heavily dependent on adequate preparation before the emergency. EMS providers living in cold environments have already learned the importance of proper clothing, including hand- and footwear. Likewise, EMS systems operating in cold environments have already learned the importance of maintaining the rescue vehicle, which includes special tires and the use of engine warming blocks.

EMS systems also must develop a system to keep their equipment at an appropriate temperature for immediate use. Medications can be kept in a portable box and carried to the vehicle for each run, but this is not practical for other equipment. Plastic endotracheal tubes and IV tubing must be kept warm enough so that they are malleable enough to use. Bags of IV fluid are of special concern because they could cause harm to the patient if cold IV fluids were rapidly infused into a patient. There are several methods to maintain the temperature of IV fluids. These include any type of electric warmer from electric blankets

TABLE D-1	*Signs and Symptoms of Hypothermia*

Neuromuscular System

Amnesia, dysarthria, poor judgment (34 degrees Celsius)

Loss of coordination, appearing "drunk" (33 degrees Celsius)

Shivering ceases (32 degrees Celsius)

Progressive decrease in level of consciousness (29 degrees Celsius)

Pupils dilated (29 degrees Celsius)

Loss of deep tendon reflexes (27 degrees Celsius)

Gastrointestinal System

Ileus

Respiratory System

Initial hyperventilation (<34 degrees Celsius)

Progressive decrease in rate and depth of respiration

Noncardiac pulmonary edema (25 degrees Celsius)

Cardiovascular System

Sinus bradycardia

Atrial fibrillation (30 degrees Celsius)

Progressive decrease in blood pressure (29 degrees Celsius)

Progressive decrease in pulse (29 degrees Celsius)

Ventricular irritability (28 degrees Celsius)

Hypotension (24 degrees Celsius)

Kidneys, Blood, Electrolytes

Cold diuresis leading to hypovolemia and hemoconcentration

Lactic acidosis and hyperglycemia

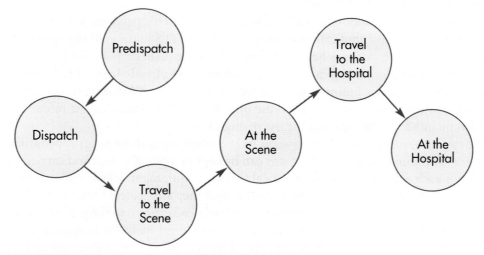

FIGURE D-1   Six stages of an ambulance call.

to small dog warmers on the rig. Obviously, the best solution is to keep the rescue vehicle in a heated garage.

Traveling to the scene, stage 3, often takes on additional meaning in the winter. The shortest route, because of travel conditions, may not be the quickest or the safest. Several EMS systems have recognized that more than one mode of travel is needed. This may include any combination of helicopter, ambulance, snowmobile, or even dogsled.

Traveling to the hospital, stage 5, may be long and arduous during winter rescue. The distances may be greater, the travel may be slower, and the vehicle more likely to break down or become stuck. Some EMS systems in North America have developed relay and backup systems for the patient. These relay systems facilitate the transfer of the patient to the nearest appropriate facility by the most appropriate mode of travel. The backup systems include a buddy system to ensure that there is someone aware of the location of the ambulance who can intervene in the event of a breakdown or a loss of communication.

Patient Assessment

Scene Size-up On-scene trauma assessment in the cold environment starts with the Scene Size-up. The hazards may not be apparent. The frozen, slippery walk or road under the snow or even the fallen power line under the snow may await the hasty rescuer. The total number of victims may not be apparent; you must look for clues to more victims. A patient left in the cold is a fatal error. It is easy to miss an unconscious, ejected patient at night or in poor visibility. The essential equipment may need to be slightly different—hydraulic equipment does not work efficiently, batteries last 25 percent as long, and flares last half as long. The phenomena of icy fog and the suspended vehicle exhaust from the rescue vehicles themselves cause decreased visibility. You must constantly reevaluate the safety of the scene, and you need the ability and backup equipment to react appropriately.

Determine the mechanism of injury. Look for clues to hypothermia. Even in a relatively warm 50 degree (10 degree Celsius) environment, the patient could have hypothermia. Consider this possibility in the aged patient, the stroke victim, or the septic patient who has been lying on the bathroom floor for hours. Consider it with the intoxicated patient who has been lying at the foot of the basement stairs for hours. In the outside environment, wet clothing and wind chill can cause rapid hypothermia in the trauma patient.

Primary Trauma Survey The ITLS Primary Survey is even more critical in the cold environment. Evaluation of the airway, cervical-spine control, and documentation of initial level of consciousness is the same. However, you must consider that the decreased level of consciousness could be a result of hypothermia in addition to any trauma or shock. The evaluation of breathing is the same; however, a decreased rate and depth of respiration may be due to hypothermia in addition to head injury or intoxication from alcohol or drugs. The treatment of an inadequate respiratory effort is the same: adequate ventilation with 100 percent oxygen. If the patient has isolated hypothermia, ventilate with warm humidified oxygen. Do not hyperventilate.

The evaluation of the circulation has the same importance that was described in Chapter 2; however, the cold environment may make it more difficult to evaluate. Note the rate and quality of the radial pulse. Check a carotid pulse if you cannot feel a radial pulse. This may take longer than usual because of the vasoconstriction caused by the exposure or because the pulse is slowed by the hypothermic state. It is important not to start chest compressions on the hypothermic patient who simply has a slow weak pulse; the compressions could induce ventricular fibrillation. The examination of the skin color and condition may be nonproductive. Because of the peripheral vasoconstriction, the skin may be pale and cool even when the patient is not hypothermic. All cold patients (except those with spinal-cord injuries) will have pale, cold extremities and delayed capillary refill. Initially, the best way to get an idea of the patient's temperature is to put your hand down the back of the neck and feel the skin of the back. This is quicker and easier to do than trying to feel down the front of the chest.

The patient in a cold environment, especially the patient who is thought to be hypothermic, cannot be exposed for a complete examination of the chest, abdomen, pelvis, and extremities. Assess the head and the neck. Application of the cervical motion-restriction device may be difficult at this time because of the patient's clothing. Palpate the patient's back with your bare hand (covered only with a latex glove) under all the layers of clothing. Palpate for tenderness, instability, and crepitation (TIC). Feel for adequate and symmetric chest wall rise. Your hand should also note the patient's temperature. If the back (or anterior chest) underneath the clothing feels in any way cool, then the patient may be hypothermic.

You may at this point decide that the patient is suffering from hypothermia in addition to the other injuries you may have found. The converse is that patients who have obviously frozen hands or feet may still be warm to touch under their clothes. (Frostbite is more common than significant core hypothermia.) Handle the hypothermic patient very gently to prevent a lethal cardiac arrhythmia. Even if the patient is hypothermic, you must complete the Primary Survey. Auscultate the lungs, and examine the neck, abdomen, pelvis, and extremities as best as you can. You should try to spend no more than 2 minutes doing this entire evaluation in the cold environment, in part to conserve body heat and to prevent further heat loss. At this point, the patient can be log-rolled and put on a backboard.

Critical Interventions and Transport Decision When the Primary Survey is complete, you have enough information to decide if the patient is critical or stable. If you find that the patient falls into the load-and-go category outlined in Chapter 2, perform critical interventions and package the patient on a wooden or plastic backboard (not metal) and immediately load into an ambulance for transport. If the patient appears stable but is in a cold environment, or if it is cool but the victim is also wet, consider this a load-and-go situation. Gently transfer the patient to the warm ambulance for the Secondary Survey, additional critical care, and the Ongoing Exams. Close the ambulance door quickly to prevent any further heat loss from the vehicle so you can remove the patient's wet clothes (if necessary). At this point, the baseline vital signs and further patient history can be obtained.

Secondary Survey When the weather is cold, you should perform the Secondary Survey in the ambulance. Remove wet and cold clothing and cover the patient with warm blankets. The patient with hypothermia must have wet, cold clothes removed in order to be rewarmed. Down clothing probably should not be cut off in the usual fashion since the heater in the ambulance will blow the feathers into the patient's wounds and the EMS equipment. Begin to rewarm the patient by both passive external rewarming with dry blankets in the warm ambulance and by core rewarming with warm (100 degrees Fahrenheit) humidified oxygen. This is usually an adequate method of rewarming for the patient with mild hypothermia (core temperature of 90 degrees Fahrenheit or greater). Do not massage or put hot compresses on the cold extremities. This may block the shivering reflex and may cause an "afterdrop" in core temperature. Rapid warming of the skin abolishes the vasoconstriction, allowing the cold blood in the extremities to return to the core causing a further lowering (afterdrop) of temperature. Patients who are still shivering have only mild hypothermia and will do fine with passive rewarming with just warm blankets. Perform the Secondary Survey as described in Chapter 2.

Critical Care and Ongoing Exam Critical care is usually performed in the ambulance during transfer. Not only is this advantageous for the patient, but also your warm hands are better able to provide the care. Advanced airway management is easier in the ambulance than in the bitter cold outside. The endotracheal tube is more malleable and is less likely to stick to the warm mucous membranes, and your glasses do not fog up in the cold. Tube placement confirmation with the colorimetric end-tidal carbon dioxide detection device may prove unreliable in the cold environment. Provide the patient with warm humidified oxygen in the ambulance; the plastic humidifier bottle can be filled with saline warmed to about 45 to 55 degrees Celsius (80–100 degrees Fahrenheit). Heated saline or water in a thermos will provide some help. Any other warming unit must be carefully checked for safety to ensure that the patient is not harmed.

Perform frequent Ongoing Exams during transport. Especially watch the pulse, blood pressure, and cardiac rhythm. The mildly hypothermic patient will often have muscle artifact (sometimes from the shivering); there may be sinus bradycardia, J or Osborne wave immediately after the QRS complex, or atrial fibrillation. These dysrhythmias require no treatment other than warming the patient. At 82.4 degrees Fahrenheit (28 degrees Celsius) core body temperature, there may be ventricular fibrillation that is unresponsive to defibrillation, and below 69.8 degrees (21 degrees Celsius) there may be asystole. Currently there is no medication that has proven effective for treating ventricular fibrillation in the severely hypothermic patient. The abdomen needs to be examined frequently. Your initial assessment may miss an abdominal catastrophe in the hypothermic patient. You should also frequently check and record the neurological exam.

You should decide about IV fluids during transport. If fluids are indicated, they should be at least the ambient temperature of the warm ambulance. Warmed fluids are preferable to room temperature fluids in the hypothermic patient but have very little effect in raising the core temperature. Fluid resuscitation may be necessary for hypovolemic shock or for hypothermia. Prolonged cold exposure causes prolonged peripheral vasoconstriction, resulting in more blood perfusing the kidney. This causes a "cold diuresis," an inappropriate diuresis of fluid induced by the cold. The patient will become hypovolemic. Patients with frostbite also benefit from warm fluids, which help the poor circulation in the vasoconstricted extremities. There is currently some exciting research going on about some new devices that may be used to warm the hypothermic patient in the field.

Contacting Medical Direction If your patient is hypothermic, it is extremely important to contact medical direction early. Even though it may take considerable time to arrive at the nearest appropriate medical facility, the facility needs time to assemble the proper trauma team or to arrange for more expeditious transfer to another facility. Medical direction needs to know how long the patient was exposed to the cold and the patient's core body temperature. Remember that axillary and skin temperatures are not closely correlated with core body temperature in the cold environment. The oral temperature is inaccurate at temperatures below 96 degrees. A tympanic membrane thermometer is the most practical method to take an accurate core temperature in the ambulance. Multiple temperature assessments must be performed. Medical direction may order the use of some IV medications, but this will depend on individual circumstances.

NOTES FOR WILDERNESS RESCUERS

If you are required to be in the cold for long periods of time (hiking or skiing in to rescue someone in a wilderness area), then remember the following:

■ *Blood is heat.* Good circulation is necessary to prevent frostbite. Drink plenty of fluids and keep your canteen under your clothing so it is warm. You can force more blood (heat) to your cold, vasoconstricted hands by "windmilling" your arms (sling your arm in a circle, forcing blood into the hands).

■ *Never go into the wilderness without a partner.* You need someone to help watch you for signs of frostbite or hypothermia and who will allow you to warm your cold hands or feet in their axilla or groin under their clothing or snuggle with you in a sleeping bag (wilderness friends are close friends indeed).

■ *Good clothing and equipment are essential* so that you maintain your temperature and don't become hypothermic or develop frostbite (don't become a victim). If you have skin areas (face, scalp, hands, etc.) exposed to the cold, not only will they vasoconstrict but they will also cause generalized surface vasoconstriction. Thus the saying, "If your feet are cold, put on a hat."

■ *Your perception of cold is related to your surface temperature,* not your core temperature. Beware the heated hand warmer that makes you feel warm while your core temperature is dropping.

BIBLIOGRAPHY

1. Auerback, P. S., E. C. Geehr. 1989. *Management of wilderness and environmental emergencies.* 2nd ed. St. Louis: C. V. Mosby.

2. Gregory, J. S., J. M. Bergstein, et al. 1991. Comparison of three methods of rewarming from hypothermia: Advantages of extracorporeal blood warming. *Journal of Trauma* 31: 1247–52.

3. Hector, M. G. 1992. Treatment of accidental hypothermia. *American Family Physician* 45(2): 785–92.

4. Ornato, J. P., J. B. Shipley, et al. 1992. Multicenter study of a portable, hand-size, colorimetric end-tidal carbon dioxide detection device. *Annals of Emergency Medicine* 21(5): 518–23.

5. Sterba, J. A. 1991. Efficacy and safety of prehospital rewarming techniques to treat accidental hypothermia. *Annals of Emergency Medicine* 20(8): 896–901.

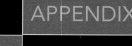
Role of the Medical Helicopter

Russell B. Bieniek, MD, FACEP

Pam Gersch, RN, CLNC

Objectives

Upon completion of this appendix, you should be able to:

1. Discuss the various roles of the medical helicopter.
2. Discuss the advantages a medical helicopter may offer over ground transport.

MEDICAL HELICOPTER SERVICES

Air medical helicopters were used extensively to transport injured servicemen during the U.S. military conflicts of Korea and Vietnam. On October 12, 1972, Flight for Life, the first U.S. hospital-based civilian air medical helicopter service, went into operation at St. Anthony Hospital in Denver, Colorado. In the years that followed, similar programs were established at multiple hospitals and various other organizations across the United States and throughout the world. According to the Association of Air Medical Services (AAMS), in 2005 there were approximately 750 helicopters dedicated to EMS use in the United States, transporting 375,000 patients per year. The structure and role of these air medical programs vary tremendously, as does their integration with the local EMS system and involvement in trauma care.

The sponsoring agency and organizational structure of a medical helicopter service encompass a wide range of models. They may be military or other government service—federal, state/province/territory, or local. They may be independent or work in cooperation with local medical care providers to provide rescue and/or transportation of injured patients. The crews may be on call and/or the helicopter may need to be reconfigured or additional equipment may need to be brought on board. The far end of the spectrum, and most common, is the fully dedicated medical helicopter that flies only critically injured or ill patients and whose interior is specifically designed and configured, always medically staffed and consistently available for a medical mission.

The role established for a specific program may be one of primary interfacility transports (hospital to hospital), scene transports (field to hospital) or, as is most frequently the case, a combination of the two with varying percentages of each type. The involvement that a medical helicopter service may have in the local EMS community may depend on its percentage of scene involvement.

The type of patient that a service transports is usually a mixture of clinical classes, including neonatal, pediatric, cardiac, maternal, medical, and trauma. The service may transport all classes of patients, may limit services to specific types of patients, or may have specific teams that accompany each clinical class of patients. The medical crew on board also varies with the specific program. The AAMS membership database in 2005 revealed that the majority of medical helicopter programs utilize two medical attendants. The credentials of the medical crew vary widely, ranging from an EMT-P to a physician. The most common configuration consists of a nurse and a paramedic, comprising 75 percent of the two-attendant crew design. The makeup of the crew also may vary by the type of specialty medical mission to which the helicopter is dedicated.

If a medical helicopter service is available in your region, it is important that you become acquainted with them and know in advance the type of cases for which you will utilize them. You also will need to know how to access them and how to involve them in your system to help improve patient care.

Multiple factors influence the availability of a medical helicopter. These include scheduled maintenance, mechanical factors, weather, and being committed on a previous mission. This resource can be very beneficial to the EMS service and the patient, but there should not be dependence on it. They may not be able to respond or have to cancel en route. Contingency plans must always be in place.

Regarding safety, there needs to be prior education and training with the medical helicopter service. This education would entail learning proper communications between ground and air, picking and describing a safe landing zone, and coordinating unloading and loading of the aircraft. In the uncommon, but possible, event of an aircraft accident, correct knowledge of the helicopter's equipment and access could be vital to crew and ground personnel. Safety must always be the first concern, as in your ITLS training: "Is the scene safe?"

THE MEDICAL HELICOPTER AND THE TRAUMA PATIENT

Caring for the trauma patient can be extremely challenging. However, it is quite rewarding to you and the patient if all the components are in place and things are done properly. As an established component and resource to an EMS service, the medical helicopter can improve patient outcome by providing assistance in two areas. The first is speed of transportation; the second is the introduction of a higher level of clinical expertise, equipment, or procedures at the scene or en route to the hospital.

Helicopters obviously are able to transport patients quicker than ground units over long distances. This involves their ability to travel at high speeds and in a straight line. They also do not have to fight road conditions, either environmental or traffic. This decreases the exposure of the general public or the caregivers themselves to the potential dangers of an ambulance rushing through busy streets with other traffic and pedestrians.

In many areas of the United States the only care available at a trauma scene is BLS. A medical helicopter would then be able to provide ALS assessment and care at the scene and en route to the hospital. Often, even in areas where ALS is available, the medical helicopter crew may be able to provide additional critical care expertise, skills, and/or equipment. Some of these may include, but are not be limited to, needle or surgical cricothyroidotomy, needle or tube thoracostomy, intraosseous needle insertion, pericardiocentesis, and various medications for such things as sedation and chemical paralysis of the head-injured patient for control of the airway and to assist in controlling increased intracranial pressure. Additional equipment might include pulse oximetry, end-tidal CO_2 monitors, positive pressure ventilators, and Doppler-assisted blood pressure monitoring devices, to mention a few. Many services also carry packed red blood cells to use in the field. The medical helicopter service personnel also usually handle a higher volume of critically injured trauma patients than the average individual provider in a rural ground system, so they may exhibit greater familiarity and comfort in working with these patients.

For interfacility transports, the patient is evaluated by the nursing and physician staffs at the referring hospital, which determine whether the patient requires additional evaluation and/or treatment at a facility with more resources available to handle the serious trauma patient. The medical helicopter provides the vehicle, crew, and speed necessary to provide a continuum of the critical care environment en route during transport.

ITLS AND THE MEDICAL HELICOPTER

ITLS provides a common language that can be used through the continuum of care for the seriously injured trauma patient. This requires coordinated education and training in a region and possibly could be an educational program offered by the medical service itself. Trauma patients would then be assessed rapidly, accurately, and completely in the field by the prehospital providers, and the decision scheme that is developed for the region on utilizing the medical helicopter service could be partly based on the results of this assessment, other specific trauma scores, types of injuries, and mechanism of injury. The medical helicopter service would then easily understand the assessment and initial treatment that was done prior to their arrival, and the report could be accomplished quickly, as they are all "speaking the same language." The helicopter medical crew can then rapidly do their ITLS assessment and begin transport with further treatments if necessary at the scene or en route.

You must constantly evaluate your skills at doing a rapid assessment of the trauma patient. When you turn your patient over to another service, such as a medical helicopter service for transport, you will not get immediate feedback on the outcome of the patient, as you do when you deliver the patient to the hospital yourself. The medical helicopter service may serve as a link between you and the hospital to help obtain this important information. When cases are reviewed, the ITLS assessment and initial management can be used as a standard to compare with the actual care given.

Medical helicopter services are one of many special tools available to you and the hospital. As with all tools, there needs to be initial and continued education and training to ensure proper and safe usage. This will improve the utilization of resources in your service area and help achieve everyone's common goal of maximizing patient outcome.

BIBLIOGRAPHY

1. Association of Air Medical Services (AAMS) Membership Database. 2005. Contact at 526 King St., Ste. 415, Alexandria, VA 22314-3143.
2. Atlas & Database of Air Medical Services (ADAMS). 2005. http://www.adamsairmed.org/

Trauma Scoring in the Prehospital Care Setting

Leah J. Heimbach, JD, RN, EMT-P

Objectives

Upon completion of this appendix, you should be able to:

1. Discuss the adult and pediatric Glasgow Coma Scale score.
2. Discuss the Revised Trauma score and the Pediatric Trauma score.

TRAUMA SCORING SYSTEMS

Trauma scoring systems consist of assigning a numerical rating or score to various clinical signs, such as vital signs or response to pain. They are used to assess the severity of injury and are especially valuable in assessment of the trauma patient with multiple injuries. Trauma scoring systems have important uses in trauma systems at all levels, including the hospital setting and the prehospital setting and in overall health-care system analysis. There are several methods of scoring severity of injury in trauma patients, including the Glasgow Coma Scale score and the Revised Trauma score (Tables F-1 and F-2).

USES FOR TRAUMA SCORING

In the hospital setting, trauma scoring systems have many uses, including the following:

- Standardizing triage between health-care facilities (deciding when it is appropriate to transfer a patient to a trauma center)
- Allocating medical resources
- Evaluating the health-care facility's overall effectiveness in providing patient care
- Conducting audits (making sure that patients who are predicted to survive their traumatic event actually do survive)
- Predicting morbidity and mortality of patients based on a particular trauma score

Although prehospital care providers should never delay transport to complete a trauma score, trauma scoring systems can provide an objective and standardized way to triage patients appropriately (including whether a patient should go to a trauma center) and to communicate injury severity, using a common language, to other members of the health-care team. Trauma scores recorded in the field are also useful in the analysis and research of EMS systems. This analysis can then be used to develop protocols for prehospital care to meet the needs of a specific EMS region.

TABLE F-1 *Glasgow Coma Scale*

Always report scores of the three components as well as the total.

Eye Opening	Points	Verbal Response	Points	Motor Response	Points
Spontaneous	4	Oriented	5	Obeys commands	6
To voice	3	Confused	4	Localizes pain	5
To pain	2	Inappropriate words	3	Withdraws	4
None	1	Incomprehensible sounds	2	Abnormal flexion	3*
		Silent	1	Abnormal extension	2**
				No movement	1

*Decorticate posturing to pain
**Decerebrate posturing to pain

TABLE F-2 *Revised Trauma Score*

Score	Score	Contribution to Revised Trauma
Total Glasgow Coma Scale score (See Table F-1)	13–15	4
	9–12	3
	6–8	2
	4–5	1
	3	0
Systolic blood pressure (mmHg)	>89	4
	76–89	3
	50–75	2
	1–49	1
	None	0
Respiration (per minute)	10–29	4
	>29	3
	6–9	2
	1–5	1
	None	0

Note: If total score is 11 or less, the patient should be taken to a trauma center.

The ITLS patient assessment includes a neurological assessment, using the AVPU scale (alert, responds to verbal stimulus, responds to painful stimulus, and unresponsive), and identifies parameters to determine whether the patient is a load-and-go case. Communicating this information along with a list of the patient's injuries to the receiving hospital will allow the hospital personnel to gather the necessary resources to optimize care.

The use of trauma scores in the prehospital setting can be confusing at a time when patient assessment, injury management, and communication to the receiving hospital need to be concise. It is recommended that you report the following information to the receiving facility.

1. Age, sex, and chief complaint

2. Mechanism of injury

3. Level of consciousness

4. What parameters led to the load-and-go decision

5. List of the patient's injuries

6. What treatment was rendered

7. Patient's response to treatment

Many EMS regions will require the use of some type of trauma score system in the prehospital setting to facilitate patient care and/or to promote prehospital research. An example of the Revised Trauma score is shown in Table F-2. An example of the Pediatric Glasgow Coma score and Pediatric Trauma score is shown in Tables F-3 and F-4. When you record and report the Glasgow Coma Scale score, always give the individual scores of the components of the scale (eye opening, verbal response, motor response) as well as the total score.

Recent literature (see references 2 and 3 in the Bibliography) questions the reliability of the Glasgow Coma Scale score (GCS) and the Pediatric Glasgow Coma Scale score (PGCS). For adults, some researchers believe that the motor component of the GCS should

TABLE F-3 *Pediatric Glasgow Coma Scale*

		>1 year	<1 year	
Eyes Opening	4	Spontaneously	Spontaneously	
	3	To verbal command	To shout	
	2	To pain	To pain	
	1	No response	No response	
		>1 year	**<1 year**	
Best Motor Response	6	Obeys		
	5	Localizes pain	Localizes pain	
	4	Flexion—withdrawal	Flexion—normal	
	3	Flexion—abnormal (decorticate rigidity)	Flexion—abnormal (decorticate rigidity)	
	2	Extension (decerebrate rigidity)	Extension (decerebrate rigidity)	
	1	No response	No response	
		>5 years	**2–5 years**	**0–23 Months**
Best Verbal Response	5	Oriented and converses	Appropriate words and phrases	Smiles, coos, cries appropriately
	4	Disoriented and converses	Inappropriate words	Cries
	3	Inappropriate words	Cries and/or screams	Inappropriate crying and/or screaming
	2	Incomprehensible sounds	Grunts	Grunts
	1	No response	No response	No response

TABLE F-4 *Pediatric Trauma Score*

Score	+2	+1	−1
Weight	>44 lb (>20 kg)	22–44 lb (10–20 kg)	< 22 lb (<10 kg)
Airway	Normal	Oral or nasal airway	Intubated Tracheostomy Invasive airway
Blood pressure	Pulse at wrist >90 mmHg	Carotid or femoral pulse palpable 50–90 mmHg	No palpable pulse <50 mmHg
Level of consciousness	Completely awake	Obtunded or any loss of consciousness	Comatose
Open wound	None	Minor	Major or penetrating
Fractures	None	Closed fracture	Open or multiple fractures

replace the GCS in outcome prediction. In children, concerns have been raised regarding the fact that current scoring systems in pediatric trauma have significant limitations because they are not age specific. It is likely that both adult and pediatric trauma scoring systems will undergo revision in the near future to more accurately predict mortality associated with traumatic injuries.

BIBLIOGRAPHY

1. Champion, H., W. Sacco, W. Copes, et al. 1989. A revision of the trauma score. *Journal of Trauma* 29: 623–29.
2. Healy, C., T. M. Osler, F. B. Rogers, M. A. Healy, L. G. Glance, P. D. Kilgo, S. R. Shackford, J. W. Meredith. 2003. Improving the Glasgow coma scale score: Motor score alone is a better predictor. *Journal of Trauma* 54(4): 671–78; discussion 678–80.
3. Potoka, D. A., L. C. Schall, H. R. Ford. 2001. Development of a novel age-specific pediatric trauma score. *Journal of Pediatric Surgery* 36(1): 106–12.
4. Rimel, R. W., J. A. Jane, R. F. Edlich. 1979. An injury severity scale for comprehensive management of central nervous system trauma. *Annals of Emergency Medicine* (December): 64–67.
5. Teasdale G., B. Jennett. 1974. Assessment of coma and impaired consciousness: A practical scale. *Lancet* 1: 81–83.

Drowning, Barotrauma, and Decompression Injury

James H. Creel Jr., MD, FACEP

John E. Campbell, MD, FACEP

Objectives

Upon completion of this appendix, you should be able to:

1. Discuss the general management of near-drowning patients.
2. Discuss which body organs are most affected by barotrauma.
3. Discuss barotrauma of descent.
4. Discuss barotrauma of ascent.
5. Discuss decompression sickness (DCS).
6. Explain why skin divers and snorkelers do not get DCS.

DROWNING

Approximately 7,000 people drown annually, making drowning the third-leading cause of accidental death in the United States. Freshwater drownings are more common than saltwater drownings, and there are more immersion accidents in pools than in lakes, ponds, and rivers. The peak incidence occurs in the warm months and most commonly involves teenagers and children under the age of 4.

Drowning is death from suffocation after submersion in the water. There are two basic mechanisms:

- Breath holding, which leads to aspiration of water and wet lungs
- Laryngospasm with glottic closure and dry lungs

Both these mechanisms can lead to profound hypoxia and death. Most adults who have drowned have about 150 cc of fluid in their lungs. The amount (2.2 cc per kilogram) is enough to produce profound hypoxia. It is thought to take about 10 times this amount to get electrolyte changes, and this is rarely seen. In the prehospital phase, hypoxia is the primary concern. Survival of the victim depends on your rapid evaluation and management of the ABCs.

Initiate management as soon as possible. Be aware of surfing/diving mechanisms that indicate potential occult cervical-spine injury. Protect the cervical spine during rescue of the patient. In water, CPR is generally ineffective. Remove the patient to a stable surface as soon as possible; then initiate CPR and the appropriate protocol. In cases in which hypothermia is responsible for the near-drowning, it appears to provide the brain, heart, and lungs some degree of protection (diving reflex) by slowing the metabolism. Therefore, no one is dead until warm and dead; do not stop CPR.

BAROTRAUMA

Barotrauma refers to injuries due to the mechanical effects of pressure on the body. We all live "under pressure" since the weight of the air in which we live exerts force on our bodies. At sea level, the weight of air pressing on the body equals 14.7 pounds per square inch (psi). Since solids and liquids are not compressible, they are not usually affected by pressure changes. The study of barotrauma is the study of the effect of pressure on gas-filled organs of the body. Gas-filled organs are ears, sinuses, upper and lower airways, stomach, and intestines.

To understand the effects of pressure changes, you must know some properties of gases. Boyle's law states that the volume of a gas is inversely proportional to the pressure applied to it. This simply means that if you double the pressure on a gas, the volume of the gas will decrease by one-half. If you halve the pressure on a gas, the volume will double. The pressure at sea level is called one atmosphere absolute (ATA). If you go up in an airplane (or climb a mountain), you have less atmosphere above you; thus the pressure decreases and the gas inside the body expands. Most commercial airliners fly at about 35,000 feet elevation (one-fifth ATA or gas volume 5 times normal) but are pressurized to a cabin pressure equal to 5,000 to 8,000 feet elevation (two-thirds to three-fourths ATA), so that gas expands to only about 1.2 to 1.4 times its original volume. Airline passengers notice no change except for "popping" of the ears as the expanding gas in the middle ears vents off through the eustachian tubes into the pharynx.

Water is much heavier than air. When one descends into saltwater, there is a change of one atmosphere for every 33 feet of depth (34 feet for freshwater). This means that at 33 feet of depth the body is subjected to 2 ATA, and gas in the body has been compressed to one-half of its original volume. Because of the pressures involved, divers are exposed to certain potential injuries during both descent and ascent.

Trauma of Descent: "Middle Ear Squeeze"

Since there is a large pressure change during the first few feet of a dive, skin divers and snorkelers as well as scuba divers are subject to trauma of descent. Let's say that a skin diver takes a breath and rapidly descends to a depth of 33 feet. All the gas in his body will decrease in volume by one-half. This includes gas in the lungs, intestines, stomach, sinuses, and middle ears. The elastic lungs, intestines, and stomach will simply decrease in size to match the volume of gas. Problems develop with the middle ears and sinuses if the pressure cannot be equalized. The sinuses (air pockets in the bones of the face and skull) each have an opening through which air from the pharynx can enter to equalize the pressure. If the openings are blocked, the skin diver will experience pain in the sinuses and may even develop bleeding and inflammation (barosinusitis). Other than the discomfort, this causes no serious problem.

Each middle ear has an opening, the eustachian tube, through which air from the pharynx can enter to equalize pressure. If the eustachian tube is blocked (mucosal congestion from allergy, infection, etc.), the pressure will push in on the eardrum and cause intense pain. This begins to be noticeable at a depth of 4 to 5 feet. If the diver cannot equalize the middle ear pressure and yet continues to descend, the pressure will eventually rupture the eardrum and flood the middle ear with cold water (even the warm waters of the Caribbean are 20 degrees below body temperature). Cold water in the middle ear causes dizziness, nausea, vomiting, and disorientation ("twirly bends"). The result can be panic and drowning or near-drowning. The diver using a self-contained underwater breathing apparatus (scuba diver) who surfaces rapidly can develop air embolism or neurological decompression sickness. Vomiting under water can cause aspiration and drowning.

Barotitis media (middle ear squeeze) requires no prehospital treatment. The pressure is relieved when the diver returns to the surface. If there is hearing loss or continued ear pain, the diver should see a physician for treatment of ruptured eardrum or bleeding into the middle ear. The conditions that you are more likely to have to manage are the near-drowning cases caused by the disorientation from water in the middle ears.

Trauma of Ascent

Injuries from expanding gas can occur as divers ascend. These injuries are much more common in scuba divers, since such injuries usually either require some time to develop (longer than a skin diver can hold his breath) or require the breathing of compressed air.

Reverse Middle Ear Squeeze If a eustachian tube becomes blocked during a dive, the gas in the middle ear will expand and cause pain during ascent. If there is enough expansion, the eardrum can rupture, with all the symptoms and dangers mentioned previously.

Gastrointestinal Barotrauma If the diver swallows air while breathing compressed air or if the diver has previously eaten gas-forming foods (e.g., beans), he may accumulate a significant amount of stomach or intestinal gas during a dive. If the diver was at a depth of 66 feet, the gas will expand to three times its original volume during ascent. If he is unable to expel this gas, he will develop abdominal pain and occasionally even collapse, and develop a shocklike state.

Pulmonary Overpressurization Syndromes (Burst Lung) These occur only in divers who have been breathing compressed air. During a dive the lungs are completely filled with air, which is at a pressure equal to the depth at which the diver is swimming. If a diver panics and surfaces without exhaling, the rapidly expanding gas will overinflate the lungs and cause one of the three overpressurization syndromes listed below. Remember, the total volume of the lungs is about 6 L. An ascent from 33 feet would cause expansion to 12 L; 66 feet, 18 L; and 100 feet, 24 L. It is easy to see how delicate alveoli can be ruptured by this expansion. The expanding air will dissect into the interstitial space, pleural space, pulmonary venules, or a combination of the three.

Air in the Interstitial Space. This is the most common form of pulmonary overpressurization syndrome. As millions of tiny air bubbles escape into the interstitial tissue, they may dissect into the mediastinum and up into the subcutaneous tissue of the neck. Symptoms may develop immediately upon surfacing or may not develop for several hours. The diver may have increasing hoarseness, chest pain, subcutaneous emphysema in the neck, and difficulty breathing and swallowing. Any diver with these symptoms should get oxygen (no positive pressure ventilations unless the diver is apneic) and transport to the hospital. While interstitial air does not require treatment with a recompression chamber (hyperbaric chamber), these patients often develop air embolism or decompression sickness. They should be observed in a facility that is capable of providing recompression treatment if necessary.

Air in the Pleural Space. If the alveoli rupture into the pleural space, a pneumothorax and possibly a hemothorax will develop. The amount of pneumothorax will depend on how much air escaped into the pleural space and how far the diver surfaced after the air entered the pleural space. A 10 percent pneumothorax at 33 feet will be a 20 percent pneumothorax at the surface. A 20 to 30 percent pneumothorax at 33 feet may be a tension pneumothorax at the surface. The symptoms will be the same as for interstitial air except the diver will now have decreased breath sounds and hyperresonance to percussion on the affected side (may be on both sides). A tension pneumothorax will also have distended neck veins and shock (and possibly tracheal deviation—a rare sign). These patients may require a needle decompression if they have a tension pneumothorax. Otherwise, give 100 percent oxygen and transport immediately.

Air Embolism. The most serious syndrome of overpressurization is pulmonary air embolism. If the overdistended alveoli rupture into the pulmonary venules, the millions of tiny air bubbles can return to the left side of the heart and then up the carotid arteries to the small arterioles of the brain. These bubbles, composed mostly of nitrogen, obstruct the arterioles and produce symptoms similar to a stroke. The symptoms produced depend on which vessels are obstructed. There will usually be sudden loss of consciousness and focal neurological signs. The symptoms almost always occur immediately when the diver surfaces. This is a very important point in differentiating air embolism from decompression sickness (which usually takes hours to develop).

The patient should be placed in supine position, given 100 percent oxygen, an IV (normal saline), and transported to a facility that can provide recompression treatment. This is one instance in which you should not hyperventilate or give positive pressure ventilations. Hyperventilation causes vasoconstriction, which will trap the bubbles. Positive pressure ventilation may force more air into the veins, worsening the injury (if the patient is not breathing, you must give positive pressure ventilation). This patient must have immediate recompression in a recompression chamber no matter how much time has passed since the injury and no matter how far away the recompression chamber may be. In a recompression chamber, the pressure is raised to 6 ATA (multiple place chamber), which will decrease the size of the bubbles to one-sixth of their previous volume. If only a monoplace chamber is available, recompression will be at 2.8 ATA. This may allow them to pass through the capillaries back to the lungs to be expelled. Air embolism may rarely affect the coronary arteries, causing myocardial infarction, dysrhythmias, or cardiac arrest.

DECOMPRESSION SICKNESS

Decompression sickness (DCS) is caused by another property of gases. Henry's law states that the amount of gas dissolved in a liquid is directly proportional to the pressure applied. This means that twice as much gas would be dissolved in a liquid at a depth of 33 feet as at sea level. It also means that gas dissolved in a liquid at 33 feet will come out of solution as that liquid ascends. This is analogous to a sealed bottle of carbonated beverage that has no bubbles as long as it is sealed but bubbles the instant that the cap is removed and the pressure is released.

Nitrogen, which accounts for about 80 percent of the volume of inspired air, is an inert gas that dissolves in blood and fat. When a diver is under water, nitrogen dissolves in the blood and fat tissue. This nitrogen is released as he surfaces, so he must surface slowly enough to allow this nitrogen to be expelled through his lungs. The U.S. Navy has developed a set of tables of no-decompression limits that give general guidelines about how long one can stay at a certain depth without going through stage decompression during ascent. There are also standard air decompression tables for those dives that exceed the no-decompression limit. Theoretically, if one follows the recommendations of the tables, nitrogen bubbles will not form in the blood during ascent. This may not always be true, because the tables were developed from a study of U.S. Navy divers, who are uniformly young, healthy, well-conditioned men who were diving in saltwater.

Today, there are 3 million recreational scuba divers and 300,000 new divers certified each year. Sport divers are not uniformly young, healthy, or conditioned. They are often older, poorly conditioned, and not always healthy. A special problem is obesity. Fat absorbs about 5 times as much nitrogen as blood or other tissue, so obese divers require longer decompression times or shorter dives. Sport divers should be very conservative when using diving tables, especially when diving in freshwater or in lakes above sea level.

The greatest danger occurs when a diver who has been submerged for a significant period of time has a diving accident, panics, and surfaces rapidly. Nitrogen bubbles will form in the blood and tissue just as carbon dioxide bubbles form in champagne. This is a different injury from barotrauma or pulmonary overpressurization syndrome, and may exist along with any of the barotrauma syndromes. It is frequently seen in divers in near-drowning situations. The symptoms are almost always delayed for minutes to hours after a dive. As a general rule, symptoms that develop within 10 minutes of surfacing are caused by air embolism until proved otherwise. Symptoms developing after 10 minutes are decompression sickness until proved otherwise. Fifty percent will be symptomatic in 30 minutes, 90 percent will be symptomatic in 3 hours, 99 percent will be symptomatic in 12 hours, and 100 percent will be symptomatic in 36 hours. A special case is the vacationing diver who is asymptomatic after a deep dive and then catches a plane home the same day. This diver may develop symptoms during flight, since the cabin pressure is only two-thirds or three-fourths ATA. These symptoms may not appear until the diver has returned home far inland from the site of the dive. All emergency providers should have some knowledge of diving injuries.

Type I Decompression Sickness

Cutaneous ("Skin Bends") Millions of tiny nitrogen bubbles may form in the microvasculature of the skin. This causes a generalized itching rash that may be red and inflamed or mottled with a central purple discoloration. It is called "marbleized skin" (cutis marmorata). This condition requires no treatment but may be an early sign of more serious decompression sickness, so the patient must be observed. Give the patient 100 percent oxygen, and transport to a facility capable of recompression therapy.

Musculoskeletal ("Bends" or "Pain-Only Bends") This is the most common presentation of decompression sickness. Over 85 percent of divers with decompression sickness will present with pain in the joints. The shoulders or knees are affected most commonly, but any joint may be affected. The pain is usually deep and aching, and there may be vague numbness around the affected joint. Characteristically, there are no physical findings and the pain may be eased by pressure such as inflating a blood pressure cuff. These patients require recompression therapy no matter how long it has been since the symptoms started and no matter how far the nearest recompression chamber may be located. Symptoms usually occur within 36 hours and most cases are obvious within 24 hours.

Type II Decompression Sickness

These syndromes are more serious and may be life threatening. This includes severe cardiopulmonary and neurological symptoms. They are emergencies that require rapid diagnosis and treatment.

Pulmonary Emergencies ("Chokes" 2 Percent of DCS Cases) Nitrogen bubbles forming in the vasculature of the lungs cause symptoms similar to the interstitial pulmonary overpressurization syndrome. The patient will develop cough, chest pain, difficulty breathing, and sometimes hemoptysis. These symptoms usually develop within an hour of surfacing (50 percent) but may be delayed for up to 6 hours and even rarely for 24 to 48 hours. Pulmonary overpressurization syndrome usually appears within a few minutes of surfacing. In either case, the patient requires oxygen and recompression therapy. Here again, be careful of positive pressure ventilation, as it may cause gas bubble emboli to the brain.

Neurological Emergencies Of DCS cases, 60 to 70 percent are now neurological. Nitrogen bubbles in the nervous system may present with any symptom from personality changes to specific localized neurological changes. By far the most common symptoms involve the lower spinal cord and often produce weakness or paralysis of the legs and urinary bladder. Bladder problems are so common that historically, urinary catheters were considered essential equipment for divers. These patients must have recompression therapy or irreversible paralysis will occur.

MANAGEMENT OF DIVING INJURIES

Patient History

- *Type of diving and equipment used.* This is very important. Remember that skin divers and snorkelers cannot get overpressurization syndrome or decompression sickness, but all divers can drown. The treatment for near-drowning is very different from that for decompression sickness or air embolism.

- *History of the dive.* You need to know where the dive occurred, at what depth, how many dives, how long on the bottom, and any in-water decompression. This information is also needed for dives during the preceding 2 days.

- *Past medical history.* Pulmonary problems that predispose to air trapping (asthma or obstructive lung disease) are frequently associated with overpressurization syndrome.

- *Exactly when the symptoms first occurred.* This may be helpful in differentiating air embolism and decompression sickness.

- *Complications of the dive.* Did the diver run out of air? Was there an attack by marine animals? Did a diving accident occur?

- *Travel after the dive.* Traveling at higher altitudes may precipitate decompression sickness.

Initial Management

- Follow standard patient assessment protocol: Primary Survey, critical interventions and transport decision, Secondary Survey, and Ongoing Exam.

- If there is any chance of overpressurization syndrome or decompression sickness, do not hyperventilate or give positive pressure ventilation. Positive pressure ventilation is indicated only for apneic patients.

- Check for hypothermia (see Appendix D) in all diving-accident victims.

- Patients with air embolism or neurological decompression sickness should be placed in supine position.

- All diving accident patients should get 100 percent oxygen.

- Shock and other injuries are treated by routine protocols.

- If a recompression facility is needed and you need information about the one nearest to your facility, you may obtain assistance 24 hours a day through the National Diving Alert Network at Duke University: (919) 684-8111.

No matter how far you may live from a large body of water, you may be called upon to manage a patient with near-drowning or diving injuries. When treating the near-drowning patient, the performance of the ABCs is most important in the prehospital phase, but do not forget the possibility of hypothermia. When treating barotrauma, you should not only follow the basic principles of ITLS, but also remember the importance of the history, patient positioning, the possibility of hypothermia, and the dangers of positive pressure ventilation.

BIBLIOGRAPHY

1. Clinchy, R. A., G. Egstrom, L. Fead. 1992. *Jeppeson's open water sport diving manual.* 5th ed. Englewood, CO: Jeppeson Sanderson, 25–49.
2. Kizer, K. W. 2003. Dysbarism. In J. E. Tintinalli (ed.), *Emergency medicine.* 6th ed. New York: McGraw-Hill.

Injury Prevention and the Role of the EMS Provider

Janet M. Williams, MD

Jonathan M. Rubin, MD

Objectives

Upon completion of this appendix, you should be able to:

1. Discuss the three components of the epidemiology triangle.
2. Discuss the three phases of an injury event as it relates to Haddon's matrix.
3. Discuss the difference between active and passive preventive interventions.
4. Discuss four ways EMS providers can help prevent injuries.

THE INJURY EPIDEMIC

Every day prehospital health-care providers serve the public by delivering quality emergency care. The ITLS curriculum has been developed to convey the principles of acute prehospital care of the injured patient. Well-trained prehospital care providers with ITLS skills save many lives of injured patients each year. Unfortunately, over 50 percent of trauma deaths occur immediately after the injury event. As a result, you often arrive at the scene only to find a patient who has died or is dying and for whom no life-saving measures can be taken. These cases illustrate the importance of recognizing injury as a preventable disease. Your role extends far beyond the acute care of the injured patient. The entire EMS community must become active in preventing injury from occurring in the first place.

Though underrecognized, injury is a major public health problem worldwide. In the United States, injury is the single greatest killer between the ages of 1 and 44 and is responsible for more years of potential life lost than cancer and heart disease combined. In the United States alone, the cost of injury is estimated to be over $210 billion annually.

Injury has been misconceived by the public as being a result of an unavoidable "act of God," an "accident," due to "bad luck," or a result of a behavioral problem on the part of the injured individual. In reality, injuries are health problems that behave like classic infectious diseases. Injuries may be characterized by demographic distributions, seasonal variations, epidemic episodes, and risk factors. In addition, they are predictable and preventable. An analogy has been made between the cause of an injury and the cause of a disease such as malaria. Table H-1 illustrates how disease causation can be applied to both of these entities.

Traditionally, medical education programs have emphasized the treatment of acute injury and have neglected the concept of injury prevention and control. It is interesting that

TABLE H-1 *An Etiologic Comparison of Injury and a Classic Infectious Disease*				
	Host	**Agent**	**Vector/Vehicle**	**Exposure Event**
Malaria	Human	*P. vivax*	Mosquito	Mosquito bite
Injury (i.e., head injury)	Human	Kinetic energy	Motor vehicle	Crash

patients presenting with cardiac symptoms are nearly always asked if they have risk factors such as history of smoking, diabetes, hypertension, hypercholesterolemia, and family history of heart disease. In addition, these patients are counseled as to how to reduce their risk for heart disease. As health-care providers, we have a responsibility to do the same for injured patients. Besides playing a vital role in the acute care of injured patients, prehospital care providers have a unique opportunity to assess risk factors for injury, to examine patients in the injury setting, to provide valuable injury information to other medical care providers, and to educate the public on injury prevention. In addition, prehospital care providers often see the "near-miss" patient who survives what could have been a fatal injury event. Such circumstances are an opportune time for prehospital care providers to give injury prevention advice.

THE INJURY PROCESS

What Is an Injury?

Injury may be defined as any damage to the human body that results from acute exposure of physical energy or from an absence of vital entities such as heat and oxygen. There are five basic forms of injurious energy: thermal, mechanical, electrical, radiating, and chemical. Roughly three-fourths of all injuries are caused by exposure to mechanical or kinetic energy during incidents such as motor-vehicle crashes, falls, and firearm discharges. Examples of injury resulting from a lack of heat or oxygen are frostbite and drowning. An individual's tolerance for injury depends on factors such as physical size, age, and presence of underlying disease.

Injury has also been defined as a disease that results from the interaction of three components of the epidemiology triangle: *host, agent,* and *environment* (Figure H-1). The host refers to the human being or victim, the agent is the form of energy involved, and the environment provides the opportunity for the agent (energy) to be transmitted to the host. The environment may be either protective and prevent injury or hostile and encourage injury (Figure H-2). The mechanism by which the agent or energy is transferred to the host is referred to as the *vector.* For example, during a motor-vehicle crash, the automobile is the vector that may transmit physical (kinetic) energy to the host if the environment is permissive.

Injury may be classified as intentional or unintentional. Intentional injuries include those such as suicide, assault, and homicide. Unintentional injuries include those that are not deliberate or planned, such as falls, motor-vehicle crashes, and burns. In some cases, it may be difficult to distinguish intentional from unintentional injury. Injury also may be categorized by the actual type of injury (such as fracture or head injury), by the mechanism or cause of injury (such as motor-vehicle crash or fall), or by the population at risk (such as pediatric, young males, or the elderly).

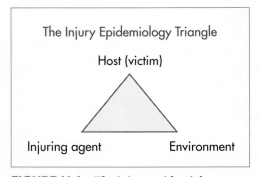

FIGURE H-1 The injury epidemiology triangle.

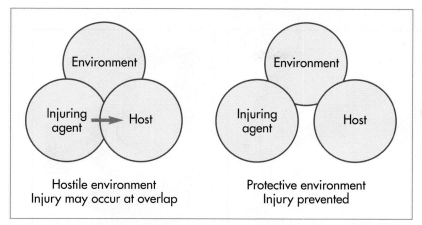

FIGURE H-2   The relationship of the environment, injuring agent, and host.

Why Do Injuries Occur?

Injury results when the victim is exposed to energy in amounts that exceed the threshold of human tolerance. In most cases, energy is transmitted as the victim is attempting to perform a specific task or action. The performance of a task refers to how well the individual executes an action, and the task demand is the amount of skill that is required to successfully perform the task. Any time that an individual's performance is below the task demand for the action, there is potential for release of injurious energy (Figure H-3). For example,

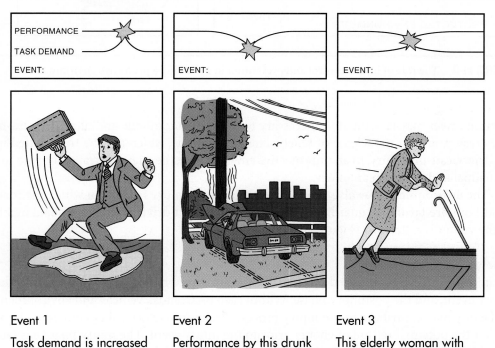

Event 1

Task demand is increased in this case as an otherwise healthy man attempts to walk over an ice patch but falls.

Event 2

Performance by this drunk driver is below the task demand, resulting in the crash.

Event 3

This elderly woman with poor eyesight and difficulty walking with subnormal performance is unable to tolerate only a slight increase in task demand such as walking over an area rug. She trips and falls.

FIGURE H-3   The relationship of performance and task demand in the injury process.

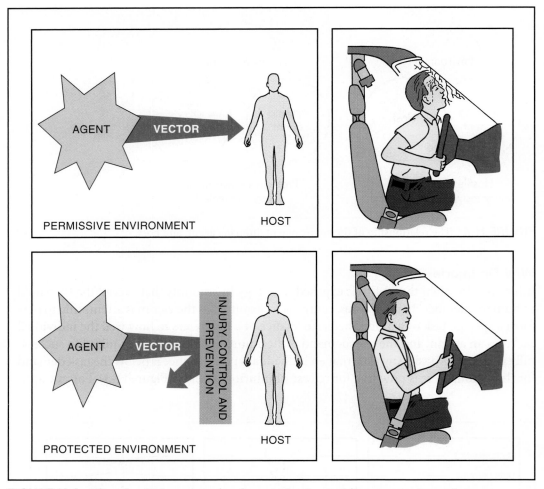

FIGURE H-4 The role of injury control and prevention in providing a protective environment.

a drunk driver may lack the skills necessary to drive an automobile and ultimately crash. The crash results in the release of kinetic energy (motion), which may be transmitted to the driver, causing injury. In an unprotective environment, the energy is transmitted to the individual and results in an injury.

The environment may also protect the victim from injury in cases in which the road conditions are favorable, guardrails are present to prevent driving over an embankment, or the victim is restrained (Figure H-4).

Analyzing Injury Events

An injury event can be analyzed by separating it into three phases: the preinjury phase, the injury event, and the postinjury phase. Within each phase, host, vehicle, and environmental factors may contribute to the injury process. Preinjury factors either contribute to or inhibit the potential release of energy prior to the injury event. The injury phase has factors that may enhance or inhibit transmission of energy to the host during the injury event. Postinjury factors tend to contribute to or diminish the severity of the injury once it has occurred. Prehospital care providers play a major role in the postinjury phase by providing rapid and high-quality care to injured victims in the field.

The analysis of the three phases of an injury event with respect to host, vehicle, and environmental factors is referred to as *Haddon's matrix*. Table H-2 provides an example of an analysis of a motor-vehicle crash using Haddon's matrix. This tool is very useful for identifying factors contributing to the outcome of an injury event, broadening the discus-

TABLE H-2 *Example Using Haddon's Matrix*

Factors

Phases	Host	Vehicle	Physical Environment	Sociocultural Environment
Pre-event	Impaired capacity due to alcohol, age, poor vision, fatigue, inexperience, poor judgment	Defective parts (brakes, tires), poor maintenance, dirty windshield/windows, improper brake lights, ease of control, speed of travel	Narrow road shoulder, poor lighting, road curvature and gradient, road surface type, weather conditions, divided highway, visibility of hazards, signalization	Attitudes about alcohol, drunk driving laws, speed limits, injury prevention programs
Event	Tolerance of body to energy, injury threshold due to aging, chronic disease (osteoporosis), etc., safety belt use	Placement hardness and sharpness of contact surfaces (dash, steering wheel), automatic restraints, vehicle size	Recovery areas, guard-rails, fixed objects (trees, telephone poles), median barriers, embankments	Attitudes about seat-belt use, enforcement of child safety seat laws
Postevent	Extent of injury sustained, knowledge of first aid, physical condition, and age	Fuel system integrity (bursting gas tank), entrapment of victim	Access to EMS, quality of EMS care, availability of extrication equipment, rehabilitation programs	Training of EMS personnel, trauma system programs
Results	Physical and mental impairment	Cost of vehicle repair	Damage to environment	Legal costs, costs to society (loss of lives and income)

sion for developing prevention strategies, and revealing that most injuries are the product of a large number of causal factors and are not just random happenings.

INJURY PREVENTION AND CONTROL

Perhaps the most important principle of injury prevention and control is that injury is a disease subject to prevention by modifying transmission of energy to the individual. The goal of *primary injury prevention* is to prevent injury from occurring in the first place. Examples include wearing a seat belt, helmet use by motorcyclists and bicyclists, and the installation of smoke detectors. Strategies that attempt to minimize further injury or death after the initial trauma or injury event has occurred are called *secondary injury prevention*. Prehospital care providers practice secondary injury prevention, or acute care, by ensuring adequate airway, breathing, and circulation as well as cervical-spine stabilization and rapid transportation to the closest appropriate medical facility.

Injury Surveillance

Injury surveillance data forms the foundation of injury control. Accurate and detailed data are needed to determine the incidence of specific injury events, the demographic distributions, the cause of an injury event, and injury risk factors, as well as other factors involved in injury. Prehospital data such as location of the injury site, mechanism of injury, host factors, agent factors, and environmental factors are required. Prehospital care providers are in a crucial position to document the mechanism of injury in great detail, including information such as the extent of damage to a motor vehicle (starred windshield or deformed steering wheel). Description of the location and conditions of the injury site also may be useful in identifying a dangerous section of road where motor vehicle crashes occur time and again or a hazardous area such as an unsafe playground where injuries occur frequently.

Risk Factors

Injuries are not random events. Some special populations, such as males, alcoholics, and certain age groups, are at higher risk for injury than others. A *risk factor* is a variable that makes an individual more likely to be injured. We can prevent injuries by reducing or eliminating risk factors. An example of a host risk factor that may predispose an individual to injury is the use of drugs or alcohol while driving a motor vehicle. A high-risk group is defined as a subset of the population that has a higher incidence of injury. This group may be exposed to hazards more frequently, may be unable to avoid a hazard, or may have a lower injury threshold. Young males are one well-known group that is at higher risk for being involved in a motor-vehicle crash than the general population.

Preventive Interventions

Haddon's matrix can be used to identify the factors affecting the extent of injury during specific injury events. Some of the factors may be amenable to prevention strategies or interventions designed to reduce the incidence or severity of injury. The three types of interventions are educational, enforcement, and engineering. Interventions may also be classified as either active or passive.

An active intervention requires a change in behavior by the individual in need of protection. Educational programs such as those that encourage seat-belt use or installation of home smoke detectors are examples of active interventions that attempt to persuade individuals to alter their behavior for increased self-protection. These programs may increase public awareness but are often ignored by those who are at highest risk for injury such as the economically and educationally deprived. Laws against drunk driving and mandatory helmet use by motorcyclists are other examples of active interventions that are aimed at changing an individual's behavior. However, the introduction of a legal intervention does not necessarily imply that it will be enforced by the authorities or adhered to by the public. Unfortunately, alcohol continues to play a part in half of all fatal motor-vehicle crashes despite laws against driving under the influence of alcohol. Active education and enforcement interventions are more effective when used together.

Passive interventions provide automatic protection and are generally more effective than active interventions, since they do not rely on human behavior change. Modifications in the engineering and design of vehicles and the environment have been very effective in reducing the incidence and severity of injuries. The incorporation of airbags and softer dashboards into automobiles has significantly reduced the incidence and severity of motor-vehicle-related injuries. Engineering improvements in road design also have been found to be effective countermeasures in preventing motor-vehicle crashes.

Designing Interventions

When developing injury prevention programs, it is critical to recognize potential pitfalls for failure as well as ingredients for success. Many intervention programs are difficult to initiate, expensive to maintain, and require the use of limited community resources. The following suggestions will be helpful in selecting injury prevention activities.

TABLE H-3 *Examples of Injury-Specific Interventions*

Injury Event	Risk Factor	Examples of Injury-Specific Intervention
Drowning	2-year-old to 5-year-old males	Install fencing around pools at least 1 meter high with self-locking door; water motion alarm; swimming lessons; prominent "no diving" notices near shallow water; easy access to EMS
Bicycle	5-year-old to 12-year-old males	Encourage helmet use; use of safety reflectors; bicycle traffic lanes; rider education programs
Poisoning	1-year-old to 5-year-old children	Package medicines in childproof containers; install safety latches on storage cabinets
Falls	Elderly with poor vision and/or unstable gait	Remove throw rugs; use nightlights; handrails on stairs; access to activate EMS

■ Target efforts toward a problem that occurs frequently or results in severe injury in your community. In some regions, this may be house fires and, for others, motor-vehicle crashes.

■ Address the problem injuries that have specific countermeasures that are known to be effective. Focus on limited, concrete solutions to specific injury events and avoid diffuse, general approaches. Examples of directed specific solutions include fire-safe cigarettes, smoke detectors for house fire prevention, and helmets for bicycle-related head injury prevention.

■ Make the intervention as simple as possible to increase public acceptance and minimize the chance of misuse.

■ Develop a critical mass of community awareness through broad-based grass-roots support, legislation, enforcement, and professional action. Prehospital care providers should take advantage of their connections with local and regional community leaders to build coalitions for effective prevention programs.

■ Promote institutionalization of programs that will last beyond the initial volunteer effort or temporary grant funding. Injury prevention programs should be designed to become a permanent component of prehospital care.

Table H-3 provides examples of injury-specific interventions that have been developed and found to be successful.

Role of the EMS Provider

Prehospital care providers are a vital link in the chain of the national injury control effort. Their interaction with the public is an opportunity to practice both primary and secondary injury prevention. As part of the medical community, EMS personnel provide information to emergency physicians and nurses, which is important in the acute care of injured victims as well as in injury control research. The injury epidemic can be addressed only through a concerted effort by the medical, community, and legislative organizations.

Following are the four areas in which prehospital personnel can make an impact and prevent injuries in their own communities.

Acute Care/Secondary Injury Prevention of the Injured Patient: Medically trained personnel, such as ITLS providers, are the initial and vital link in the trauma care system. By providing prompt and appropriate care, many lives are saved each year.

Community Education/Primary Injury Prevention: As respected and credible members of the community, prehospital care providers have a unique opportunity to practice primary injury prevention, since they interact directly with injured patients and their families. Less severely injured patients and their families and friends can be counseled about how the present and any future injury could be prevented. Examples include advising the public to wear helmets when riding bicycles, motorcycles, and all-terrain vehicles, as well as wearing seat belts and using child car seats in automobiles.

By assessing the scene of the injury, prehospital personnel may identify specific injury prevention strategies for a given family, such as how to "childproof" a home or ways to make the home of an elderly person less risky for falls. As community spokespersons, prehospital care providers often interact with groups such as the local parent–teacher association and the rotary club. In doing so, community leaders will become more aware of the important concepts of injury prevention and work toward developing a safer community.

Public Policy: Seat-belt and fire-safe cigarette legislation are two examples of regulations that have been instituted with the support of EMS personnel. Seat-belt legislation has been very effective in increasing the number of people who wear seat belts and decreasing the number of highway deaths. For those states without seat-belt laws, EMS personnel can be effective in encouraging the passage of such legislation. Similarly, it was prehospital care providers who found that the most common cause of fatal house fires is cigarette smoking. With their support, a fire-safe cigarette has been developed. Prehospital care providers may be the first to recognize a new injury pattern or high-risk group for a specific injury. By reporting this type of information to local and state authorities, injury prevention strategies may be put into place by legislators in hopes of reducing fatal and serious injuries.

Research/Injury Surveillance: Accurate documentation of the circumstances surrounding injuries such as demographics, location, mechanism of injury, and associated risk factors is important in identifying problem injuries and designing and implementing prevention strategies. Providing reliable information to local community leaders, legislators, and physicians—such as the location of the "dangerous intersection," the poorly supervised quarry, and the "unsafe" playground—can lead to the development of effective injury prevention strategies and a safer community.

BIBLIOGRAPHY

1. American College of Emergency Physicians. 1992, September 16. *Guidelines for trauma care systems*. Dallas: The College.

2. Baker, S., B. O'Neill, M. J. Ginsburg, G. Li. 1992. *The injury fact book*. New York: Oxford University Press.

3. Centers for Disease Control and Prevention. 1992. *Setting the national agenda for injury control in the 1990s: Position papers from the third national injury control conference*. Atlanta: The Centers.

4. Centers for Disease Control and Prevention. 1993. *Injury control in the 1990s: A national plan for action*. Atlanta: The Centers.

5. Christoffel, T., S. P. Teret. 1993. *Protecting the public, legal issues in injury prevention*. New York: Oxford University Press.

6. Committee on Trauma Research, Commission on Life Sciences, National Research Council, and the Institute of Medicine. 1985. *Injury in America: A continuing public health problem*. Washington, DC: National Academy Press.

7. Kaalbfleisch, J., F. Rivera. 1989. Principles in injury control: Lessons to be learned from child safety seats. *Pediatric Emergency Care*, 131–34.

8. Martinez, R. 1990. Injury control: A primer for physicians. *Annals of Emergency Medicine* 19: 72–77.

9. The National Committee for Injury Prevention and Control. 1989. *Injury prevention: Meeting the challenge*. New York: Oxford University Press.

10. Wilson, M. H., et al. 1991. *Saving children, a guide to injury prevention*. New York: Oxford University Press.

Multicasualty Incidents and Triage

David Maatman, NREMT-P/IC

Roy Alson, PhD, MD, FACEP

Jere F. Baldwin, MD, FACEP, FAAFP

John T. Stevens, NREMT-P

Objectives

Upon completion of this appendix, you should be able to:

1. Compare and contrast the definitions of the terms *disaster* and *multicasualty incident.*
2. Define the term *span of control.*
3. List the responsibilities of the medical director, triage supervisor, transport supervisor, treatment supervisor, and staging supervisor.
4. Describe the Initial Assessment.
5. Identify Priority 1, 2, 3, and 4 patients.

DISASTERS AND MULTICASUALTY INCIDENTS

Definitions

- *Disaster (major).* Any natural catastrophe that causes damage of sufficient severity and magnitude to warrant major disaster assistance.
- *Incident Command System (ICS).* The combination of facilities, equipment, personnel, procedures, and communications operating within a common organizational structure, designed to aid in the management of resources during emergency incidents. It is used for all kinds of emergencies and is applicable to small as well as large and complex incidents.
- *Multicasualty Incident (MCI).* An incident involving a large number of persons injured in which the EMS system is unable to manage the situation utilizing day-to-day procedures. An MCI may be classified as a disaster, but not all disasters are MCIs.
- *Paper Plan Syndrome.* Having a written MCI/disaster plan without training the individuals who would most likely activate and work it.
- *Span of Control.* The number of individuals a supervisor is responsible for, usually expressed as the ratio of supervisors to individuals. (Under the NIMS, an appropriate span of control is between 1:3 and 1:7.)
- *Triage.* To prioritize or sort injuries or the injured, usually into four categories: Priority 0, 1, 2, and 3 (Black, Red, Yellow, and Green).

The Role of EMS

It is not uncommon for EMS to have more than one patient at a trauma scene. However, most day-to-day operational procedures are designed for the single-patient incident. Safety, organization, and communication are paramount in all EMS activities. When faced with multiple patients, this need is even greater. It is essential that these components be effective and that all entities of the emergency system work from the same plan.

An effective and efficient way to obtain this unity is to have Emergency Medical Services operate as a branch of the Incident Command System (ICS). Primary functional components of the medical branch include the medical director, triage, treatment, transport, and staging. (Even with a single-patient incident, these four components exist, but one person usually is responsible for the functions of all components.) There is a medical director in charge of the patient care (team leader), injuries are triaged (prioritized assessment), treatment is provided for the patient, a transport decision that includes destination and mode of transport is made, and deployment of on-scene vehicles is determined from a point of safety, ingress, and egress (staging).

By having the medical branch function as part of the ICS, it provides EMS with dependable, reproducible results when faced with multiple-casualty incidents. As with the other components of an ICS, the medical branch must be simple enough for new users but expandable enough to provide the necessary structure to manage large incidents.

Incident Command System

In the early 1970s the ICS was developed in southern California under FIRESCOPE (FIrefighting RESources of California Organized for Potential Emergencies). Though originally developed to assist in the response to wildland fires, it was quickly recognized as a system that could help public safety responders provide effective and coordinated incident management for a wide range of situations.

Multiple variations of the FIRESCOPE ICS have been developed to include Fire Ground Command System (FGC) and National Fire Protection Association (NFPA) 1561, which was then called Standard on Fire Department Incident Management System.

FIRESCOPE ICS and its variations served as the basis for the National Incident Management System Incident Command System (NIMS ICS). The NIMS ICS was developed, under the Department of Homeland Security (DHS) Federal Emergency Management Agency (FEMA). Additional information about NIMS can be found online at www.fema.gov/NIMS

The typical on-scene components of the Operations Section of an ICS are Command, Fire Suppression, Rescue/Extrication, Law Enforcement, and Medical (Figure I-1). The structured flexibility of an ICS enables it to be adapted to all types of emergency incidents: fire, rescue, law enforcement, and multicasualty incidents. Because of its modular design, the structure of the ICS can be expanded or compressed, depending on the changing conditions of an incident. It must be staffed and operated by qualified personnel from an emergency service agency.

If an on-scene incident command system is not immediately established, other rescuers will take independent actions, which will frequently be in conflict with each other. These independent actions (freelancing) may be dangerous and disruptive in an environment that requires organization and accountability. Without organization and accountability, chaos will occur and too many people will attempt to command the incident. If you do not control the situation, the situation will control you.

Medical (Emergency Services) Branch

One branch of the operations sector of an on-scene ICS is the medical branch, which is broken down into manageable components (subfunctions or groups). The five primary

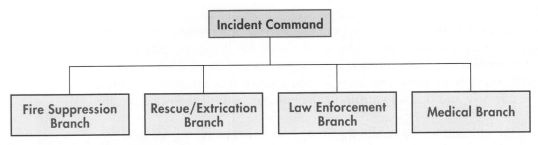

FIGURE I-1 On-scene incident command structure.

positions of the medical branch are the medical director, triage group, treatment group, transport group, and staging group (Figure I-2). It may not be necessary to have one person in each position, but it is necessary to ensure the function of each position is executed. At a scene with multiple patients, it may be necessary to have more than one person take on the function of these components. When considering the need to expand or condense the medical branch of the ICS, the best indicator is current or anticipated span of control. The general rule is to have one person oversee five subordinates. Some latitude may be given due to the complexity of the situation. A highly complex or difficult situation may require a span of control of 3:1, or a simple situation may allow up to 7:1.

All participants of an ICS need to know their responsibilities. Following are ideas and suggestions used in determining the responsibilities of the medical branch of an ICS.

- ■ *Medical Director*
  - Establishes liaisons with on-scene Incident Command
  - Establishes a working branch with appropriate groups
  - Ensures that proper rescue/extrication services are activated
  - Ensures law enforcement involvement as necessary
  - Ensures that helicopter landing zone operations are coordinated
  - Determines the amount and types of additional medical resources and supplies
  - Ensures that area hospitals and medical control authorities (MCAs) are aware of the situation so they can prepare for casualties

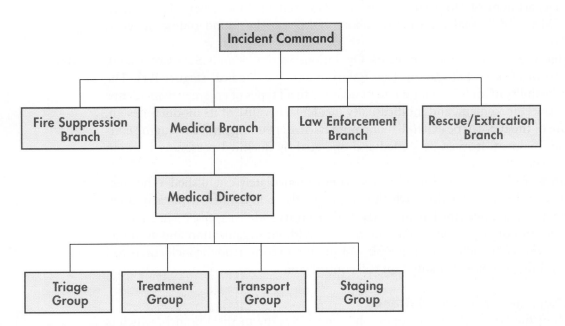

FIGURE I-2 Medical branch of the ICS.

- Designates assistance officers and their location
- Maintains an appropriate span of control
- Works as a conduit of communications between subordinates and the Incident Commander

■ *EMS Staging Supervisor*
- Maintains a log of available units and medical supplies
- Coordinates physical location of incoming resources (i.e., ambulances and helicopters)
- Coordinates incoming personnel who wish to aid at the scene
- Provides updates to the medical director as necessary

■ *Triage Supervisor*
- Ensures proper utilization of the Initial Assessment triage system or other local protocol
- Ensures that triage tags or other visual identification technique is properly completed and secured to the patient
- Makes requests for additional resources through the medical director
- Provides updates to the medical director as necessary

■ *Treatment Supervisor*
- Establishes suitable treatment areas
- Communicates resource needs to the medical director
- Assigns, supervises, and coordinates treatment of patients
- Provides updates to the medical director as necessary

■ *Transport Supervisor*
- Ensures the organized transport of patients off-scene
- Ensures an appropriate distribution of patients to all local hospitals to prevent hospital overloading
- Completes a transportation log
- Contacts receiving hospitals to advise them of the number of patients and condition (may be delegated to a communications leader)
- Provides updates to the medical director as necessary

TRIAGE

As a triage person, you should spend less than 1 minute doing the Initial Assessment to determine the priority of a patient. It cannot be overemphasized that the person doing the triage does not render any treatment to a patient. Treatment is to be done by the treatment group of the medical branch of the ICS. A triage person begins treatment of victims is no longer doing triage, and the function of triage must be reassigned. Once the medical priority of a patient has been determined, using the ITLS Triage Decision Tree (Figure I-3), the triage person should affix an appropriately completed triage tag (Figure I-4) or other visual identification technique to the victim and move on to the next victim to be assessed.

Patient Assessment

In triage, patients typically are prioritized into four categories.

■ *Priority 0.* Black tagged; dead or alive, but nonsalvageable (Some EMS systems will group the "alive but unsalvageable" patients in the Priority 1 category and work on them as long as resources are available and it does not take away from the needed resources for a salvageable patient.)

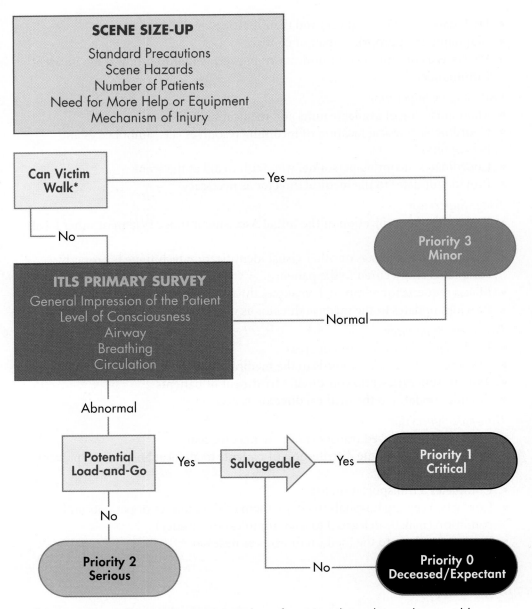

FIGURE I-3 ITLS Triage Decision Tree. This decision tree reflects the steps of initial triage. Subsequent and more detailed assessments should occur throughout patient care.

- *Priority 1.* Red tagged; critical condition, unstable but salvageable (load and go)
- *Priority 2.* Yellow tagged; serious condition, potentially unstable
- *Priority 3.* Green tagged; stable condition, minor injuries, "walking wounded"

Although there is a tendency to over triage, one must refrain from this because of its impact on the resources available to the EMS system. We need to be as accurate in our triage assessment as possible. Three basic human systems need to be quickly evaluated to determine the patient's medical priority: neurological system (LOC), respiratory system, and circulatory system. By utilizing the ITLS Initial Assessment during the triage phase and the Rapid Trauma Survey or the Focused Exam in the treatment phase, we will be accurate

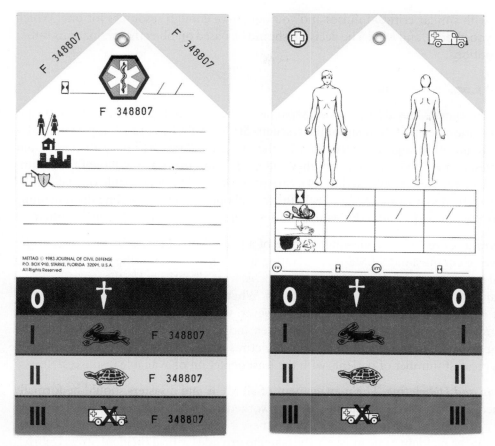

FIGURE I-4   Triage tag, (a) front and (b) back.

in our assessment and make the best use of resources by providing the greatest amount of good to the greatest number of patients. The general steps are as follows:

- General impression (patient overview)
  - Victim's approximate age?
  - What position is the victim in?
  - What is the victim's activity (aware of surroundings, anxious, in distress)?
  - Does the victim have adequate perfusion (skin color)?
  - Are there any major injuries or bleeding?
- Level of consciousness
- Airway
  - Is it open and self-maintained?
  - Is it compromised?
- Breathing
  - Is the victim breathing?
  - What is the approximate rate (fast, slow, normal), quality and effort?
- Circulation
  - Is there a pulse?
  - What is the approximate rate (fast, slow, normal), quality, and regularity?

Once the Initial Assessment has been completed and you have figured in a "survivability factor," you have a good idea how to prioritize the patient. An example of applying the survivability factor would be if you were presented with a geriatric patient and a pediatric patient with similar critical injuries and you only have enough resources for one. Which one do you choose, and why? The decision should be based on objective evaluations rather than emotions.

Special Considerations

Injured Rescuers Many ICSs provide a separate medical component at the scene of the incident for the care and treatment of the rescuers. Structurally, this branch is part of the logistics section of a large ICS structure. In the event of illness or injury to one of our colleagues, we need to be assured that they will not fall into the triage system of the victims of the incident. We are obligated to take care of our own. This will enable our fallen colleague to return to duty quicker and help the overall operation by providing the remaining rescuers the peace of mind of knowing that their fellow rescuer has not been forgotten.

Standard of Care When reviewing the care of a patient of an MCI, we have to consider the adverse circumstances EMS was operating under at the time of the incident. During normal day-to-day operations, standard protocols treat all patients for the worst-case scenario and thus many patients are overtreated. When manpower and resources are available, it is prudent to provide such care. However, when working in an MCI or disaster environment, the inefficient use of manpower and resources may be catastrophic. The guiding principle in triage and treatment of victims of an MCI is to do the greatest good for the greatest number of patients with the least depletion of available resources.

Critique and Debriefing The management of all MCIs and disasters should be formally critiqued. Primary focus should be on what worked and what did not. An MCI/Disaster Plan is a dynamic document, modified when there is a problem. In addition to taking time to critique the incident, time must also be taken to provide Critical Incident Stress Debriefing (CISD) for the participants of an incident. The mental health of EMS professionals is as important as their physical health.

Other Triage Schemes

The term *triage* is used in many different ways. Although the definition of the term is essentially the same (to sort), the mechanisms to sort and the application varies.

The START (Simple Triage and Rapid Transport) system developed by the Newport Beach Fire and Marine Department and Hoag Hospital in Newport Beach, California, and JumpSTART developed by Dr. Lou Romig from Miami Children's Hospital in Miami, both utilize algorithms that require a quantitative assessment (actual count) of respirations. This provides a "hard point" for determination of priority or continued assessment. However, the algorithms do not provide for a qualitative assessment, the use of a general impression, or opportunity to determine if the victim is salvageable.

Sacco Triage Method (STM) developed by Dr. Bill Sacco utilizes mathematical computations to determine a physiological score that predicts survival. Patients are triaged on anticipated outcome in conjunction with transport and treatment resources. The use of precise mathematical formulas in the initial phase of an incident may be considered overwhelming and not aid in the on-scene resource management. This scheme claims to be evidence based and shows promise for development of regional impact plans.

The American College of Surgeons Committee on Trauma (ACS COT) developed "field triage criteria" that is specific to trauma patients and aids in the determination of transport destinations to trauma centers. This algorithm assesses vital signs and level of consciousness, anatomy of injury, mechanism of injury, and comorbid factors. Based on these findings, it recommends a transport destination. This triage scheme is detailed and may not be applicable for the initial phases of on-scene triage to determine which patients should be treated and transported first.

ITLS RECOMMENDATIONS

The priorities of any incident, no matter how small or large, should be safety, organization, and then patient care. To provide the most effective and efficient patient care, one must approach it in a safe and organized fashion.

To have an effective medical branch of the ICS requires its use in day-to-day operations, including the routine, small emergencies. The rehearsal of the standardized structure of an ICS on smaller situations will develop proficiency and allow for a smooth transition into the larger, more complex incidents. Activating the ICS only when an incident reaches a high level can result in a lack of familiarity with its use. Routine activation of the system develops confidence in its use for all levels of command and agencies involved. To avoid the paper plan syndrome, the regular implementation and review of an MCI/disaster plan is paramount to having successful operations.

An ICS is not a magic wand that will save lives by itself, nor will it replace the common sense and good judgment required of experienced EMS professionals. There is no Holy Grail for effective triage in all situations. It is necessary to have a plan, communicate, and execute it. It may be necessary to blend multiple triage schemes to capitalize on the best outcome. Successful management of a situation still requires properly trained people who know what to do and how to do it. ICS properly utilized can increase the overall effectiveness of the participants by providing a proactive approach to management. If you do not manage the situation, the situation manages you. The key to effective performance in a leadership role is not necessarily rank, but the understanding of the duties of that position and the ability to properly function at that level.

For large-scale incidents an operation may last for days or even weeks and will require additional resources. As part of the disaster plan, an ICS provides the structure for the necessary administrative, planning, financial, and logistical support.

BIBLIOGRAPHY

1. http://www.jumpstarttriage.com (created 2006; revised December 30, 2006)
2. http://www.start-triage.com/ (accessed January 31, 2007)
3. http://www.sharpthinkers.com (accessed January 31, 2007)
4. http://www.facs.org (revised January 10, 2007; accessed January 31, 2007)
5. http://www.fema.gov/nims ICS-100: Introduction to ICS, September 2005
6. Maatman, D. V., S. A. Huisman. 2005. *T-4, Triage treatment & transport training.* Grand Rapids, MI: D&D Publications.

Agricultural Rescue Course Overview

Davis Hill, EMT-P

S. Robert Seitz, MEd, RN, NREMT-P

Objectives

Upon completion of this appendix, you should:

1. Be aware of the need for EMTs and rescue personnel in rural agricultural areas to have coordinated training in rescue and treatment of victims of farm injuries.

2. Know how to obtain access for this type of training.

RESCUE ON THE FARM

The term *rescue* is defined as actions to set free from danger. Rescue is needed when someone or something is in danger, and action is taken to either stop or remove a person or thing from that danger. It is the desire and expectation that after the rescue intervention, the person or thing will be removed from the danger with the minimal amount of additional injury. Consider the following scenario.

A northeastern dairy farmer was found pinned under his tractor late one October afternoon, just at dusk. The temperature was in the low 50s. He was alert and oriented and in considerable pain, but could not feel his lower extremities. He was pinned under the rear wheel at his pelvis and both legs. He remembers overturning the tractor and believes it happened in the early afternoon, although he really could not recall the timing clearly. He was found by his wife and son who promptly called for emergency services by contacting 911.

This rural community was served by a local volunteer fire service and BLS ambulance. By the time emergency responders arrived on-scene, several family members and neighbors were present and obviously very anxious. The fire chief called for a medical helicopter and a ground ALS unit was dispatched earlier. As soon as the tractor was secured from further movement, EMTs on-scene began a patient evaluation.

The patient's vitals were surprisingly stable for his condition and they determined that initially his most serious condition appeared to be crushing injuries to the lower extremities and pelvis. They urged the fire service members and the fire chief who was incident commander (IC) not to extricate until ALS units arrived on-scene for further evaluation. This request was backed up by both incoming units, as their arrival time was estimated to be between 10 and 15 minutes. However, due to the family's demands and the fact that the outside temperature was dropping, the IC ordered the extrication to take place and stated that the patient could be treated by ALS in the ambulance. As the tractor was lifted from the patient, his condition deteriorated rapidly. When ALS providers arrived on-scene, the patient had arrested and could not be resuscitated.

RURAL RESCUE

Rescue is a relatively new term in rural communities. To truly be proficient in rescue techniques, individuals need to be knowledgeable and competent with mechanical skills as well as advanced patient care techniques. While such skills training may be more readily available to career personnel, obtaining it can be very difficult or near impossible for volunteers. This type of training may be hard to justify in areas that have very few true "rescue" calls. Requiring every fire/rescue member to be a paramedic or experienced EMT and trained in multiple aspects of agricultural rescue is unrealistic with the existing constraints of personnel, finances, training, and competency requirements. Thus, performing rescue in rural communities requires teamwork between the people doing the mechanical work (normally firefighters) and the people doing the patient care work (EMS providers). The time to realize this is not at a scene as described above, but during a training exercise that involves both parties.

FARM TRAUMA IS UNIQUE

Farm trauma may be very different from other trauma that rural emergency responders are trained to handle in an everyday manner. Farm trauma can be equated to victims caught in building collapses, with similarities to time of discovery or type of treatment. On the farm, it may be several hours before a victim is even missed, since most farmers work alone in very remote areas. Victims of a building collapse can be crushed for several hours or more before SAR personnel get to them. Should the quality of care each victim receives be different?

In the rural community, probably the most common occurrence that brings fire and EMS personnel together is a motor-vehicle crash. The majority of MVCs are discovered soon after occurrence so responders quite often are presented with victims in a compensated state. These individuals may be able to survive in spite of poorly coordinated care. However, when an extended period of time has elapsed before the victim is found or the rescue requires extended time, the patient may have exhausted his or her ability to compensate for injuries, and without close coordination between rescuers and EMS, the victim may not survive.

TEAMWORK TRAINING

Traditionally, rescue training involves teaching mechanical techniques such as shoring, door and roof removal, high angle and confined space techniques, hazmat management, and so on. Little discussion takes place about patient care during the rescue process, short of the very basic levels of support necessary to keep the patient alive until the patient was brought to the EMS providers. There is certainly benefit to adding a module to each rescue curriculum dealing with injury management specific to each type of rescue and encouraging participation by those responders who will provide patient care. This is why Pennsylvania State University developed a true rescue training program (Agricultural Rescue Course) designed to bring both rescue personnel and EMS personnel together in the same classroom to learn how to manage trauma patients injured in agricultural accidents. The Pennsylvania State University has united with ITLS in the development of the medical components for several agricultural rescue training modules.

Many rural EMS responders are not members of the fire service so their participation in fire "rescue" training courses is infrequent. Even when EMS is part of the fire service, there is often not a solid partnership between personnel. For a successful rescue to take place, all individuals regardless of rescue function should understand the role of other rescue personnel and work together as a team to facilitate the best patient outcome possible.

TRACTOR AND MACHINERY INCIDENTS

Tractor overturns and machinery entanglements account for about two-thirds of all farm deaths and serious injury on farms. It is not uncommon for an injured farmer to be found (usually by the family) several hours after the incident occurred. With this delay in time, traditional treatment protocols may need to be modified depending on the extent of injury. This is one type of rescue where advanced life support measures must be delivered to the patient prior to extrication activities. Severe crushing injuries (similar to those found in building collapse victims) may need to be treated prior to other rescue activities.

Crushing injuries can occur when a tractor operator is pinned under a tractor for an extended time. They also commonly occur when the farmer becomes entangled in a rotating shaft or a machine's rollers or augers. Another complication to machinery incidents is hydraulic injection injuries. Hydraulic pressures on farm equipment are typically 1,500 to 3,000 psi (pounds per square inch). If a pinhole leak develops in a hydraulic line, pressure of the oil exiting the leak can exceed 7,000 psi, which when injected into the body can cause serious tissue and structure damage.

Rural EMS responders need to be methodical in assessing the patient's condition and potential injuries. Likewise, those actions involving stabilizing the machine and extrication activities (lifting, dismantling, cutting, etc.) become so technical that fire personnel need to concentrate on those actions and not be concerned with in-depth patient care needs. EMS responders should understand the issues faced by the fire personnel but will not need to be involved in their actions.

FARM CONFINED SPACES

There are a host of confined spaces on farms that farmers enter on a regular basis. High among them are silos, which are structures used to ferment and store high-moisture forages. Many "rescue" people would argue that EMS care is not normally provided within a confined space, rather the patient is removed to a safe area for treatment. However, one of the leading causes of involvement in a silo entrapment is entanglement in the unloading auger. Crushing injuries and potential amputations (along with surgical amputations) are factors that may be encountered. Again, protocols and techniques that work well for other types of incidents need to be revisited when dealing with farm trauma.

Emergency responders must realize that the majority of farmers in the United States are not obliged to follow OSHA confined-space standards that other industry workers must follow. This fact should suggest that those procedures designed to protect the worker may not be in place on the majority of farms.

Rescue personnel should not take for granted a backup plan for rescuing someone who is involved in a confined space is in place. The farmer will rely on the local emergency responders whether they are trained or not. As confined-space rescue is a specialization itself, rural EMS responders should also be encouraged to become trained in confined-space entry to be able to work hand in hand with the personnel trained to perform entry, initiate patient care, and assist with extrication activities.

AGRICULTURAL RESCUE—AN OPPORTUNITY

Agricultural rescue as defined should combine patient care with the mechanics of access, disentanglement, and extrication. As both disciplines are extremely technical in and of themselves, to expect responders responsible for stabilization, disentanglement, and extrication to also provide the level of medical intervention that may be needed has a potential to overburden those few personnel who may be cross trained and experienced. Farm incidents happen so infrequently that proficiency comes slowly. Specializing in each aspect of "rescue" is a must. This should start with the training programs that acknowledge the importance of all resources necessary and identify and promote an understanding of various roles, integrate rescue practice with patient care, and increase communication between all rescue personnel involved.

For more information on the Agricultural Rescue Course and availability of courses, please contact the ITLS International Office at 888-495-4857 (international calls: 630-495-6442).

BIBLIOGRAPHY

1. Hill, D., S. R. Seitz. 2006. *Farm rescue course.* University Park: Pennsylvania State University.

ITLS Access Overview

Roy Alson, MD

Objectives

Upon completion of this appendix, you should:

1. Be aware of the need in certain localities for EMTs to have skills in crashed vehicle entry techniques using basic equipment.

2. Know how to obtain training in these skills.

Motor-vehicle collisions remain a major cause of multiple trauma. Studies have shown that the sooner a trauma patient reaches definitive care, the better the outcome for that patient. The goal of ITLS is to provide the responder with the tools and training to assess, stabilize, and rapidly transport the trauma patient to the appropriate medical facility. Before beginning assessment and treatment of the trauma patient, the responder must first be able to access the patient. In most locales, EMS resources respond to motor-vehicle collisions accompanied by fire and/or rescue personnel or have rescue personnel immediately available. Often in more rural and isolated areas, there are situations in which rescue equipment and personnel are not available or may require prolonged times to respond. Those EMS responders may be faced with gaining access with whatever equipment they can carry on their ambulance or rescue vehicle.

To assist the EMS responder in gaining access to entrapped victims, ITLS has developed the ITLS Access Course. This training gives the responder the knowledge base to safely reach the victim of a motor-vehicle collision and begin applying the principles taught in the ITLS course, thereby saving some of the Golden Hour. The techniques taught in Access Course involve use of very basic, inexpensive tools and equipment that can be carried on any ambulance or rescue vehicle. This hands-on course also teaches where and how to use those tools to rapidly stabilize and then gain access to a crashed vehicle.

The first and foremost principle on any accident scene is that of safety. The appropriate use of personal protective equipment (PPE) to prevent injury, as well as contamination with blood or body substances, cannot be overemphasized. Each one of us on the scene is a safety officer and we must remember that our own safety and that of our colleagues is paramount. If we become injured, we cannot help the victim.

Assessment of the scene begins with dispatch and the information provided. As you approach the scene, begin to assess for hazards and look at the mechanism of injury. Are there issues with fuel spills, dangerous cargos, downed lines, and so forth? Remember that unless you have the appropriate equipment and training, you should not handle downed power lines. You should always assume a line is live until instructed otherwise by power company personnel. You should place your vehicle in a safe location and be sure that it is safe for you to enter the scene. In a hazmat or other type of call, without appropriate PPE, you may not be able to safely enter the scene. For many of us, that could be the most difficult decision of our lives. Yet if we rush in without proper protective equipment, we may forfeit both our lives and those of the victims.

How many victims? What other resources are needed? To where should those resources respond? All of these questions must be answered and transmitted back to the dispatch center. At this point, one of your crew members must take control of the scene and serve as the incident commander until relieved or the incident ends. We do this informally on most calls but on a major event, this must be determined and initiated promptly.

You should sweep the scene—looking both toward the incident and away, to locate victims. Once you have located the victims, are any still in the vehicle? If so, how do you render the vehicle safe? Even on the wheels, unless it is made stable, a vehicle can roll over a responder or further injure a victim. Even after the wheels are chocked, unless it is cribbed, the vehicle can still move on the suspension. If the vehicle is on its side or roof, it is even more unstable and must be rendered stable prior to making entry to assess the patient. You can use materials from the scene, such as jacks or spare tires, etc., to stabilize the vehicle, until additional support arrives.

Once you have stabilized the vehicle, entry can be made. Ideally you can open the vehicle doors to extricate the patient(s). For vehicles not on their wheels or with damage to the doors, you may have to make entry by other points. The simplest way to breach the car structure is to make entry through the windows. Side glass on most passenger vehicles is made of tempered glass. When the surface tension is broken, the glass shatters into tiny but sharp pieces. If you must breach the window, try to do so as far as possible from the victims. Take every effort to protect them from debris, using blankets, coats, and so on. Use of a center punch in the corner of the window will quickly break the window. Once cleared of glass, you can enter and begin patient assessment and management, beginning with the ITLS Primary Survey.

Be sure that you are wearing the appropriate PPE, as you may need to stay with the patient during the process of disentanglement and extrication. That process is often complicated by the fact that the patient will need spinal motion restriction, thus making it necessary to create a larger path for egress than if the patient were exiting the vehicle under his or her own power. During this process it is your responsibility to maintain support of the patient's airway and other vital functions.

Team effort is required for the process of extrication to work. You should be thoroughly familiar with the tools needed and the techniques required. This is best accomplished through frequent practice under realistic conditions, followed by a frank and detailed review to identify areas for improvement.

For more information on ITLS Access and availability of courses, please contact the ITLS International Office at 888-495-4857 (international calls: 630-495-6442).

BIBLIOGRAPHY

1. Alson, R., B. Patterson. 2006. *Access*. 2nd ed. ITLS.

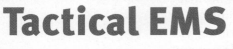

Tactical EMS

Walter J. Bradley, MD, MBA, FACEP

John Wipfler, MD, FACEP

William Pfeifer, MD, FACS

Bill Bozeman, MD, FACEP

Martin Greenberg, MD

Objectives

Upon completion of this appendix, you should be able to:

1. Describe the goals of tactical emergency medicine support (TEMS).
2. Explain the need for TEMS.
3. Describe the purpose of a TEMS provider.
4. Discuss when the ABCs should be changed to CAB.

INTRODUCTION

Tactical EMS is a growing subspecialty of Emergency Medicine and Emergency Medical Services that is increasingly more prevalent in the United States. The dangerous atmosphere faced during law enforcement tactical training and operations often results in significant risk of injury to police officers, hostages, suspects, bystanders, and others, including medical personnel that may be involved. Unfortunately, the nearest available prehospital medical care is too often staged with an ambulance several blocks away, waiting for the scene to become "safe." Their efforts are too often uncoordinated, unprepared, and too late. This older "traditional" method of utilizing standard EMS providers can expose prehospital personnel to great danger. In addition, traditional arrangements that do not integrate the medical team into the tactical unit often disrupt or endanger the law enforcement tactical mission.

Law enforcement agencies are increasingly recognizing the need to have emergency medical care immediately available and integrated with their units. To meet these needs, carefully selected and specially trained and equipped prehospital medical personnel and emergency physicians are increasingly supporting tactical units, also known as special weapons and tactics (SWAT) units. This subspecialty is rapidly expanding and is called tactical emergency medicine support (TEMS). It is well established in many cities and is increasingly prevalent throughout the world. Medical personnel who provide TEMS ideally are equipped, trained, and have developed unique skills to meet the demands presented by operational support of law enforcement tactical teams. This chapter will discuss these unique aspects and provide a foundation of knowledge regarding tactical EMS.

WHAT IS TACTICAL EMS?

The definition of tactical emergency medicine support (TEMS) is as follows:

> The delivery of emergency medical services at law enforcement and military special operations, and the provision of comprehensive health care to members of tactical units on an ongoing basis, maintaining their physical and mental health to optimize the performance of the tactical team.

The goal of TEMS is the same as the goal of special weapons and tactics (SWAT) units: to accomplish the law enforcement mission without injury or death resulting from the team's intervention, and the preservation of life and safety of everyone.

Modern SWAT Teams

The general public sometimes has a negative image of tactical teams, due perhaps to television shows and movies that unrealistically portray SWAT teams as simply showing up and "blowing away" the bad guys. In fact, modern tactical teams are comprised of highly trained, experienced, and reliable "cream of the crop" law enforcement officers who do everything they can to resolve dangerous situations without anyone getting hurt. The fact is, SWAT units save lives. Approximately 95 percent of SWAT callouts are resolved peacefully. Practically speaking, a SWAT team is organized as both a crisis intervention and rescue team with assault and negotiation capabilities.

The following positions are usually incorporated in the tactical team.

■ *Incident/Unit Commander*—supervises the entire operation from the command post.

■ *Team Leader*—directs the team personnally and may enter with entry team in third or fourth position.

■ *Entry Tactical Officers*—usually a minimum of two entry teams (three to six officers each) are involved and possible third backup rescue team.

■ *Medic/Tactical EMS Provider*—offers immediate medical support to ill/injured team members, suspects, victims, or bystanders; other roles include preventive medicine.

■ *Negotiations Team*—usually communicate via telephone or throw phone systems. Crisis negotiations resolve an overwhelming majority of SWAT operations.

Evolution of Tactical EMS

The beginnings of TEMS started with the armed services. Napoleon is recognized as having the first modern field medical evacuation system integrated into units engaged in combat. Clara Barton helped show the benefits of providing medical stabilization of a wounded soldier before and during transport from the site of injury. Her philosophy of treating soldiers as soon as possible ("treat them where they lay") led to present-day military and civilian prehospital care systems.

For years, military special operations units have included medical support in their organizational structure, as they have recognized that this support, especially in covert or tactical operations, can enhance the probability of a successful mission.

Significant historical events led to an increased interest in specially trained tactical units: the University of Austin clock tower shootings (15 people killed, 35 wounded by a single shooter on August 1, 1966) and the Los Angeles Watts Riots of 1965 and 1992. These events shook civilian law enforcement agencies and forced them to consider how they would react to these violent acts in their own jurisdiction.

Why Tactical EMS Is Needed

The reasons for TEMS are easily explained. Terrorist bombings, kidnappings, bank robberies with hostages, riots, drug dealers utilizing fully automatic weapons, emotionally disturbed persons with weapons, and other violent acts have increasingly filled newspapers and become a part of life in the United States. The citizens of our communities expect law enforcement agencies to resolve these incidents promptly and safely. These agencies usually have a team of highly trained individuals who respond to these potentially violent emergencies, and officers (and others) are at high risk for injury and death. In addition, the 1999 Columbine school shooting/bombing incident, the 2005 Beslan Russia school attack, and other critical incidents occur throughout the world with increasing frequency. When they occur, the response by law enforcement personnel is urgently needed, and officers who respond increasingly need medical support. The concept of TEMS is supported by the facts in Table L-1.

Roles of Tactical EMS

Tactical EMS providers typically provide support for civilian law enforcement tactical teams and other law enforcement teams such as riot squads and bomb squads. The prehospital medical providers involved in this field have a simple goal—to contribute to mission success by preventing injuries and illness and by safely providing the best medical care possible when illness and injuries occur. The medical support is provided in three key areas as listed here.

- ■ Before a mission
  - Provide general medical support for team members during training that maximizes performance. This includes preventive medicine, health maintenance, and injury control (team "doc").
  - Provide immediate medical care to team members who become injured or ill during training (a significant number of major injuries suffered by tactical officers occur during training sessions).
  - Teach tactical officers self-care and buddy combat medical care.
  - Participate in mission planning and medical threat analysis (MTA).
  - Prepare a MTA.
  - Provide appropriate medical advice while keeping missions confidential to avoid any information leaks.
  - Prepare the TEMS team to deal with pertinent medical threats and hazards expected at a scene.

TABLE L-1 *Justifications for Tactical EMS*
— An integrated TEMS unit may function with less risk and more benefits for the tactical team.
— The security of tactical operations is enhanced when the medical support team is integrated.
— Time lag occurs if regular EMS care is used ("wait until scene is safe" is often too late).
— Preventive medicine in training and callouts by TEMS results in decreased injury and illness.

- During a mission
  - Primarily provide immediate medical care to tactical team members and law enforcement officers.
  - Secondarily provide emergency care to bystanders, suspects, or others in need on-site.
  - Advise the command staff of developing medical concerns, and be available for medical consultation.
  - Perform remote assessment medicine (RAM) of any downed victims in exposed positions.
  - Remain a liaison with the local EMS system, hospitals, and officials from other public safety and law enforcement agencies.
- After a mission
  - Perform incident review and assist command staff with analysis of the operation/training event.
  - Document and review all medical records relevant to operational or training missions.
  - Appropriately optimize treatment, rehabilitation, and mental health for injured officers through involvement with hospitals, physicians, family, and police department officials (while respecting patient confidentiality regulations).
  - After review and analysis of the incident, provide advice to improve policies.

TACTICAL EMS MODELS

A number of different models of TEMS units have evolved over the years. A common theme is that there is no single "best" tactical EMS model that will meet the needs of all agencies. All of the models have their own strengths and weaknesses, and each program must be tailored to fit the needs of specific agencies using the available resources.

Provider Models

Who is the ideal person to be a "tactical medic"? In general, it is easier and less costly if the TEMS provider is primarily employed in a medical profession, and then secondarily trained in law enforcement/tactical medical support. The 1,000 or more hours it takes to train and maintain skills as a paramedic makes it expensive and impractical for a law enforcement agency to train one of their own officers to be able to perform advanced life support (ALS) medicine. Conversely, a medic/paramedic may take a shortened law enforcement training course to learn the basics of law enforcement supplemented by tactical EMS training courses that will provide a foundational TEMS knowledge base. The advantage of this approach is that the medic or other medical professional is performing medical work on the normal job every workday and is thus able to maintain medical skills and also more easily comply with state EMS regulations and credentialing.

Some law enforcement agencies have trained and certified their tactical officers in basic life support (BLS) as an EMT-Basic or EMT-Intermediate and utilized them for TEMS. This approach at least improves the level of emergency medical care training, decreases the potential for accidental "leaks" of important information, and eliminates the presence of a "civilian" on the tactical team. If this method is used, however, it is still important to designate several tactical officers as "TEMS—medical only," a role that most officers will try to avoid (as they prefer to apprehend or neutralize suspects). Although not mandatory, many TEMS providers will arrange to be designated or certified as some type of law enforcement officer (usually auxiliary, certified part-time police officers, or, rarely, full time). This arrangement may allow liability and insurance benefit coverage to be extended to the individual TEMS officers and allows for increased law enforcement training opportunities.

The ideal situation is debatable but, in general, the TEMS unit is better integrated and supported if medics can become part-time or auxiliary police officers/deputies. This arrangement allows the TEMS members to receive additional training, adds to "esprit de corps," and allows most liability concerns to be addressed. Medical malpractice may or may not be covered by the municipality and each situation will vary. Several states have successfully passed legislation that indemnifies medical professionals when they assist or provide medical support to law enforcement officers.

Deployment and Positioning

Where is the best location for a tactical medic? This is a debatable topic, but in general, when a tactical operation begins and the SWAT unit makes entry, the optimal location for the TEMS providers is the safest position that is close enough to allow a fast (less than 30-second) response time to the tactical team's location, and to any wounded officers. Ideally, this is a location that allows the medics to visualize the tactical team's exact entry point. This concept is known as the "point of relative safety." If the scene is not secured, but conditions allow the injured to be moved to the medics and hard cover, they may be moved to obtain stabilizing first aid. Each situation will vary, and there may be circumstances that require the TEMS provider to come forward to assist downed officers.

In general, during the initial SWAT callout organizing stages, the medical team is best located at the command site (tent, vehicle, room), where they are relatively safe, yet can provide medical support and input into resolving the incident as needed, as well as get a good grasp of the details of the operation. When the tactical team moves into position, the TEMS providers may move forward to the point of relative safety to stand by behind hard cover until needed. However, some teams keep their medics at the command site, and others will bring properly trained medics inside on their entry team.

There are pros and cons of these systems and each unit will need to decide for themselves given the preferences of the involved persons and departments. Overall, each TEMS unit will need to work closely with the tactical unit to define policy and procedures regarding the deployment location of their medical officers. There are several locations where the TEMS officer can be positioned. In a traditional civilian EMS prepositioning system, the SWAT team has no tactical EMS support and they simply call the local ambulance squad and place them at a safe place nearby, perhaps several blocks away. This, unfortunately, continues as the sole medical support for many SWAT teams. The newer tactical EMS model utilizes medical personnel inside the outer perimeter, and often within the inner perimeter. The exact location of TEMS personnel will vary according to the local tactical unit's preference, the type of tactical callout, and the level of TEMS training. The three classic zones are described as follows:

- *At the outer perimeter (cold zone).*   This is frequently the best place for TEMS personnel to be located initially and is also the usual location of the incident command center, or tactical operations center (TOC).

- *Outside of inner perimeter (warm zone).*   As above, this is a good location once the SWAT team has moved into the inner perimeter. The TEMS unit usually approaches the building or structure with the tactical team, and then when a close observation point with hard cover is reached (i.e., a brick wall or other cover that stops bullets), the TEMS providers may remain there, ideally along with one or two law enforcement officers who can provide security.

- *Inner perimeter with the SWAT entry team (hot zone).*   This is controversial and may depend on the level of the TEMS additional training and/or experience. Some SWAT teams have a highly trained paramedic or EMT present on the actual "stick" entry team, and thus actually go inside the building initially as the fourth or fifth person on the entry team. This has the advantage of immediate medical care, but at a relatively higher risk to the TEMS medical personnel. A safer method for smaller buildings or single-unit houses is to keep the medical team nearby but behind cover, and to call the TEMS officers forward *only* if the need arises.

There is one exception to the inner perimeter zone, which is extremely rare, but remains a possibility and thus all tactical teams should and usually do train for this contingency. This type of incident would include a large building with multiple rooms and levels, in which there are known injured victims and the suspect(s) potentially remain inside the building. In this type of incident many TEMS units train to function on the rescue team and work with tactical officers to clear the building and simultaneously provide medical care to any injured persons found.

Extrication and Transportation

TEMS personnel may or may not have their own patient transport capabilities. If they do not, they may require interfacing with the local EMS system for transportation of injured SWAT team members or non–law enforcement personnel. This consideration must be kept in mind during the planning of protocols and procedures, especially the location of the TEMS unit and coordination of transportation efforts.

Armed Versus Unarmed Controversy

Should the tactical medic be allowed to be properly trained and authorized to carry a firearm for personal protection of self and patients? It is controversial for some agencies, while other agencies gladly take the time and effort to arm their medics for the dangerous tactical environment. The official position by national training institutions is neutral on this issue. For those TEMS providers who are not allowed or choose not to be armed, it is absolutely essential that they make arrangements for reliable security to protect and watch over them during SWAT callouts. It is important that any efforts to create a new TEMS unit *not* let this controversy block the formation and development of the unit. Many teams have been successful in starting a working TEMS relationship and then dealing with the firearm issue after mutual respect and understanding is better developed.

SPECIFIC TEMS EQUIPMENT AND TACTICS

Equipment and Supplies

Uniforms, Protective Equipment, and Medical Supplies: The uniforms, protective gear, medical equipment, and medical supplies will vary among individual TEMS units, but Table L-2 presents some ideas for consideration. These are simply "things to think about," and every unit will carry a slightly different variation of each item.

Specialized Equipment: The medical gear/medications to provide medical support may be organized and/or carried in many different ways. Generally, each unit does it differently. Some TEMS units have adopted this simple philosophy: "If it's not attached to you, you won't have it there when you need it." For example, some TEMS units utilize a three-level system. Two remain with the TEMS officers at all times, while the third (Large Advanced Medical Bag) typically remains secured nearby or in a vehicle.

■ *Level I: Tactical Medical Vest with Belt, Holster, Airway (Leg) Pack*
  • Stethoscope, nitrile rubber gloves, face mask with eye shield or goggles
  • Airway management kit: cricothyroidotomy hook, scalpel, pocket mask, tension pneumothorax decompression kit, hemostats, ET tube (6.5 and 7.5), stylet,

<table>
<tr><td>

■■□
□■□ **TABLE L-2** *Personal Uniform/Protective Equipment*

— Uniforms (appropriate agency uniform for training and callout missions)
— Boots (good ankle support, good all-around traction, waterproof, and body-fluid resistant)
— Ballistic vest (level III preferred, with side protectors and ceramic plates [level IV] considered)
— Helmet (Kevlar) with stable suspension system
— Black Nomex balaclava (protect identity at scene, prevent facial burns)
— Eye protective goggles with side shielding (clear polycarbonate lenses to protect from flying debris/trauma)
— Ear protection (foam plugs, shooting muffs)
— Gloves (rubber gloves [nitrile ideal], and leather or Nomex external gloves)
— Medical standard precautions protective gear: face mask/shield, gloves, hazmat gear if needed
— Gas mask (with optic inserts if needed)
</td></tr>
</table>

oropharyngeal airway, size 28 nasopharyngeal airway, laryngoscope with #3 blade, BVM or oral ventilation system
- Compression trauma bandages (3), cloth tape, small roll of duct tape
- Tourniquet (2 or more)
- Hemostatic agent (QuikClot 1st Response sponge or Celox) (2)
- Asherman penetrating chest trauma seal (2)
- Minor wound medical kit: steri-strips, benzoin, betadine, neosporin ointment, bandaids, 2x2 bandages
- Common medicine for common complaints: ibuprofen, acetaminophen, antacids, etc.
- Handcuffs, holster and defensive weapon (pistol), ammo, extra magazines as needed
- Trauma scissors, knife—folding style utility
- Communications: radio with headset, cellular phone, pager
- Tactical flashlight
- Small binoculars for remote assessment and observation; consider night vision monocular/headset
- Digital camera (for evidence preservation, documentation, interesting cases)
- Metal detector (handheld, silent vibratory type) for identifying hidden weapons or needles

■ *Level II: Tactical Medical Backpack*
- A second (backup) advanced airway management kit, which includes a second set of above airway supplies, bag-valve mask, Magill forceps, laryngoscope #1 and #3 blades, full assortment of ET tubes (adult and pediatric)
- Large curved hemostats, scalpels
- Two 1-liter IV LR fluid bags/IV starter kits with two blood tubing IV lines/pressure IV bag
- Disposable hot packs (to keep IV fluid warm in cold weather operations)
- 7-French change-out catheter set (for cut-downs/IV access)
- Additional trauma dressings, gauze bandages
- ACLS medications: atropine, epinephrine, lidocaine, D50

■ *Level III: Tactical Medical Advanced Emergency Medication Pack.*   This pack may be kept locked in a controlled environment at the base hospital. The contents may include controlled substances, which must be properly stored, controlled, and monitored per DEA requirements (Table L-3). In addition, it is important to prevent exposure to high heat due to the sensitive medications contained. Many hospitals will "restock" this bag every 6 months and recycle the medications prior to expiration, allowing the net "cost" to be very low. Additional items included in the Advanced Medical Supply Kit include the following:

- Syringes and needles, alcohol wipes
- Suture kits (2) and minor surgical emergency supplies—gauze, basin, sterile gloves, suture material, betadine swabs
- Additional IV fluid and IV lines, IV starting kits
- Anderson blast gauge
- Sterile saline (2 bottles) for irrigation/cleaning wounds
- Dental kit: mirror, dental floss, clove oil, topical anesthesia, tongue blades, stoma wax, temporary filling material
- Additional trauma supplies: antiseptic towelettes, compression elastic bandage, trauma pads, eye dressing, Q-tips, SAM splints, triple antibiotic ointment, band-aids, tape, nonstick gauze, gauze pads, moleskin/blister kit, irrigation syringes/solution, Betadine and Hibiclens scrub brushes, cold packs, heat packs, cling wrap, two tension pneumothorax kits
- Extra stethoscope, pen light, trauma scissors, knife/paratool
- Latex gloves, sterile and nonsterile; face mask/shield
- Pencil marker, waterproof paper, medical records of unit members
- Patient ID/triage tags, emergency thermal blankets (2), strobe light
- Medical waste bags, disposable sharps hard plastic container
- Thermometer (regular and special hypothermia)

Training Considerations

There is a significant body of knowledge that is integral to the practice of tactical medicine that is entirely separate from standard prehospital and emergency medical training. These topics come from a variety of medical disciplines and law enforcement/military operations. They are taught by numerous high-quality training agencies that specialize in tactical medical training (Table L-4). It is in the best interest of the TEMS provider to complete a formal TEMS educational course and then utilize the unique skills and knowledge in routine training with the tactical unit, to gain familiarity and mutual respect of individual roles and abilities.

Special Tactical Medical Procedures

There are several topics important for the TEMS provider to be aware of, and proficient in, during law enforcement support.

Make the Scene Safe by Disarming Before Treating: If the officer is seriously injured, first remove weapons (do not forget backup guns, any explosives, chemical munitions). If the injured officer is lightly wounded, alert, and under fire, or still facing a threat, then consider allowing the officer to keep his weapon to protect himself and TEMS personnel.

All criminals should be considered to have hidden weapons, handcuff keys, hypodermic needles, and other hazards. Always get help when removing weapons from a suspect/criminal. Always use caution!

Trauma Combat Casualty Care: During a SWAT callout, a TEMS provider may be called upon to care for someone who is shot or otherwise injured. The tactical commander and team must focus on completing the mission safely, including calling for additional help if needed, establishing fire superiority, abolishing threats, and preventing additional casualties. These are analogous to making the scene safer. Medical care provided in this situation

TABLE L-3 *Example of One TEMS Unit's Advanced Kit**

Symptom/Category	Medications
Colds/Flu Symptoms	Cough drops Entex PSE decongestant (20) Neosynephrine nasal spray (1 bottle)
Minor Pain Control	Ibuprofen 400-mg tablets (30) Tylenol 500-mg tablets (30)
Severe Pain Control	Morphine for IM/IV use
Allergy/Anaphylaxis	Epinephrine 1:1000, (3) 2-cc ampules Benadryl 25 mg capsules (20) Prednisone 20 mg tablets (10) Albuterol inhaler (1) (used for asthmatics also)
GI Ailments	Immodium tablets (20) Peptobismal tablets (approx 20) Mylanta tablets (approx 20)
Unresponsive Patients	Ammonia capsules (2) Dextrose 50%, (1) 50-cc syringette Oral glucose syrup, (1 tube) Narcan, (2) 2-mg ampules
ACLS Drugs	Lidocaine 1%, (2) 10-cc syringettes Atropine, (2) 1-mg syringettes Epinephrine 1:10,000, (4) 1-mg 10-cc syringettes Nitroglycerine S.L. spray Baby aspirin, 81 mg (chest pain use)
Seizure Control	Diazepam for IV/IM use, (1) 10-mg vial
RSI (Rapid Sequence Intubation) Meds	Diazepam, 10-mg vial Etomidate for IV use—sedation Ketamine for IM/IV use (1 bottle) Vecuronium (Norcuron), 10-mg powder Rocuronium (Zemuron), (2) 5-cc vials Normal saline, 25-cc bottle (to reconstitute Norcuron)
Ear/Eye Ailments	Gentamycin ophthalmologic ointment (2 tubes) Gentamycin opth. drops (2 bottles) Cortosporin otic suspension (1 bottle)
Skin Ailments	Lotrizone cream, 10 gm (3 tubes) Triamcinolone 0.1% cream, 10 gm (3 tubes) Sunscreen, 30–SPF (1 tube)
Infection Treatment	Cephalexin, 500-mg tablets (10) Levaquin, 750-mg tablets (10) Ancef (2 gm, IV/50-cc bag) Rocephin (2 gm, IV/50-cc bag)
Other Medications	Oralgel (dental analgesic) (1 tube)

*For use only under the direction of a physician.

TABLE L-4 Specialized Tactical EMS Topics

- Operational Considerations
  - Indications for Tactical Unit Callout
  - Leadership Roles and Responsibilities
  - Tactical Unit Entry Strategies: Dynamic Versus Stealth Entry
  - Crime Scene Operations
- Deployment Considerations of a TEMS Unit/Operators
  - Staging, Integration with EMS
  - Scene Safety in the Tactical Environment
  - Tactical Movement with Light and Sound Discipline
  - Weapons Familiarization and Safe Removal and Handling
- Communications
- Emergency Medical Care in a Tactical Environment
  - Care under Fire and Modifications of Standard Protocols
  - Downed Officer Scenarios—Immediate Action Drills
  - Medical Threat Analysis (MTA)
  - TEMS Extrication and Evacuation Considerations
  - TEMS Transportation Considerations and EMS Interface
- Other Medical Care Topics
  - Preventative Care and Health Maintenance
  - Posttraumatic Stress Debriefing and Mental Health
- Considerations for Lethal Threat Management and Self-Defense
  - Recognition/Management of the Violent or Potentially Violent Suspect
  - Criminal Countertactics and Threats; Communications and Tactics
  - Use of Force Continuum
  - Lethal Force Considerations for the TEMS Provider
- Management of Other Specific Threats in a Tactical Environment
  - Terrorism and the TEMS Operator
  - Biological Terrorism
  - Chemical Terrorism
  - Blast and Burn Injuries and Explosive Terrorism (suicide bombers)
  - Penetrating Trauma—Ballistics
  - Clandestine Drug Labs/Methamphetamine Labs

is abbreviated and the need for intervention must be carefully weighed against the need for safety of the medical providers.

Priorities of Combat Casualty Care: The classic approach to trauma care involves sequential assessment of the ABCs in a safe environment. In an unsafe situation, and in recognition that *uncontrolled extremity bleeding* represents 80 percent of preventable trauma deaths in combat environments, there is a temporary modification of this approach when providing care in the tactical setting prior to securing the scene. It is called the CAB approach. Circulation (C) is addressed first, with immediate application of a compression bandage or tourniquet to control life-threatening external hemorrhage, followed by rapid assessment of airway (A) and breathing (B).

Military-style combat dressings such as the Israeli dressing/emergency bandage can be highly effective in this setting. Several easily applied and effective tourniquets are available and appropriate for tactical EMS use. Remember to expose gunshot or knife wounds by removing body armor and clothing to visualize the wounds, allowing more accurate assessment and placement of compressive dressings, chest seals (Asherman or other one-way valve-type dressing), and other hemostatic agents. Several new hemostatic agents and dressings (QuikClot and Celox) have been developed and deployed by the military for a treatment of last resort for exsanguinating hemorrhage. Their use should be considered in civilian TEMS systems as well.

If a patient has obvious signs of severe injury, and there are no signs of life, then further medical care is futile. If critically injured officers without a pulse or spontaneous breathing are found inside the inner perimeter under *immediate hostile threat*, responders should remember that they are *dead*. In a *hostile environment* CPR is never indicated unless the officer, suspect, or other can be safely removed or all threats neutralized.

Rapid Evacuation: As soon as practical, evacuate victims to a safe area to provide advanced medical care and initiate transport to a medical facility. This is where planning and immediate action drills are essential. Have a plan, know where to go, which roads to take to get there, and know what type of vehicle you will use, and what medical care can be provided along the way to the hospital. This will help saves lives.

Important Do's and Don'ts of TEMS: No one desires to provide medical care in an unsafe situation. Any situation whereby a victim requires medical care must be carefully evaluated for the risk involved in providing medical care. If the patient is safe and relatively stable, then let the person lie there until the threat is neutralized. If the patient is critically injured and dying *now,* but is isolated from medical help and is trapped by gunfire, then difficult decisions must be made: What are the risks of getting to and treating that patient? What are the benefits of treating that victim now (versus dragging the victim to other safer areas), and what are the chances of having an additional dead provider? This decision is difficult, but several guiding principles exist. The important principles for treating all tactical casualties are as follows:

- The TEMS operator must always assess the tactical situation. Do not endanger yourself or your team members. If the perpetrator(s) remains a direct immediate threat, keep behind or under hard cover until the threat is neutralized.
- Approach the casualty by whispering or saying "Rescue," to inform him of your purpose for touching him. Quickly evaluate/remove the person from danger if possible. This should be to a point of relative safety.
- When you are presented with a tactical casualty: **LOOK—LISTEN—THINK—ACT!**

There have been very few injuries or deaths to tactical medical operators. There are many mistakes made. The following are four common errors made by tactical medical officers.

- *Failure to recognize threats.*   Do not underestimate the potential for violence in female suspects, mentally unstable suspects, senior citizens, and drug addicts.
- *Improper search or no search.*   Never trust the search of a fellow officer; search again prior to treatment and transport; be aware and watch for improvised and concealed weapons.
- *Failure to call for backup.*   Never enter a building or structure alone. About 20 percent of police officers who die from firearms are killed with their own guns.
- *No operational plan.*   Do you and your partner have a contingency plan? Have you made a plan with your partner for hostage situations? Who will cover who if you lose your SWAT officer escort?

In addition, tactical medics should remember the following:

- Prepare for the unexpected (it will happen).
- Predetermine hard cover.
- Recognize the medical problem.
- Triage accurately and rapidly.
- Maintain emotional composure.

TEMS Medical Threat Assessment

Medical threat assessment (MTA) refers to the gathering of medical intelligence that can have an impact on the physiological and psychological health and performance of the tactical team and others for which the team is responsible. All tactical operations require medical threat assessment, including high-risk warrant service, barricaded suspects, training exercises, and protection details.

Remote Assessment Medicine

RAM is a unique aspect of tactical medicine in which an injured officer or suspect/bystander is assessed from a distance, without direct contact. Usually binoculars are the optic device that is used, but a spotting scope or rifle scope may be used as well.

Medicine Across the Barricade

One situation in which a SWAT unit is often called for is the barricaded suspect such as a bank robbery with hostages inside. These are resolved peacefully more than 90 percent of the time, but often the hostages may have medical problems that are exacerbated by the stressful situation, or may be shot or injured and in need of stabilizing medical care. If the suspect can be talked into it, hopefully these people may be released. However, if the injured or ill victim must remain inside the "barricaded bank," then medical care directions may need to be given to the fellow citizens inside.

Special Medical Procedural Techniques

- *Intubation modifications.* Due to the limited access to potential patients, the TEMS provider must practice and be prepared to intubate the victim while in unique situations, such as lying on the ground next to the victim (keep a low profile) and using digital intubation skills and special bends of the endotracheal tube in order to place it properly.

- *Resuscitation limitations.* Each scenario is different. The decision of whether to pronounce a person dead or not is complex and involves many factors. The TEMS officer must be prepared to quickly decide that a person is deceased or has injuries incompatible with life.

- *Light discipline.* Night operations may result in a tactical situation where the suspect is firing upon any police officer flashlight/light source, but there are shooting victims who need medical care, all lying within eyesight of the suspect's gun. These situations will require that the rescuers perform their work in the dark, with no visible light seen. Low-light or no-light medical care will require tactile use of the hands in assessing the patient, as well as use of instruments and treatment without light.

- *Noise discipline.* Similar to above, if the suspect has a weapon and may shoot in the direction of noise, it is important to be very quiet. Communications may be limited to hand signals or quiet radio microphone use.

Medical Aspects of Sustained Operations

If a SWAT unit is called out, and the situation is resolved in 4.5 hours (actual average time to resolve situations), then the team members are generally able to return to their normal duties without great stress to themselves or their families. However, during prolonged tactical operations (i.e., more than 12–18 hours) the SWAT unit members become fatigued, hungry, sore, impatient, bored, homesick, cold, or hot. It is important in prolonged operations for the TEMS providers to provide support and preventive medical care to the best of their abilities. It is in the prolonged scenario that medical personnel can be a huge asset. In addition to being prepared to treat the following ailments or possibilities, the TEMS officer can advise the incident commander of the *prevention* of heat or cold casualties (use proper clothing or gear), fatigue (rotate officers fairly and often), and dehydration (provide good water or rehydration sources).

Contingency plans should be made beforehand with the Red Cross, disaster support agencies, and local restaurants and supply stores. Prepackaged kits with necessary supplies for extended operations should be made and available if needed. Consider delegation of TEMS providers to specific tasks, and also consider sending any extra help home to stay rested and return 12 hours later to replace and rotate out the initial TEMS providers.

EVIDENCE PRESERVATION

It is imperative that any evidence that is identified and collected be done with a strict, well-documented chain of evidence, and it must be stored in proper containers that will be upheld in court. In general, TEMS officers should avoid becoming involved in this chain of evidence due to the often insufficient training, and future time and court appearance requirements.

TOXIC MATERIAL HAZARDS

One of the growing threats throughout the nation (especially in rural areas) involves the "meth lab," or clandestine drug lab (CDL). It is possible to purchase $100 worth of chemicals and illegally produce a synthetic type of methamphetamine that can then be sold for $100,000. Due to this fact, the addiction potential of this drug, and the relative ease to acquire the materials and equipment needed for this production, law enforcement agencies are increasingly finding these CDLs. These labs are often booby-trapped and are associated with dangerous criminals, many of whom are armed with fully automatic weapons. This makes the recovery and investigation of these labs a very dangerous occupation. Therefore, it is important for TEMS officers to be familiar with the unique hazards associated with CDLs, and be prepared (knowledge and medical treatment gear) to deal with hazardous material–associated injuries, flame burns, inhalation injuries, acid burns, penetrating trauma, and blast victims.

If known about prior, most law enforcement agencies will get the DEA (Drug Enforcement Administration) involved to investigate and clean up the toxic CDL. However, sometimes these labs are discovered accidentally during house fires or during a tactical entry. If practical, the tactical team should immediately withdraw and contain the area while waiting for the DEA to deal with the lab.

SPECIAL ISSUES

Anyone involved with a TEMS unit should be aware of a number of special issues related to TEMS that are beyond the scope of an introductory chapter. There are many important support, legal, and administrative issues, some of which are medical direction and administrative considerations for TEMS providers; administrative considerations for forming and maintaining a TEMS unit; expanded scope of practice protocols; and unique training considerations for the tactical physician assistant, nurse, and physician. These topics are discussed in depth in textbooks elsewhere.

ADDITIONAL RESOURCES FOR TEMS TRAINING

The increasingly hazardous environment faced by special law enforcement and military tactical units may be partially offset by the provision of close-up tactical emergency medical support, or TEMS. The recent growth of this subspecialty acknowledges the unique knowledge, equipment, and skill set required of tactical medicine operators. In an ever-changing world challenged by criminals, drugs, the methamphetamine drug lab epidemic, school violence, terrorism, and other incidents, today's military and law enforcement special operations units are increasingly arranging for TEMS providers.

This addendum provides an introductory awareness of the many important issues and topics that the tactical medicine provider must be aware of and prepared for. The unique knowledge, skills, equipment, and teamwork that are required must be optimized for the well-prepared team of TEMS providers. Mutual respect and understanding will develop as medical personnel train routinely with their own community's law enforcement tactical unit or military special operations unit. Modifications of standard civilian EMS treatment protocols are mandatory, given the unique "hot zone" threats that must be appropriately dealt with in the priority necessary to help save lives.

The EMS provider who wishes to learn more about or delve into the challenging tactical medicine arena is best served by seeking qualified educational courses and resources, some of which are listed in Table L-5. A baseline education in the principles of TEMS is important for a foundation on which to build your skills but equally important is the routine monthly tactical training and integration with the provider's local law enforcement tactical unit. It is during repetitive realistic training, drills, and eventual actual callouts that the TEMS provider will become recognized as a trustworthy professional with much to add, and help accomplish the mission of resolving the crisis in as safe and injury-free fashion as possible. Before, during, and after a mission, the TEMS provider can be a valuable asset that should lead to on-site prevention of illness and injuries, rapid emergent care if needed, and efficient and safe evacuation of casualties that will lead to more lives saved.

TABLE L-5 *Tactical Emergency Medical Support Schools*

1. EMT-Tactical School

   This school has several courses offered, and is associated with Integrated Force Health Protection (IFHP), formerly part of the CONTOMS program (Counter Narcotics and Terrorism Operational Medicine Support). The EMT-T School/CONTOMS program is a five-day, 58-hour TEMS course offered to EMTs, paramedics, nurses, physician assistants, and physicians who are affiliated with law enforcement agencies. To contact: 301-295-6263 or www.casualtycareresearchcenter.org

2. International School of Tactical Medicine

   The course is directed by Dr. Lawrence Heiskell, who is one of the pioneers of TEMS. The Basic and Advanced TEMS courses are five-day courses, taught semiannually by board-certified emergency physicians and medics who are actual participants in TEMS units throughout the United States. To contact: 760-325-2591 or www.tacticalmedicine.com.

3. Tactical Operations Medical Support course

   Cypress Creek TEMS located in Houston, Texas, offers six-day basic and five-day advanced courses. To contact: 281-440-9650 or www.ccems.com

4. Alabama Terrorism and Tactical Operations Medical Support Course

   This is a five-day course. Contact Blake Strickland at 205-387-0511, extension 5730.

5. Tactical EMS Course

   National Tactical Officers Association (NTOA) offers a 3-day course. To contact: www.ntoa.org/tems

6. International Tactical EMS Association

   This organization maintains a listing of other TEMS courses and also hosts an annual conference as well as an online newsletter and *Journal of Tactical EMS*. To contact: www.tems.org

BIBLIOGRAPHY

1. Campbell, J., J. Smith, et al. 2007. *Homeland security and emergency medical response.* New York: McGraw-Hill, Inc.
2. DeLorenzo, R., R. Porter. *Tactical emergency care.* Upper Saddle River, NJ: Prentice Hall.
3. Kolman, J. 1982. *A guide to the development of special weapons and tactics teams.* Springfield, IL: Charles C. Thomas.
4. Wipfler, J., J. Smith, et al. 2007. *Tactical EMS—The essentials of tactical emergency medicine.* New York: McGraw-Hill, Inc.

abrasion scraping or abrading away of the superficial layers of the skin; an open soft-tissue injury.

abruptio placenta early separation of the placenta from the uterus.

acidosis a condition caused by accumulation of acid or loss of base from the body.

adventitia the layer of loose connective tissue forming the outermost coating of an organ.

aerobic requiring oxygen.

air bag a passive restraint system in automobiles and other vehicles.

alkalosis a pathologic condition resulting from accumulation of base or loss of acid in the body.

anaerobic lacking oxygen.

anoxia absence of oxygen supply to the tissue.

asphyxia a condition due to lack of oxygen; suffocation.

aspirate taking foreign matter into the lungs during inhalation.

assessment to evaluate the condition of a patient.

ATV all-terrain vehicle.

AVPU a description of the level of consciousness. AVPU stands for: A—alert, V—responds to **v**erbal stimuli, P—responds to **p**ain, U—**u**nresponsive.

avulsion an injury in which a piece of a structure is torn away.

axial loading compression forces applied along the long axis of the body. *Example:* a fall in which a victim lands on his feet and force is transferred up his legs to his back, causing a compression fracture of a lumbar vertebra.

bag-valve mask a system of artificial ventilation in which the oxygen inflow fills a bag that is attached to a mask by a one-way valve.

Battle's sign swelling and discoloration behind the ear caused by a fracture of the base of the skull.

beta agonists medications such as Albuterol that stimulate the beta receptors in the smooth muscles of the bronchi causing bronchodilatation. They are used to treat asthma and bronchospasm.

BIAD blind insertion airway device, such as the esophageal tracheal Combitube.

BLS burns, lacerations, swelling. Can also mean basic life support.

body surface area (BSA) percent of a patient's body affected by a burn.

bronchospasm contraction of the smooth muscle of the bronchi.

Broselow tape a tape used to estimate the weight of a child by measuring her length.

BVM (bag-valve mask) a system of artificial ventilation in which the oxygen inflow fills a bag that is attached to a mask by a one-way valve.

caliber the diameter of a bullet expressed in hundredths of an inch (.22 caliber = 0.22 inches); the inside diameter of the barrel of a handgun or a rifle.

capillary blanch or refill test for impairment of circulation: pressure on tip of the nail will cause the bed to turn white, if it does not turn pink again by the time it takes to say "capillary refill," the circulation is impaired. The test has been found to be unreliable for early shock.

carbonaceous sputum sputum that is "sooty" or black.

carbon dioxide monitor a device used to monitor or confirm endotracheal tube placement by measuring expired carbon dioxide. These devices either measure expired carbon dioxide (capnographic) or show a color change when carbon dioxide is present (colorimetric).

carina the lowest part of the trachea, where the trachea divides to form the two mainstem bronchi.

catecholamines a group of chemicals of similar structure that act to increase heart rate and blood pressure.

C-collar (cervical collar) a device to limit movement of the neck.

central cord syndrome an injury to the spinal cord that produces more loss of sensory and motor function in the arms than in the legs.

cerebral perfusion blood flow to the brain.

cerebral perfusion pressure (CPP) the pressure moving blood through the brain.

CNS central nervous system; the brain and spinal cord.

CO_2 monitor a device used to monitor or confirm endotracheal tube placement by measuring expired carbon dioxide.

comminuted fracture fracture in which a bone is broken into several pieces.

compartment syndrome muscle ischemia that is caused by elevated pressure within an anatomic fascial space.

compliance the "give" or elasticity of the lungs and chest wall. This influences how easy it is for the patient to breathe.

concussion a jarring injury to the brain resulting in disturbance of brain function.

constricted to shrink or contract.

contracoup an injury to the brain on the opposite side of the original blow.

contralateral situated or affecting the opposite side.

contusion bruising; the reaction of soft tissue to a direct blow.

COPD chronic obstructive pulmonary disease. The end result of asthma, chronic bronchitis, or emphysema.

copious large amount.

coup an injury to the brain on the same side as the original blow.

crepitation feeling of crackling; the sensation of fragments of broken bones rubbing together.

Cushing's reflex a reflex whereby the body reacts to increased pressure on the brain by raising the blood pressure.

DCAP deformities, contusions, abrasions, penetrations.

DCAP-BTLS deformities, contusions, abrasions, penetrations, burns, tenderness, lacerations, swelling.

DCAPP deformities, contusions, abrasions, penetrations, paradoxical movement.

deceleration to come to a sudden stop, decreasing speed.

decubent position the position assumed when lying down.

delivered volume the amount of air that you actually deliver to the lungs with each breath when you perform artificial or assisted ventilation.

denatured to destroy the usual nature of a substance.

dermis the inner layer of the skin, containing hair follicles, sweat glands, sebaceous glands, nerve endings, and blood vessels.

diaphoresis perspiring profusely.

diffuse axonal injury type of brain injury characterized by shearing, stretching, or tearing of nerve fibers with subsequent axonal damage and edema of the brain tissue.

diuretic an agent that promotes the excretion of urine.

doll's eyes oculocephalic reflex; a test of brain stem function that is never performed in the prehospital setting.

dura the tough fibrous membrane forming the outermost of the three coverings of the brain.

ecchymoses blue-black discoloration of the skin due to leakage of blood into the tissue.

EGTA esophageal gastric tube airway; an improved esophageal obturator airway.

EKG electrocardiogram.

EMS emergency medical services.

endotracheal intubation the insertion of a tube into the trachea to assist or control ventilation.

EOA esophageal obturator airway.

epidermis the outermost layer of skin.

epidural outside the dura; between the dura and the skull.

erythema general reddening of the skin due to dilation of the superficial capillaries.

ETA estimated time of arrival. An estimation of when you will arrive at the receiving hospital.

etiology the cause of a particular disease.

ET tube endotracheal tube.

evisceration the protruding of internal organs through a wound.

expeditious quick, speedy.

exsanguinate to bleed to death.

extrication removal of a patient from a dangerous position or situation.

FROPVD flow-restricted, oxygen-powered, ventilation device. An artificial ventilation device that provides 100% oxygen at a flow rate of 40 L/min at a maximum pressure of 50 ± 5 cm water.

full-thickness burn third degree burn.

gastric insufflation the filling of the stomach by air when performing positive pressure ventilation.

GCS (Glasgow Coma Scale) a method used to measure the severity of a head injury.

genioglossus muscle the muscle that pulls the tongue out of the mouth.

grunting a deep, guttural noise made in breathing; a sign of respiratory distress in small children.

Hare splint a type of traction splint.

Heimlich maneuver a method of dislodging food or other material from the throat of a choking victim.

hemiparesis partial paralysis affecting one side of the body.

hemoptysis to spit up blood or blood-stained sputum.

hemothorax the presence of blood in the chest cavity within the pleural space, outside the lung.

hypercarbia high blood carbon dioxide level.

hyperresonant giving an increased vibrant sound on percussion; tympanic.

hypertympany hyperresonant.

hyperventilation increased rate of breathing; 20 breaths per minute for an adult.

hypoventilation decreased rate of breathing, 10 breaths per minute for an adult; insufficient respiration demonstrated by an elevated blood carbon dioxide level.

hypovolemic shock hemorrhagic shock; shock caused by insufficient blood or fluid within the body.

hypoxia a deficiency of oxygen reaching the tissues of the body.

ICP intracranial pressure. The pressure inside the skull.

impaled object a penetrating object that is still in place in a patient's body.

Initial Assessment part of the Primary Survey. This is a rapid exam of airway, breathing and circulation. It is performed on all patients.

intra-abdominal within the abdomen.

intracranial within the skull.

intrathoractic within the chest.

IPPV intermittent positive pressure ventilation.

ipsilateral situated on or affecting the same side.

JVD jugular vein distention. Distended jugular veins in the neck.

kinematics the phase of mechanics that deals with possible motions of the body.

labial angle corner of the mouth.

laryngeal mask airway (LMA) an invasive airway device to assist ventilation.

lateral decubitus position position assumed when lying on one's side.

lesion an injury or abnormal condition of a part.

LMA laryngeal mask airway. An invasive airway device to assist ventilation.

LOC level of consciousness.

MAP mean arterial blood pressure.

MAST military antishock trousers. Also called pneumatic antishock garment (PASG). A device that applies circumferential pressure to the legs and abdomen to raise the blood pressure in hypotensive patients.

MCI multicasualty incident. An emergency situation in which there are multiple injured patients.

mean arterial blood pressure diastolic blood pressure plus 1/3 (systolic minus the diastolic blood pressure).

medial toward the middle.

minute volume the volume of air breathed in and out in 1 minute. This varies from 5 to 12 liters per minute.

mortality frequency of death or death rate.

MVC motor-vehicle collision.

nasopharyngeal airway an artificial airway positioned in the nasal cavity.

necrosis the death of tissue.

neonate newborn infant.

nonrebreather mask an oxygen mask that allows the patient to breath oxygen at a concentration close to 100%.

NP airway nasopharyngeal airway. An artificial airway positioned in the nasal cavity.

occult injuries injuries hidden or concealed from view.

OLMD on-line medical direction.

OPIM other potentially infectious material (other than blood).

oropharyngeal airway an artificial airway positioned in the oral cavity to keep the tongue from occluding the airway.

osteomyelitis inflammation or infection of a bone or bones.

pallor paleness, absence of skin color.

palpate to examine by touch.

paradoxical motion the motion of the injured segment of a flail chest, opposite to the normal motion of the chest wall.

parenchymal the essential elements of an organ.

paresis slight or incomplete paralysis.

paresthesia abnormal sensation; a "tingling" sensation.

partial-thickness burn a burn that does not injure the full thickness of the skin. A first degree burn involves only the epidermal layer. A second degree burn involves the epidermis and part of the dermis.

PASG pneumatic antishock garment. Also called military antishock trousers (MAST). A device that applies circumferential pressure to the legs and abdomen to raise the blood pressure in hypotensive patients.

patent open.

pathophysiology the basic processes of the disease.

perfusion the passage of blood or fluid through the vessels of an organ.

personal watercraft (PWC) a small motorized watercraft that one or two persons can ride. Much like a motorcycle except it travels on water.

pia mater innermost of the three layers of tissue that envelop the brain.

placenta previa an abnormal location of the placenta, so that it covers the opening of the uterus (cervical os).

PMS pulses, motor function, and sensation. Description of the exam of an injured extremity.

pneumothorax the presence of air within the chest cavity in the pleural space, but outside the lung (collapsed lung).

pocket mask a small face mask for performing assisted ventilation. It is made to be carried in the rescuer's pocket.

potential space a space that does not exist except under abnormal circumstances. *Example:* Normally the lungs completely fill the chest cavity so that the pleural space (between the lungs and the chest wall) is only a potential space. If the pleural space contains blood it is a hemothorax.

PPE personal protection equipment such as gloves, face shields, and impervious gowns.

Primary Survey a brief exam to find immediately life-threatening conditions. It is made up of the Initial Assessment and either the Rapid Trauma Survey or the Focused Exam.

pulse oximeter a noninvasive device that monitors the oxygen saturation of the blood hemoglobin.

pulse pressure the sensation given by the heart contraction to the palpating finger on an artery.

PWC personal watercraft.

raccoon's eyes swelling and discoloration around both eyes; a late sign of basilar skull fracture.

respiratory reserve lung tissue over and above the body's need to provide oxygenation for the body.

rhabdomyolysis disintegration (lysis) or dissolution of muscle; this releases myoglobin into the blood, which can precipitate in the kidneys, causing renal failure.

RTSS radio telephone switch station; a type of radio that accesses the telephone lines.

Sager splint a type of traction splint.

SAMPLE history the least amount of information needed on a trauma patient. S—symptoms, A—allergies, M—medications, P—past medical history, L—last oral intake (last meal), E—events preceding the injury.

scaphoid shaped like a boat. When used to describe the abdomen, scaphoid means sunken in.

scuba diver a diver who is able to remain under water by breathing compressed air from a breathing apparatus needing no connection with the surface. SCUBA stands for self-contained underwater breathing apparatus.

Secondary Survey a comprehensive head-to-toe exam to find additional injuries that may have been missed in the brief Primary Survey.

Sellick maneuver a maneuver (posterior pressure on the cricoid cartilage) to prevent gastric insufflation and vomiting.

sheering forces forces that occur in such a direction to cause tearing of an organ.

sibling brother or sister.

skin diver a diver who holds his breath when swimming under water. He uses no artificial breathing methods.

SMR spinal motion restriction; the act of stabilizing the spinal column to prevent as much motion as possible.

snoring to breathe in a hoarse, rough noise, usually with the mouth open.

snorkeler a diver who uses a short tube (snorkel) in order to float on the surface and observe underwater life. When diving, a snorkeler must hold her breath.

spontaneous pneumothorax collapsed lung caused by the rupture of a congenitally weak area on the surface of the lung.

standard precautions procedures used to prevent contamination by a patient's body fluids. This usually entails gloves and possibly a gown and face shield.

stridor breathing that has a high-pitched, harsh noise; a sign of impending airway obstruction.

stroke volume the amount of blood pumped by the heart in one beat.

subcutaneous emphysema the presence of air in soft tissues, giving a very characteristic crackling sensation on palpation; the Rice Krispies feeling.

tachypnea adult respiratory rate of 24 or more breaths per minute.

tamponade compression of a part of the anatomy, as the compression of heart by pericardial fluid.

TBI traumatic brain injury.

tension pneumothorax a condition in which air continuously leaks out of the lung into the pleural space, increasing pressure within the space with every breath the patient takes.

Thomas' splint a type of traction splint.

TIC tenderness, instability, crepitation. An acronym for the description of the exam of a bony area.

tidal volume the amount of air that is inspired and expired during one respiratory cycle.

traction the action of drawing or pulling on an object.

trajectory the direction a missile takes in flight or after striking a body.

transected to cut transversely.

Trendelenburg position supine with lower body elevated about 30 degrees.

vallecula the space between the base of the tongue and the epiglottis.

vasomotor affecting the size of a blood vessel.

venous pressure pressure of the blood in the veins.

viscera any large interior organ in any one of the three great cavities of the body, especially the abdomen.

volatile a substance that evaporates rapidly at room temperature when exposed to air.

wheezing whistling sounds made in breathing; a sign of spasm or narrowing of the bronchi.